Bad Men Do What Good Men Dream

*A Forensic Psychiatrist
Illuminates the Darker Side
of Human Behavior*

Bad Men Do What Good Men Dream

A Forensic Psychiatrist
Illuminates the Darker Side
of Human Behavior

By Robert I. Simon, M.D.

Clinical Professor of Psychiatry
Director, Program in Psychiatry and Law
Georgetown University School of Medicine
Washington, DC

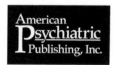

American
Psychiatric
Publishing, Inc.

Washington, DC
London, England

To buy between 25 and 99 copies of this or any other APPI title at a 20% discount, please contact APPI Customer Service at appi@psych.org or 800-368-5777. To purchase 100 or more copies of the same title, please e-mail us at bulksales@psych.org for a price quote.

Manufactured in the United States of America on acid-free paper
12 11 10 09 08   5 4 3 2 1
First Edition, Revised

Typeset in Adobe Baskerville

American Psychiatric Publishing, Inc.
1000 Wilson Boulevard
Arlington, VA 22209-3901
www.appi.org

Library of Congress Cataloging-in-Publication Data
Simon, Robert I.
  Bad men do what good men dream: a forensic psychiatrist illuminates the darker side of human behavior / by Robert I. Simon. − 1st ed., rev.
      p. ; cm.
  Includes bibliographical references and index.
  ISBN 978-1-58562-294-8 (alk. paper)
  1. Antisocial personality disorders. 2. Mentally ill offenders. 3. Psychopaths. 4. Acting out (Psychology) 5. Good and evil–Psychological aspects. 6. Shadow (Psychoanalysis) I. Title.
  [DNLM: 1. Personality Disorders. 2. Forensic Psychiatry. WM 190 S596b 2008]
  RC555.S57 2008
  616.85'82–dc22

                                                                              2008004459

British Library Cataloguing in Publication Data
A CIP record is available from the British Library.

To Ann

Your goodness has made many things possible
and everything worthwhile.

The heart has its reasons which reason does not understand.

—*Blaise Pascal, Penseés*

Contents

Foreword

Tout comprendre, c'est tout pardonner.

Madame de Stael

A recent movie entitled *Mr. Brooks* tells the story of a vicious serial killer with a long history of murdering strangers. The movie begins, paradoxically, with Mr. Brooks receiving a "Citizen of the Year" award. This paradox is at the heart of this book by Robert I. Simon, M.D., in which this experienced, outstanding clinician and forensic psychiatrist describes in often chilling detail the "wolves disguised to live among the sheep." But his analysis carries us further: to the wolf in everyone.

Sociologists have made the point that the human psyche has been subject in its history to three great blows to its narcissism. The first was delivered by Nicolaus Copernicus, suggesting that the earth, humankind's home, is not the center of the universe. The second, delivered by Charles Darwin, was that humanity is not even a unique species but has evolved from precursors. The final blow was delivered by Sigmund Freud, who suggested that human beings are not even in conscious charge of their own minds, impulses, and decisions, but were influenced, if not controlled outright, by unconscious forces.

This last point brings us to the subject matter of this book. By demonstrating the parallels between the actions of "bad men" and the uncensored dreams of the rest of us, Simon has presented what amounts to a bid for tolerance and understanding, in the form of a forensic review of individuals he has so carefully and thoughtfully studied. He counsels—and, more meaningfully, demonstrates—the value of empathically understanding the "bad" in order to better appreciate and accept our own dark natures. He and I are of similar minds about this: Simon kindly quotes me as teaching—in regard to the most regressed, psychotic, or perverse patient my trainees are striving to treat—the maxim: "There, but for the grace of better defenses, go I."

There seem to be two major dimensions to Simon's thesis. The first is that unmistakably "bad" persons may seem very much like the rest of us. Leston Havens, M.D., notes that the differential diagnosis of a person labeled "psychopath" includes the label "normal." Such individuals excel at social mimicry, blending into the population and revealing their true nature only when caught and exposed; the extreme version is the impostor psychopath, who may convincingly forge an entire false identity and live that second life without detection. The modern literary versions of this story are no improvement on Thomas Mann's classic, *Confessions of Felix Krull: Confidence Man*.

This mimicry accounts for the fact that psychopaths are found in all walks of life, not just in incarcerated populations. Law school, business school, medical school, divinity school—none can successfully screen out psychopaths, since these institutions select not for character (impossible in any case), but for competence, and many psychopaths are both extremely competent and highly manipulative in achieving their ends.

The second dimension of Simon's thesis is the commonality of "the rest of us" with the various sinners and criminals he describes. By encouraging recognition and acceptance of our own dark sides, Simon strives not only for empathy but for an end to the polarization "we are good and they are bad." This polarization, Simon makes clear, leads to the whole spectrum of problems from self-righteous egocentrism to genocide. Many mentally ill persons see the world in sharp black-and-white, all-or-none ways; Simon proposes the more mature viewpoint that acknowledges shades of gray.

Perhaps a comment closer to the mark of Simon's intent in this work comes from noted psychiatrist Harry Stack Sullivan, who commented that the schizophrenic is more nearly human than otherwise. Even with this most serious of mental illnesses, capable of profoundly altering the person's mind, emotions and behavior, Sullivan encouraged looking beyond symptomatology to the essential humanness beneath. Simon has a similar goal: to reveal the humanistic core all humans share, even those distinguished by seemingly inhuman behavior.

In expansion of this latter theme, Simon points out the evils done by "good" men who are not enslaved by mental disorders: the *petit fonctionnaires,* the petty bureaucrats, for example, who kept meticulous business records of the victims sent to the Nazi death chambers, providing the embodiment of Arendt's banality of evil. Sadly, we need not look as far back as the Second World War to find ordinary people apparently treating alleged terrorist detainees with probably illegal inhumanity, seemingly with the same psychological rationalization that Simon describes: "These are the enemy and deserve no better."

For those who, even after reading this work, remain resistant to the idea of a "dark side" in ordinary people, we might note the current public fascination with serial killer narratives, police and crime scene procedurals, and similar materials in books, films, and television programs. These varied art forms likely provide vicarious gratifications of the impulses and fantasies that Simon so evocatively details.

In the end, this book should be read not only for its fascinating, riveting, and disturbing case histories, but also for its essential humanity in encouraging understanding of the most deviant of human behavior and in accepting the ubiquitous evils of which most of us, fortunately, only dream.

Thomas G. Gutheil, M.D.

Preface

The proposition that not very much separates "good" and "bad" persons is difficult for many people to acknowledge. To some who consider themselves good, the very idea is an abomination. But I view the belief that we are good and that badness exists outside of ourselves as a fiction—the fiction that drives the engines of prejudice and discrimination, and, on a larger scale, of terrorism, wars, and genocides. It destroys the healing potential of empathy, not only for others but also for ourselves. Denial of mankind's dark side, and projection of it, allows demonization and extermination of others, of whole countries. The serial killers, the evildoers, the psychopaths described in this book justify their criminal acts by calling their victims "trash," as the Green River Killer declared. The reality is that "good" persons are not always good and that "bad" persons are not always bad. There are no saints among us.

Throughout this book, I try in various ways to answer the difficult if not impossible question: Why do bad men do what good men dream? Dostoyevsky recognized that this was a conundrum when he observed, "While nothing is easier than to denounce the evildoer, nothing is more difficult than to understand him." In my analysis of the evildoers in this book, the answer to the "why" question is evident in some cases, at least to some extent, but in most others a definitive answer continues to be elusive.

The book's purpose goes beyond that analysis. It is predicated on the notion that once we acknowledge that no great gulf exists between "good" and "bad" men, we can properly look inward instead of outward. The mass of humankind live unexamined lives of what Thoreau called "quiet desperation." But men's demons luxuriate in darkness. To illuminate them is a hard task. What makes us quintessentially human is the ability to turn our minds back upon ourselves, to shine a light on our demons, and thereby to harness them and put them to productive work. Evildoers cannot do so; they fail spectacularly at self-reflection and self-control. We who consider ourselves "good" people have choices. We can continue to curse the darkness or we can celebrate the human spirit by striving to engage our dark side in the pursuit of an enlightened destiny, not only for ourselves but also for all of humanity.

Robert I. Simon, M.D.

Acknowledgments

One of the pleasures of writing a book is acknowledging those persons who assisted in its creation. Robert K. Ressler, a former FBI special agent and a foremost expert on serial killers provided critical insights for the chapters on workplace violence and serial killers. I value his contribution greatly. I also consulted Albert M. Druktennis, M.D., J.D., a forensic psychiatrist, on the essential subject of this book, humankind's darker side. I found his penetrating illumination of this topic to be uniquely incisive and extraordinarily sensitive. Tom Shachtman was my editorial consultant. His encyclopedic knowledge and expertise as a writer were extremely helpful.

I am grateful to American Psychiatric Publishing, Inc., to Robert E. Hales, M.D., M.B.A., editor-in-chief, and John McDuffie, editorial director, for their foresight and willingness to break new ground in publishing and updating a book of the forensic genre for informed laypersons and mental health professionals. A special thanks goes to the publisher's editor, whose painstaking review greatly improved the quality of this book. When I embarked on this project, the outcome was far from certain. I was permitted freedom to pursue and refine my topic.

Finally, I want to express my thanks to my former secretary, Ms. Susan Breglio, for her faithful and competent assistance. Ms. Breglio being one of the most wholesome persons I have ever met, her fascination with serial killers caught me briefly by surprise. For my wife, whose patience and support made this book as well as so many other things possible, words fail me in expressing my deepest gratitude and affection.

1

Illuminating the Darker Side of Human Behavior

Know then thyself, presume not God to scan;
The proper study of mankind is man.

—Alexander Pope

Humankind has a dark side, and its existence ought not to come as a surprise to those who think of themselves as good people. Most religions conceive of humankind as bad, unregenerate, and in dire need of redemption. The story of Adam and Eve depicts man's fall from grace and descent into a desperate condition. From that day on, the history of the world has been filled with violence.

Today, newspapers, television stations, and the Internet hawk their inventory of human tragedies. Interpersonal violence is a staple of local television news—"Grisly Murder at 11." In the past 30 years, tens of millions of people in the United States have been injured by criminals; every 22 seconds, someone is beaten, stabbed, shot, robbed, raped, or killed. In the era of random violence, nobody feels safe. Overseas, the horrible *ethnic cleansing*—genocide by another name—continues unabated. In Somalia, tens of thousands of people starved to death while feudal warlords fought among themselves, then turned their violence against the very people who came to save the Somalis from starvation. In Darfur, since 2003, many thousands have been raped, tortured, and starved to death, while the government and rebels fight each other.

Glimpses of the demons that peek out from the dark recesses of our minds come from some of the greatest writers, such as Goethe,

1

Dostoyevsky, Poe, Stevenson, and Shakespeare, who have written classic tales about humankind's darker impulses. La Rochefoucauld observed that "We would often be ashamed of our best actions if the world knew the motives behind them." Joseph Conrad wrote in *Heart of Darkness* that "A man's most open actions have a secret side to them." Examples abound in real life: for instance, a sadistic little boy might grow up to be a renowned surgeon. Such sadistic little boys are the subject of William Golding's novel *Lord of the Flies*, which explores the *beast* within us: English boys marooned on a tropical island degenerate into vicious savages, illustrating the point that violence is often released in the absence of restraining, civilized structures. Sigmund Freud delved deeply into just this notion in many of his works: *Civilization and Its Discontents* viewed the human being as a creature driven by powerful instincts of aggression and primal passions that lead to rape, incest, and murder, imperfectly contained by social institutions and guilt.

We are frightened and yet fascinated by the dark side. Millions of upright citizens are avid consumers of movies, television programs, videos, books, and articles that portray murder, rape, and other forms of violence. The Internet has become another medium through which stalkers, sexual exploiters, and other evildoers can pursue their victims. Interactive video games are a multimillion dollar industry. One particularly violent game, *Halo,* in its three editions has sold tens of millions of copies. Its credo is "Thou shalt kill," and players must shoot it out with others to conquer space. Many video games are devoted to violent adventures that reward the player's ability to kill and kill quickly. One of every eight Hollywood movies has a theme of rape. By the time the average American reaches the age of 18, he or she will have viewed 250,000 acts of violence, including 40,000 murders on television. Mystery writers can count on making a good living by exploring the theme that almost anyone can be driven to kill. The reach of these violent images has been greatly extended by the proliferation of electronic communications—the Internet, DVDs, even cell phones, to which the young seem addicted.

What about the good people among us? Most humans go about the daily business of life without robbing, raping, or committing murder. Yet, after 40 years of work as both a treating and a forensic psychiatrist, I am absolutely convinced that there is no great gulf between the mental life of the common criminal and that of the everyday, upright citizen. The dark side exists in all of us. There is no "we-they" dichotomy between the good citizens, the "we," and the criminals, the "they." Who among us has not had the wish or felt the urge to do something illicit? If we could press a button and eliminate our rivals or enemies with impunity, how many of us would resist? In fact, if this were possible, probably very few people would be left standing. One cannot listen for so many years as patients and criminal defendants reveal their inner lives without coming to the conclusion that bad men and women do what good men and women only dream about doing.

But good men and women are far from perfect in their behavior. We are neither all good nor all bad. To varying degrees, we are a combination of both. An unexpected situation may become the occasion for one side or the other to win out. Combat, for example, may incite the same person to acts of heroism or cowardice, depending on the circumstances. In peace time, a former sadistic concentration camp guard may slip into the role of the respected but feared cop on the beat.

The basic difference between what are socially considered to be bad or good people is not one of kind, but of degree, and of the ability of the bad to translate dark impulses into dark actions. Bad men such as serial sexual killers have intense, compulsive, elaborate sadistic fantasies that few good men have, but we all harbor some measure of that hostility, aggression, and sadism. Anyone can become violent, even murderous, under certain circumstances. Therapists who have undergone their own psychoanalysis or insight psychotherapy have a humanistic recognition of the universality of human intrapsychic experience. These therapists acknowledge in themselves many of the same psychological struggles they find in their patients and in others. It is hoped that therapists handle their personal problems better more of the time, but this is not necessarily so. Dr. Thomas G. Gutheil, Professor of Psychiatry at Harvard and a famed forensic psychiatrist, candidly acknowledges what most therapists know about themselves: "There, but for the grace of better defenses, go I."

This idea is very difficult for many people to accept. Perhaps our dark side comes from our evolutionary heritage, in which aggression ensured our survival. Maybe it is the result of faulty wiring in our brains. The depletion of certain brain neurotransmitters, such as serotonin, has been found to parallel aggressive behavior. Our brains are wired for aggression and can short-circuit into violence. All of us have aggressive impulses. His Holiness Tenzin Gyatso, the 14th Dalai Lama of Tibet, and the winner of the 1989 Nobel Peace Prize, spoke of the dark side of his dreams to an interviewer:

> In my dreams, sometimes women approach me, and I immediately realize, "I'm *bhiksbu,* I'm monk"—so you see, this is sort of sexual.... Similarly, I have dreams where someone is beating me, and I want to respond. Then I immediately remember, "I am monk and I should not kill."

It is difficult to underestimate most people's allegiance to the belief that good men and bad men are fundamentally different or that bad men are "crazy." Even as you read this book, you may say to yourself, "Not me. I would never do such things." You may never have considered the acts committed by the persons depicted in these pages, or, if you did consider any of them, you quickly rejected the notion as "sick." Yet psychiatrists know that if people are removed from their normal world, without their usual external controls and surroundings, they may take liberties that previously they could only have imagined. For example, after a major disaster, there is always looting. Many looters are people who never before considered robbery. Usually, there are so many looters that the authorities must institute martial law to regain control of the situation. Members of a crowd act in ways that they would not consider as individuals. Being part of a crowd does not eliminate an individual's thinking or control as much as it can nullify the person's conscience. Who can forget the televised scenes of looting following the Katrina disaster?

People's antisocial impulses are opportunistic. After major disasters in the United States, fake and inflated damage claims cost the insurance industry tens of billions of dollars. Similarly, thousands upon thousands of ordinary folk regularly cheat on their income taxes or fail to file altogether. Polygraph operators who conduct preemployment examinations of *normal* persons for industry soon discover that an incredible number of illegal acts, sexual deviations, addictions, and all manner of unimaginable, bizarre activities are admitted to by the examinees. During fraternity initiations or in the hazing of cadets at military academies, extremes of behavior occur. Atrocious acts are routinely reported—some that even result in deaths. These tortures are not acts perpetrated by devilish people but by our privileged, "normal" young men and women—those we consider to be our hope for the future.

I mention these seeming contradictions because I believe that you, the reader, can derive the most benefit from this book if you do not fall prey to the good man–bad man illusion—the belief that good men and women do not have a sinister dark side. Nothing could be further from the truth. It is likely that among the deviant behaviors portrayed within these covers, you will grudgingly recognize aspects of your own human condition. For some, that realization may be personally threatening—it may even make them want to put the book down and go no further with it. I hope that will not happen to you. I hope that the knowledge gathered in this book will cause you to change, to be more accepting of your humanity and that of other people. But if, after reading this book, you still believe that good men and bad men are worlds, maybe even universes apart, will you also continue to curse the darkness and thereby deny your own humanity? Or will you simply lose an opportunity to gain insight into recognizing, harnessing, and productively channeling the dark side we all share? This book presents an opportunity. If I can help you realize that this opportunity must be seized rather than denied, then I will have succeeded in an important task, and it is hoped I will have enriched your life.

Two Perspectives

In a courtroom, I am invariably asked about my *bona fides*—why I am qualified to give an opinion—and I want to answer the same question here by suggesting that as a forensic psychiatrist and as a treating psychiatrist, I am able to bring two different perspectives to the subject of humanity's darker side. In my forensic practice, I have often been asked to evaluate men charged with exhibitionism. Most exhibitionists are generally passive men who feel inadequate about themselves, particularly in the way they relate to women. They are outwardly anything but macho, "Rambo" types, though they may still be dangerous and may ultimately progress to more aggressive sexual behaviors. What the exhibitionist attempts to accomplish when he exposes himself to a woman is basically to demonstrate that he is not inadequate. The shock he hopes for in the woman's surprised or stunned expression is aimed at reversing his own fears and inadequacies. By exposing himself, the exhibitionist attains a fantasized dominant position that reduces his anxiety.

In my consulting practice, I see a steady stream of male patients who are struggling with the same underlying problem as the exhibitionists—feelings of inadequacy—but who manifest these feelings in symptoms of impotence, or premature or retarded ejaculation. The exhibitionist has lived out his fantasies, whereas the patient has grappled with similar demons and has instead developed dysfunctional sexual symptoms and inhibitions. The "good" man has come for treatment, whereas the "bad" man has psychologically assaulted and traumatized women. Why the exhibitionist acts out his problem while the patient only develops symptoms is a clinical and theoretical conundrum that psychiatrists have long pondered. It is a question to which there is no easy answer, only a case-by-case analysis.

Forensic psychiatrists often examine criminal defendants who have committed all manner of antisocial acts, persons that they would not generally see in private practice. We evaluate defendants for competency to stand trial. One of our duties is to assist the judicial system in determining whether a defendant was sane or insane at the time of the crime. Forensic psychiatry is involved at all levels of the criminal process, from assessing a person's competency to confess to a crime to the extremely controversial matter of evaluating competency to be executed. We make pre-sentence evaluations, offer recommendations for disposition and treatment, and advise judges, parole boards, and other law enforcement agencies.

Forensic psychiatrists are also active on the civil side of the system, consulting with attorneys on malpractice cases, in child custody disputes, in personal injury litigation such as that resulting from auto accidents, and in cases involving worker's compensation, insurance matters (accidental death versus suicide), wills that are being contested, and myriad other litigation matters at the fascinating intersection of psychiatry and law. On administrative matters, forensic psychiatrists are asked to give testimony at legislative hearings—for instance, prior to the enactment of laws governing the sexual misconduct of professionals and the right of an individual to refuse treatment.

As a treating psychiatrist, I see patients with a wellness rather than a litigation agenda. Patients come to us because they are suffering mentally. They are depressed or anxious; they have feelings of panic and unbidden thoughts and actions, as well as personality problems that interfere with their day-to-day functioning and quality of life. Although some of these patients may, from time to time, put their problems into action, in the main their personal difficulties are contained within themselves, manifested only as unpleasant, painful symptoms and inhibitions that often interfere with their personal relationships. Yet, in my experience as a forensic psychiatrist, their dreams can be thematically similar to those of criminal defendants.

That there is an intimate and reciprocal connection between symptoms and destructive acting-out behavior is brought home again and again to the treating psychiatrist. For example, a patient who has been harmfully acting out personal conflicts comes into treatment and simultaneously stops those behaviors, but in their place starts to experience anxiety and depression. These "new" symptoms and their underlying causes then become the focus of treatment. Sigmund Freud insisted that the object of psychoanalysis was to substitute ordinary human unhappiness for neurotic misery. And that is a sensible objective. After all, psychotherapy does not promise utopia. What it does, really, is encourage patients, through the trusting support of the psychiatrist, to face and conquer their personal dragons and to make sense out of their mental difficulties.

Let us be clear about this: at one time or another, most of us will struggle with our personal demons. No one can run from them for very long. One cannot escape them by sticking one's head in the sand or by retreating into various addictions, because these actions can be as painful as or more disabling than the original problems. I have treated patients who have sought geographical cures to their problems by moving hither and yon, only to reexperience and repeat their problems in a new venue. Psychiatrists aim to empower their patients by helping them to discover alternative, more adaptive problem-solving techniques. To get away from being stuck in automatic ways of thinking, feeling, and behaving, patients learn mental manual overrides and other new ways of dealing with their problems. In a successful treatment, autonomy and responsibility for one's own life replace previous helplessness and destructive repetitions.

Mad or Bad?

Society, religion, and the law all take moral positions about right and wrong, about the acts of "bad" men, often labeling such persons and their behavior as evil. Medically trained and wedded to the scientific method, psychiatrists do not ordinarily apply the term *evil*, even to the aberrant destructive acts they are sometimes called upon to understand and explain. Psychiatrists look at causes and effects in human behavior and try not to make moral judgments. What society labels evil behavior, the psychiatrist seeks to understand within the framework of the psychopathology of mental illness or even of everyday life. Although the law holds that each of us has the free will to choose between right and wrong, psychiatrists generally see the human being as a creature who is affected by powerful internal forces and not always free to make rational decisions.

For many people, Jeffrey Dahmer seems the personification of evil. The details of the 17 serial sexual killings associated with him, as brought out by media reports, shocked and sickened many people around the world. Dismembered body parts were found in his apartment. Decomposed torsos floated in acid-filled vats. A refrigerator contained human heads, a freezer held a heart and male genitals. Dahmer confessed that he had drugged and strangled his victims, had sex with their dead bodies, then dismembered them, smashing the bones into small pieces with a sledgehammer. He boiled the heads to remove the skin so he could paint the skulls white, and made meals of the various body parts. Dahmer commented that a bicep tasted like steak.

Was Dahmer inherently bad, or was he mad? The law allows an exception to the rule that a defendant is responsible for a criminal act if, as a result of mental illness, the defendant did not know what he or she was doing or that the act was wrong, or was not able to control the behavior, even if aware that it was wrong. In Dahmer's trial, the defense claimed that Dahmer could not stop killing because he was mentally ill. Because of a "sickness he discovered, not chose...he had to do what he did, because he couldn't stop it." His own attorney described Dahmer as "a steamrolling killing machine" on the track of madness. The forensic psychiatrists at the trial all found some form and degree of mental disorder in Dahmer—how could anyone display such outrageous, sexually violent behavior and not be abnormal? But they differed on whether Dahmer had been able to control himself.

The Milwaukee jury dismissed both the arguments that Dahmer had been mentally ill and that he lacked the substantial capacity to control his murderous behavior, convicting him of 15 murders. In essence, the jury decided that Dahmer was bad and that whatever the degree of his madness, his vile behavior could not be excused by society. Punishment, not treatment, was the message in the jury's verdict. The judge sentenced Dahmer to 15 consecutive life sentences, roughly 950 years in jail, with no possibility of parole. Dahmer was murdered in prison.

The "Normality" of Evil

Jeffrey Dahmer indeed seems to be the personification of evil, and thus to provide strong evidence against the thesis of this book, which is that bad people do what good people dream. Yet the sadistic traits seen in such serial killers as Jeffrey Dahmer have their tamer counterparts in patients who will never commit a sexually sadistic crime of any kind, who are respectable persons, good mothers and fathers, successful professionals.

I have treated solid citizens who mentally torture their spouses, children, elderly parents, and themselves but would not dream of raising a finger to physically harm anyone. Sexual sadism, dominance, and submission have long been part of the spectrum of human behavior. Power and aggression can be identified as factors in all sorts of human courting and mating behaviors, whether in primitive cultures or in modern and presumably civilized ones. Such behaviors occur along a continuum that stretches from intense fantasies and private, noncriminal sexual acts between consenting partners to the more publicly deplorable behaviors of rape and the baroque and bizarre sexual fantasies that lead to ritualized serial sexually sadistic murders.

The Dahmers of this world are rare, but sadism and power motives are common to all human beings. Patients who are able to be extremely candid about their fantasies will often reveal a rich variety of sexually sadistic fantasies that underlie dysfunctional symptoms and behaviors. Even those who are not so candid prove capable of channeling their sadistic impulses into other, less personally destructive activities. Have you enjoyed watching a professional football game lately? How about boxing or professional wrestling? Horror movies, extreme TV medical dramas, and the constant drum of violent crimes on the local news command large audiences.

In this book I try to dispel a basic fallacy—that destruction and violence reside only in the acts of bad men and women and not in the thoughts of good people. We must all struggle with the dark forces. In the Middle Ages, ecclesiastical thinking held that aggression and violence were caused by foreign, evil spirits besetting an individual. In the twenty-first century, those of us who exclusively ascribe aggression and violence to sickness fall prey to the same inherently flawed perception of man as did the clerics of the Middle Ages. Although there is no doubt that some of the dramatic violence described in this book is attributable to psychopathic personalities and psychotic individuals, much of it is not. Most of the violence and mayhem in this world are committed not by the mentally ill but by individuals and entire societies not considered to be sick, at least not by any known measure of mental illness. The answer to why such violence occurs lies beyond the psychopathology of evil. No competent psychiatrist is so arrogant as to think that human motivation and behavior can be fully explained by current medical and psychological theories. Only God knows the human mind and heart.

I shall never forget the forensic examination of a woman who was terribly traumatized by witnessing an execution-style killing. During a robbery of a fast food establishment, she witnessed from a back room the shooting of a coworker who was on her knees begging for her life. The coworker's murderer was a 13-year-old boy. As she related the horrible scene and her personal horror, I became aware of my own acute discomfort. I clumsily commented that the boy himself must have been victimized in some way. I was brought up short by her quick retort: "You must realize, doctor, that there is real evil in this world." Unfortunately, human history is replete with the "real evil" of atrocities, wars, mass killings, and genocides. Adolf Hitler and the Nazis exterminated perhaps as many as 10 million people. It is estimated that Joseph Stalin and his henchmen deported and murdered 20 million of their countrymen. In addition, the twentieth century saw the Turkish genocide of Armenians, estimated at 1 million people, and the killing of 2 million Cambodians by the Khmer Rouge. In 1994, more than 500,000 people were slaughtered in the Rwandan genocide. As this book goes to press, hundreds of thousands are being slaughtered in Darfur.

But Stalin did not pull the trigger of each gun, nor did Hitler turn on the gas cock in every extermination room. Were all the enabling participants in their murders mentally ill? Consider Adolf Eichmann, the Nazi bureaucrat who directed the deportation of millions of people to concentration and extermination camps. Even though he had perpetrated unconscionable evil, a half-dozen psychiatrists certified him as normal.

The term *banality of evil*, used by Hannah Arendt in describing Nazi atrocities, refers in part to the infrastructure that subserves genocidal execution. For every paid sadistic functionary who tortures his or her victim, at least 50 "administrators" provide support by answering the phones, driving cars, keeping records, and performing other ordinary, day-to-day tasks. It is just another day at the office. No better example exists of how great evil can be perpetrated by ordinary people, performing ordinary tasks and living ordinary lives. Also appalling is the knowledge that, unlike mass-produced state torture, ordinary individuals devilishly and exquisitely tailor their torture to the intimately known vulnerabilities of their victims, behind the closed doors of millions of workplaces and homes throughout the world.

Many among the Nazi executioners went home after a day of exterminating women, children, and old men to resume quite comfortable and normal lives in the bosoms of their families. They ate good food, listened to classical music, read a refined book, made love with their wives, coddled and embraced their children. How could the mind of an executioner juxtapose an evening of domestic bliss against the atrocities he perpetrated during the day? Was it mental illness that allowed such a duality?

Many murderers and torturers have been facilitated by an infrastructure of compliant, enabling supporters who were in all likelihood certifiably normal. And I stress that in all of the cases of mass killings and sadistic acts such as those of the Nazis, there must have been dramatic failures of empathy and enormous excesses of projection of their own unacceptable thoughts and feelings that permitted the perpetrators to conceive of the victims as detestable, nonhuman objects.

The mental states that permit such immense cruelties evolve out of ordinary psychological processes. For example, an ordinary psychological defense observed in the psychiatrist's office and in everyday life may shed some light on humankind's worst inhumanities. The vehement criticism of others, on closer scrutiny, often turns out to be a disturbing self-criticism. It is far easier to see our problems in others than to acknowledge them in ourselves. To look inside and discover unacceptable impulses can be a very troubling experience. For some people it is intolerable. These individuals, and sometimes whole societies, need to attribute their dark sides to others and then dehumanize them as a prelude to victimization.

But these immense cruelties and monstrous acts—and the fact that "normal" people are implicated in them—also force us to think. We must consider the possibilities. Could it be that the evils of this world that are perpetrated by human beings result from an innate, natural, self-centeredness? Might this self-centeredness be the psychological counterpart to the instinct for survival? Might it push us to give greater importance to ourselves and interfere with our ability to consider others as worthy human beings? Could it be that virulent forms of self-centeredness and entitlement can account for the overvaluation of the perpetrator's self, producing contempt and devaluation of others that becomes the psychological engine for these atrocities and mass killings? If so, then how do people reach that point at which lethal self-centeredness overrides any tendency to be decent to others? Psychiatric concepts fail us miserably here.

On a more personal scale, can we figure out whether, when, why, and how an element of destructive self-centeredness enters into our everyday social intercourse and causes hurt, misunderstanding, and psychological harm to others? The Golden Rule is an intuitive recognition of the connection between self-centeredness and evil. In adjuring us to do unto others as we would have others do unto us, it exhorts us to sublimate our natural selfishness into empathy for others.

The Hitlers, Stalins, and other mass murderers and torturers are on the extreme end of the continuum of violence and sadism that is common to all of mankind. They know what they are doing. But their counterparts, the most deranged, violently mentally ill criminals, do not conceive and perpetrate horrible crimes while in other regards maintaining "normal" lives. Many are incarcerated in institutions for the criminally insane. Over a million other prisoners populate American jails. The majority of them are not considered mentally ill by current diagnostic standards, though many of them have committed violent acts. Yet there is a surfeit of violence in our society; it may not hold the headlines of history in the way that Hitler's atrocities do, but terrible things go on daily, such as the psychological and physical maiming and murder of children.

To think that these events have nothing to do with people considered to be normal is to refuse to look at the evidence for my basic thesis: we are all human beings and capable of a grand spectrum of behaviors, both that which is considered good, and that which we know very well to be bad. Although most people are able to curb their sadistic, destructive dark side, that side continues to be present and operative to varying degrees by day and by night. Primitive humans thought that when the moon waned, part of it ceased to exist. Today, we know that the dark part of the moon, though not visible, is still there. We are made up of many goods and bads, and we had better face that fact. Indeed, it is one of the aims of this book to help us do so.

As I review in my mind the experience of treating and evaluating literally thousands of people, I find that I cannot generalize about them. Rather than containing two strands, one good and the other bad, each individual is like a rope with intertwining psychological strands of immense complexity. For the patient, the difficult but often rewarding work of psychotherapy is unraveling some of the more troublesome strands. It is far better to grab hold of one's rope than be hung by it. To attempt to cast out violence by attributing it to "them" and not to "us" will only enslave us to a greater and more psychologically damaging myth of safety. We must stare our demons in the eye and learn to control them, so that our darkest dreams will never be translated into terrible actions.

The Dalai Lama articulates with beautiful simplicity a major theme of this book: "Many people today agree that we need to reduce violence in our society. If we are truly serious about this, we must deal with the roots of violence, particularly those that exist within each of us. We need to embrace 'inner disarmament,' reducing our own emotions of suspicion, hatred and hostility toward our brothers and sisters."

That all men and women must struggle with their dark side is not reason to despair. Love and kindness are also fundamental parts of ourselves and find expression every second, everywhere on earth. The grand catastrophes of humankind, such as the Holocaust, and the evils of our everyday lives, reveal that the greatest danger comes from denying that there is a beastly part of our humanity. If we can acknowledge the beast and attempt to control it, the beast is less likely to leap out when we least expect it.

"A Light Unto My Path"

A few years ago I was asked by a young psychiatrist to supervise her therapeutic work with a difficult patient. During the course of the supervision, she reported to me an incident with the patient that was deeply troubling her. Therapy sessions with this patient, a single, middle-aged woman with chronic depression, had begun 8 months earlier and were characterized by the patient's anger and complaints about her life. The patient seemed to find the minor problems in life to be very wounding. My colleague traced these reactions to the patient's sense of self-importance and entitlement. After the conclusion of an especially difficult therapy session, full of bitter, tearful complaints and recriminations, the patient went into the bathroom of the waiting room area. A few moments later, my colleague opened the door from her office to the waiting room to greet the next patient, but that one had not yet arrived. The previous patient, still in the bathroom, had left her purse on a waiting room chair. My colleague was jolted by an impulse to take something from the patient's purse. Astounded and ashamed of this impulse, she closed the door and shut herself back in her office to contemplate her urge to steal from the patient.

Later that day, she and I had a regularly scheduled supervisory session. She told me of the incident and felt comfortable enough to examine the unbidden impulse to steal. She had been turning over in her mind what it might possibly mean. It was not money or anything in particular she wanted from the purse, the psychiatrist told me, it was that she just wanted something back from the patient. This deeply self-centered patient was an inveterate taker, giving nothing in return to any of her relationships. After a time people would drop her, leaving her with a numbing sense of rejection, isolation, and chronic depression. Now, after 8 months of treating the patient, the psychiatrist was experiencing feelings of emotional depletion and reacting against being treated as an object. This patient, of course, aroused similar feelings in nearly everyone with whom she came into sustained contact. The psychiatrist knew that these were also feelings the patient had experienced at the hands of a distant, depressed, rejecting mother and an indifferent father.

But why had she wanted to steal or to possess something from this patient now? After examining her own feelings, the psychiatrist recognized the extent of desolation and emptiness in the wake of the recent breakup of her unhappy marriage. Also, the failure of the marriage had triggered unresolved feelings of loss and loneliness from her childhood, following the sudden death of her mother. Now my colleague realized that she had been subconsciously looking to her patient for nurture and sustenance at a time of her own personal crisis. In this paradigm, the patient stood both for the psychiatrist's lost mother and her more recently lost spouse, and her yearnings for both of them.

With the insight she had gained about her own mental and emotional situation through examining the singular impulse to steal, the psychiatrist then returned her therapeutic attention to the patient. For the first time, the psychiatrist felt empathy for the patient and pointed out to her the pattern of feelings the patient aroused in others, which enabled the patient to see how she was reversing and reenacting the distant, cold relationship she had experienced with her mother. This insight proved to be of great assistance to the patient.

My colleague's breakthrough with the patient was made possible because she was willing to face directly the black pain of her own losses and to insist on understanding why it had erupted as a wish to steal in this particular situation. The ability to face, hold, and examine antisocial thoughts and feelings is not just a requirement for psychiatrists and their patients. It is necessary for everyone. I am not naïve enough, however, to believe that the vast majority of humankind can or will examine their darker impulses, consciously control these brooding forces, or harness them for good purposes. History suggests the unlikelihood that most of us will perform that task. This book is for the few who can look inward.

Restraint of antisocial impulses is learned from the cradle, within the family and through many other social structures. Parents and caretakers help children internalize the ethical, philosophical, cultural, and religious values that also restrain antisocial impulses. Later on, a society's political system attempts to ensure through law and custom that destructive tendencies remain curbed—and largely unexamined. But even the healthiest genes, the warmest parents and family, the most morally unassailable community, the best education, and the most humane society cannot eradicate the dark and destructive forces in our personalities. Nor should they, for our dark side is an inextricable part of our humanity. When it is denied or run from, there is always some price to be paid. Moreover, the darker side of men and women cannot be snuffed out by building more prisons and carrying out more executions. This is not society's purpose; rather, its goal is to deter, punish, restrain, and reform.

As in the first law of thermodynamics, which explains the conservation of energy, our darker side can neither be created nor destroyed; it can only change form. It can be retained in thoughts and feelings, it can be rechanneled into productive activity, or it can be acted out in a destructive way. In my work with patients, I have learned that we essentially have two courses to follow: either struggle to recognize, control, and channel our basic conflicts and impulses, or allow them to luxuriate and perhaps to dominate us. Unfortunately, much of humankind takes the latter road, which is strewn with many of life's perturbations and miseries.

It is far better to choose, as my colleague did, to walk in the path that leads to the light, to confront the dark side, and to work through it. In that particular instance, the light was revealed reasonably swiftly. But as psychiatrists know from working with patients, insight and intuition for self-discovery is not accessible to everyone, neither is it an unmitigated good, whenever it does become accessible. For some, psychological insight can be a peak transforming experience. When our antisocial impulses are buried alive, like vampires, they can emerge to harm us. Exposing our dark side to the light does not make our personal vampires disappear as in legend. But doing so offers the possibility that we can develop constructive options once we are clearly able to see the inhabitants of our dark side. This empowering idea is expressed in John 7:28: "For you shall know the truth and the truth shall make you free."

In a sense, our patients are never the same after an insight is achieved—it is hoped they are changed for the better. For others, insight may be undesirable. For still others, it is ineffective in alleviating certain behaviors. To add insight to the injury already present may worsen some patients' conditions. The American poet Robinson Jeffers wryly observed that most people would rather face a tiger on the road than confront the truth. We must remember that the majority of people get by passably well in controlling their most dangerous and antisocial impulses through reasonably effective internal controls and such pragmatic restraints as the police officer on the next corner.

But when we walk the path of light, we are able to see where we are going. We will recognize the landscape around us for what it is, be it beautiful or threatening. My colleague, willing to shed noonday light on a dark corner of the road, channeled a destructive impulse into a constructive growth experience that helped her and her patient. The path that leads to the light is open to anyone who has a native capacity for insight, intuition, and a natural curiosity about his or her behavior. Along this path, we shed light on our demons and discover our humanity. We may understand that dark impulses can be channeled and used to enrich and empower our lives through art, literature, humor, athletics, or simply through the sheer zest and enjoyment of the hurly-burly of life that comes from channeled aggression. In fact, much of life's work and play involves controlling and redirecting aggressive impulses. It is a path that permits us to take responsibility for our actions by facing and acknowledging our feelings. Because it discards disabling myths and illusions, it enables us to make freer choices. It is a path that, like this book, leads through patches of darkness so we may better understand and appreciate the light. One of the greatest, most ennobling human characteristics is the ability to turn one's mind back upon itself in a momentous act of personal discovery. We can celebrate, with the psalmist's song of praise, that personal knowledge is "a light unto my path."

2

Human Killing Machines and Us

A Psychology of Evil

There is no sin, no crime I could not be guilty of.

—*Johann Wolfgang von Goethe*

The Serial Killer Next Door

Why are people fascinated by serial killers? The plethora of books, movies, and television documentaries about them attests to the public's obsession with these human killing machines. Yet compared to the number of spouses who kill their partners, or drunken drivers who commit vehicular homicide, there are relatively few serial killers: the FBI estimates that at any given time, between 200 and 500 serial killers are at large and that they kill 3,500 people a year. (See Chapter 11 for an in-depth discussion of serial killers.)

My hunch is that people are fascinated by serial killers because of their perceived resemblance to Dr. Jekyll and Mr. Hyde. As with Dr. Jekyll, most serial killers appear outwardly quite ordinary, like your neighbor or mine, living normal everyday lives in which, just as we do, they fill the car with gas, hold down a job, pay taxes. Then, from behind this veneer of ordinariness, their Mr. Hyde personality, representative of the darkest aspect of humanity, jumps out to kill their victims—and to transfix us.

Prime examples uphold the stereotype. They all hid in plain sight. Dennis Rader worked for 14 years as a security company employee,

19

then as a census taker, and for another 14 years as an animal control and zoning employee of his Wichita, Kansas, suburb. He had been married for decades, had two grown children, was a long-term member of his Lutheran church, and had served as president of its congregation council, as a member of the zoning board of appeals, and as a Cub Scout leader. He looked harmless, neighbors exclaimed when he was arrested as the "BTK" killer in 2005, but soon he confessed to having murdered 10 people in incidents dating back to the 1970s. BTK, which he had suggested as one of the names by which he could be called, was used in taunting letters and missives to the police and the media; it stood for Bind, Torture, and Kill. The packages he sent contained dolls bound in plastic as well as graphic evidence of the murders.

Alexander Pichuskin, dubbed the Chessboard Killer, worked as a grocery store clerk in Moscow for a dozen years before being arrested and charged with 49 murders in 2007. He had been planning, he told a court, to commit a total of 64 murders, one for each square on an imaginary chessboard.

John Wayne Gacy was a building construction contractor, twice married, active in community projects, and a member of civic organizations. In 1967, he was voted the Jaycees' Outstanding Member. Joining the Jolly Joker Club, he created the character of Pogo the Clown and, costumed as Pogo, went into hospitals to cheer up sick children. In 1978, Gacy was director of the Polish Constitution Day Parade in Chicago, and during the festivities was photographed with First Lady Rosalynn Carter. But as Gacy once said, "A clown can get away with murder," and he did—raping, sodomizing, torturing, and strangling to death 33 young men over the course of more than a decade.

Theodore Robert "Ted" Bundy's mother considered him an ideal son. His political friends were convinced he was on the fast track in the legal profession and would one day be a governor or a senator. Dashingly handsome, intelligent, and witty, Bundy was a romantic dream come true for many women. Some described him as an attentive, tender lover who sent flowers and penned love poems. A photo shows Bundy immersed in happy domesticity, opening a bottle of wine as he sits with a girlfriend. At the moment the photo was taken, Bundy had already abducted and murdered 24 women and committed necrophilia with their bodies.

How is it possible for someone who appears to be the guy next door to commit multiple horrific murders? And why are we so fascinated with those who commit such crimes? People have always been gripped by the dark side of human behavior. Our minds follow an inescapable syllogism: "I am human. Serial killers are human. Am I, like them, capable of monstrous deeds?" Most people, having posed this question to themselves, conclude that the answer is "No, I am not even capable of thinking about such evil."

The Rope of Evil

As with pornography, most people recognize evil when they see it. Reaching a universal definition of evil, however, is impossible. Evil is a complicated concept, akin to a thick rope of many strands in which philosophers and theologians become entangled. Evil is in the eye of the beholder, influenced by social, political, religious, philosophical, psychological, and other factors. For example, combatants frequently demonize their enemies as evil, even while each side is certain that God is on its side. The 9/11 terrorists believed that murdering thousands of innocent people would ensure their entrance into Paradise. Antiabortionists who kill doctors or other abortion clinic personnel contend that they are killing murderers. As a psychiatrist and forensic psychiatrist, I will tug at just one strand of the rope of evil, the psychological strand.

Here, in psychological terms, is a working and admittedly imperfect definition: Evil is the intentional, gratuitous, or, on occasion, unintentional infliction of harm by individuals, committed against other individuals, groups, or entire societies. I include unintended acts in the definition because heedless self-indulgence may lead to negligent deeds that produce unintended harm, as when drunken drivers cause deadly accidents. I exclude wars in which millions of people are killed, and which are declared "just" or "unjust" by participants on one side or the other, both praying for victory and convinced that God is with them and not with their enemies. My purpose is to isolate and focus on the inner psychological mechanisms that play essential roles when humans harm each other.

Evil is interpersonal. If you doubt that, read the Ten Commandments: their admonishments and strictures apply to the evils that beset our relationships with man and with God, but mostly with man. Evil is the exclusive province of human beings; it does not take place among animals. Harm directed at inanimate objects is not considered evil unless there is a concurrent element of human suffering. Thoughts that are considered evil invariably deal with doing harm to other human beings.

Psychiatrists are medically trained in and wedded to the use of the scientific method, so they avoid applying the term *evil* to the aberrant or horrible acts they are sometimes called upon to understand and explain. Psychiatrists observe causes and effects in human behavior and try not to be judgmental about them. The determination that a particular behavior is or is not evil is a moral judgment, and what society may label as evil behavior the psychiatrist tries to understand within the framework of mental illness and the psychology of daily life.

Nonetheless, the insight that evil involves acts of interpersonal harm opens the door to analysis of the psychological interaction between perpetrator and victim. That analysis depends on the concept of empathy. The presence or absence of empathy is key to determining an individual's capacity to maintain constructive, collaborative relationships with others; empathy is the ability to put oneself in another's psychological shoes, to sense what the other may be thinking and feeling. But empathy without caring is empty. Psychopaths (remorseless predators) are very skilled at divining what other people feel and think, but they do so in order to manipulate them. They do not care one whit about other people, whom they regard as morsels to be consumed, with the remnants to be thrown away as trash. Serial sexual killers will unblinkingly take a life in order to have an orgasm.

Edmund Edward Kemper III was a necrophilic serial killer who treated his victims as totally discardable objects. After being imprisoned, he was quite clear about his intentions toward his victims: "I'm sorry I sound so cold about this, but what I needed to have was a particular experience with a person, and to possess them in the way I had to, I had to evict them from their bodies."

Suspension of empathy is necessary in order to intentionally harm other people, and it is usually accompanied by the psychological mechanisms of devaluation and projection. Individuals intent on committing harm first dehumanize others and then project onto these others—their victims—their own disavowed, unacceptable traits and inner conflicts. These same mechanisms are involved in prejudice and scapegoating.

Serial sexual killers demonstrate spectacular failures in empathy and equally egregious use of devaluation and projection to rationalize their terrible crimes. In interviews with John Wayne Gacy, it was learned that during his childhood and adolescence, his father voiced contempt for Gacy's illness (psychomotor epilepsy) and for the pampering by Gacy's mother. The father also warned Gacy's mother that John was "going to be a queer," and heaped scorn on John by calling him a "he-she." Years later, after Gacy's killing spree, Gacy referred to his victims as "worthless little queers and punks." It is not difficult to perceive in Gacy's attitude toward his victims echoes of the contempt and verbal abuse his father inflicted on him.

Ted Bundy expressed contempt toward victims. He professed surprise that society was making a fuss over "these girls" that he had murdered, and that their families so deeply mourned their losses. "What's one less person on the face of the earth?" Bundy asked, and referred to his victims as "cargo" and "damaged goods." Gary Ridgway, the Green River Killer, referred to his victims as "trash."

Rader, Ridgway, Gacy, Bundy, and Kemper are all serial sexual killers, a distinct subcategory of serial killers. Not all serial murderers are serial sexual killers. Some kill for reasons other than sex, such as money, jealousy, revenge, power, or dominance. Serial sexual killers enjoy torturing their victims (sadism) for one reason only: to obtain a maximal orgasm that they are unable to achieve in any other way. Most serial killers, regardless of type, are not psychotic; that is, they have not lost their grip on reality.

We consider entire societies that act like serial killers to be evil. But were all the members of the Nazi party during World War II psychopathic? —Yes and no. Some leaders and chief sadists undoubtedly were, but most of the compliant members who took part in the killings were ordinary non-psychopathic citizens who rationalized the atrocities they were committing by the mechanisms of empathic failure, devaluation, and projection. Adolf Eichmann, the Nazi bureaucrat who directed the deportation and extermination of millions of Jews and other peoples, used these mechanisms as well. Interestingly, Eichmann was certified as normal by a half-dozen psychiatrists, even though he had perpetrated monstrous, unconscionable evil. The psychiatrists' diagnosis was reinforced by an odd incident that took place at his trial. A former concentration camp inmate had been waiting for years to testify against him, yet when he stood before Eichmann at the tribunal, the former inmate unexpectedly passed out. Upon being revived, the would-be witness explained his fainting at such a crucial moment by saying, "Eichmann looked so normal."

The first deliberate, systematic genocide of the twentieth century occurred with the extermination of an estimated 1.5 million Armenian men, women, and children by the Ottoman Turks. On the "killing fields" of the Khmer Rouge, in Cambodia, between 1.7 and 2.3 million people died in just a few years. In 1994, 800,000 people were murdered in three months in Rwanda. More recently, tens of thousands have been murdered in Darfur.

Were the perpetrators of such horrific acts sadistic psychopaths? Assuredly some were, but it is also certain that their acts were facilitated and condoned by an infrastructure of compliant supporters, whom psychiatric evaluation would in all likelihood have diagnosed as normal. For every paid killer or torturer in these mass murders, there were "administrators" who participated in the killings by answering telephones, keeping records, driving cars, and performing other day-to-day tasks so that the business of torture and murder could go on—just a regular part of an administrator's ordinary day at the office.

The point is that in all cases of mass killings and sadistic acts, dramatic failures of empathy and caring must take place, and enormous excesses of projection of unacceptable thoughts and feelings must occur, to permit the perpetrators to perceive their victims as detestable human rubbish.

Us, More or Less

What about us, the more or less law-abiding, responsible, respectable folks? Qualification is necessary because we are human beings; nature has built into us the instinct to survive, and in order to do so we are (and must be) adaptively self-centered. To overempathize with others would make us inattentive to our basic needs and expose us to danger. The nineteenth-century philosopher Arthur Schopenhauer wrote, "If we were not so excessively interested in ourselves, life would be so uninteresting that none of us would be able to endure it." Perfect empathy is the province of saints, and as George Orwell observed, "Saints should always be judged guilty until they are proven innocent." For the rest of us, more or less ordinary human goodness is good enough.

We are all self-referential. But there is a fundamental difference between adaptive and maladaptive self-reference. Healthy self-esteem is the foundation stone for the positive regard and empathy we are able to feel toward others. People who do not like themselves are often critical of others and reject them. As a psychiatrist, I have found that it is individuals unable to accept themselves who make vehement criticisms of others, and that these are often self-criticisms. Serial sexual killers have extremely low self-regard, which they project onto their victims. The serial killer, in his perverse empathy, corrupted by self-loathing and cruelty, puts his hated self in the shoes of his victim, then tortures and kills the victim.

Most of us live between the extremes of serial killer and saint. We all participate in what I call *the evils of everyday life*; feeling our lives and needs to be the most important of all. In our cravings and strivings to accomplish our personal goals, we inevitably bump up against others who are similarly striving, and we may intentionally or unintentionally harm them.

Underlying some of these trivial evils of everyday life are the same failures in empathy, devaluation of others, and projection of the dark side onto others that can be observed at full throttle in serial killers. To forget a spouse's birthday or anniversary causes hurt and is a reflection of a failure of empathy, and perhaps even a measure of devaluation and projection.

What can we do to turn around our natural self-centeredness? To defeat envy, for instance, we can work at identifying and empathizing with the good fortune of others. The scenario that envy usually follows is this: You have something that I want but do not have. I feel resentfully deficient and angry. I must destroy what you have (or you). But empathic identification with the good fortune of others allows us to put ourselves in their shoes so that we share in their happiness. This is healthy self-centeredness. We more or less healthy people can do this; serial sexual killers cannot.

Our capacity for empathy, though it may reach glory in compassion, is limited. We can only absorb so much pain from the lives of others, and certainly cannot encompass the monstrousness of genocide. We are unable to mentally put ourselves in the shoes of hundreds, thousands, or millions of people who have been tortured and murdered. Joseph Stalin, one of the worst genocidal killers of the twentieth century, knew this; he was reported to have said, "One death is a tragedy; 20 million deaths is a statistic."

The extreme depravity of serial sexual killers is also beyond the conscious mental life of most people. I cannot fully explain why "bad

men" act out antisocial impulses while "good men" channel potentially destructive psychic forces into constructive action. But I can and
must ask: Have you been mentally torturing anyone lately, perhaps
subtly—maybe even yourself? Have you manipulated others for
personal advantage? When you slowed down to rubberneck at an accident, what were you trying to see? Was that your dark side peeking
at gore and death?

We must no longer permit ourselves to doubt that "bad men" do
what "good men" dream. All men and women struggle with their dark
sides, but that is not reason to despair. One of humanity's greatest
achievements is the ability to turn the mind on itself to achieve insight
and growth. If we can acknowledge and channel our demons, we are
able to harness a powerful force.

M. Sindy Felin, acclaimed for her first novel, *Touching Snow*, observed, "I always thought I was destined to be either a serial killer or
a mystery writer." The serial killer, however, is incapable of transforming the basic drives that we all have into higher, life-affirming
attitudes and behaviors. Theirs are failures of sublimation. Their
pathological self-centeredness is in large measure the consequence of
unsocialized, unchanneled sexual and aggressive impulses. Against
the primitive drives that constantly demand self-gratification, the conscience of the serial killer is no match. Driven to gratify his deadly desires, the serial sexual killer has no joy in his life, only a transitory sexual release at the death of a victim, a release that soon requires the
torture and death of a new victim. Instead of engaging in passionate
relationships and work interests, as mentally healthy people do, this
killer pursues the domination and submission of others. Instead of
having the commitment to life goals and progress that characterize
mentally healthy people, the serial killer is doomed to repeat a never-
ending cycle of compulsion, death, and more compulsion. Beyond
envisioning murder and sadistic gratification, the imagination of the
serial killer is blind.

The ability to examine unacceptable antisocial thoughts and feelings without translating them into action is not just a requirement for
psychiatrists or their patients. Most people are able to curb or modify
feral instincts, often with the help of knowing that a policeman stands
on the corner. An enormous difference exists between thinking evil
and doing evil, and although some religions do not accept this distinction, the law does. If it did not, all of us who occasionally have anti-

social thoughts would be in jail, perhaps on death row. As the pioneering psychoanalyst Theodore Reich observed, "If wishes were horses, they would pull the hearses of our dearest friends and nearest relatives. All men are murderers at heart."

Jeffrey Dahmer killed and cannibalized 17 young men. His father, Lionel Dahmer, wrote in his book that, as a youth, he himself had awakened at times with the feeling that he had committed murder. The difference was that Jeffrey had actually done what Lionel had only feared having done: "I had awakened in a panic that consciousness soon ended. Jeff had awakened into a nightmare that would never end." Lionel Dahmer worried that he had passed on to his son a killer gene that had caused Lionel's murderous dreams to burst full force into Jeffrey's brain and actions. Various theories emphasize different combinations of environmental, biological, and genetic factors in serial killers, but no one knows why Lionel's dreams stayed as dreams and Jeffrey's were acted out as murders. We can only echo the prophet Jeremiah (17:9), who concluded, "The heart is deceitful above all things, and desperately wicked; who can know it?"

We may not be able to know the heart, but we can discern that big and little evils occur when we ascribe our unacceptable thoughts and feelings to others through the processes of dehumanization and projection. If we can acknowledge the beam in our own eye, we will be less likely to stigmatize the mote in the eye of others. To have, to hold, and to recognize the universality of the darker side that we each have within ourselves can be the key to enhancing our ability to experience a shared humanity rather than yield to the impulse to persecute others for our frailties. An important element of what the world calls *evil* is our failure to see an aspect of ourselves in others' behavior, especially in their bad behavior. The mote in his eye is the beam in mine, and to acknowledge that is essential to achieving ordinary human goodness.

Understanding and insight about our psychological mechanisms, such as projection, dehumanization, and the ability (or inability) to empathize, permit us to exercise options rather than be bound by reflexive behaviors. We have the ability to learn about ourselves from multiple sources, from everyday experience, especially tragedies; from education; from arts and literature; from our relationships, whether constructive or destructive; from personal therapy; and from the myriad other ways that life can teach us. But self-knowledge and insight are not enough. Some people in this world understand themselves quite well but have neither the desire, the ability nor the character to harness their antisocial impulses.

"Man is born unto trouble as the sparks fly upward," Job laments, yet, remarkably, there are very many "good" people in this world, able to rise above the destructive impulses that we all possess.

It is the human condition to have dark demons and to struggle against them. When we acknowledge the dark side of our humanity, when we locate the possibility of evil within ourselves, when we attempt to tame our demons by channeling them into fantasies, dreams, and creative achievements, we are doing what humanity as a whole has done in taming fire—even though, inevitably, sparks will still fly and will be infinitely dangerous. By striving to harness our demons, we express the undaunted aspect of the human spirit, the urge to pursue and fulfill our destiny as individual human beings.

3

Psychopaths

The Predators Among Us

They are absolutely the world's best manipulators, liars, and fabricators of truth. They do so convincingly because they believe their own lies. After all, their life is nothing but a lie, a sham, how can we possibly assume they know anything different.

—Hervey Cleckley, M.D.

When FBI supervisor Robert Philip Hanssen was arrested in February 2001 and charged with selling government secrets to the U.S.S.R. and then to Russia over a 15-year period, for $1.4 million in cash and diamonds, his espionage was termed "possibly the worst intelligence disaster in U.S. history." The son of a Chicago police officer, Hanssen was reported to have been emotionally abused in childhood. He has said that he decided to betray his country at age 14. He studied dentistry and Russian and received an M.B.A. degree, but then went to work in the Chicago police department as an internal affairs investigator. Joining the FBI at the age of 35, he rose quickly to supervisor in the counterintelligence bureau in Washington, D.C. He began spying for the Soviets in the mid-1980s, compromising U.S. agents and double agents. His espionage was attributed, in part, to his belief that his FBI colleagues did not appreciate his brilliance and refused to accept him as a peer and friend. Hanssen refused to be considered for a higher position in the FBI because he would have been required to take a lie detector test, which he suspected he would fail. A convert to Catholicism, he attended mass almost daily, was a member of the secretive Opus Dei sect, and seemed devoted to his wife and six children. At one point, his wife confronted him and demanded he confess his crime to a priest; the priest directed him to hand over to charity, as penance, some of the money he had received for his espionage.

Insight into Hanssen's complex psychological makeup and his reasons for the espionage has been limited by his imprisonment and a gag order forbidding him to speak to the public. However, the personalities and early lives of a previous group of very damaging spies, the Walker family, are better known.

For 17 years, John Anthony Walker, Jr., used his position and knowledge as a career Navy Chief Warrant Officer to gain access to top-secret naval communications involving U.S. nuclear submarines. He sold these critical military secrets to the Soviet Union. To assist him, he recruited his son, his brother, and his best friend, Jerry Whitworth, all of whom were also in the Navy. He also tried to enlist his daughter's help when she was in the Army, but she refused. It has been alleged that he strapped a money belt on his unsuspecting mother to bring spy payments back from Europe. The Walker spy ring jeopardized the lives of all Americans and, possibly, everyone in the free world. It inflicted enormous damage to the military security of the United States, with economic costs estimated in the high millions, if not billions of dollars. John A. Walker received about $1 million from the Soviet Union for his treachery. Of that amount, he paid his son only $1,000.

In my opinion, John A. Walker, Jr., displayed many of the antisocial behaviors typically found among psychopaths. Because I have not examined Walker personally, I cannot make a diagnosis of antisocial personality disorder. But there is plenty of detailed information about Walker's childhood and family in Pete Earley's book *Family of Spies,* from which the following account is drawn.[1] John Anthony Walker, Jr., was born on July 28, 1937, the second of three sons. "Jack" became his mother's favorite. A special bond between them grew stronger over

---

[1]From Pete Earley, *Family of Spies.* Copyright ©1988 by Pete Earley. Used by permission of Bantam Books, a division of Bantam Doubleday Dell Publishing Group, Inc.

the years. His father was severely alcoholic, a man who held and lost a succession of jobs. The family was often impoverished. The parents fought constantly. During the father's drunken states, he often beat the mother and sometimes abused the Walker children.

By approximately age 10, Jack had conceived an intense hatred toward his father and determined to kill him. His plan was to thrust a cast-iron rollaway bed down the stairs as his drunken father was staggering up them. If the resulting fall did not kill his father, Jack planned to finish him off with a baseball bat. The plan went awry when the father returned to the house as expected, but passed out before he could get up the stairs. Jack fell asleep while waiting for him to continue his climb. The antisocial side of Walker's personality became more evident as he moved through adolescence. A childhood best friend recalled that "what you see on the surface with Jack is not what you get. Trust me. I knew him like a brother, better than anyone else. Jack is cunning, intelligent, clever, personable, and intrinsically evil."

As an adolescent, Jack and his friends stole eggs and used them to pelt streetcars. They rolled used tires down hills at cars that passed below. They threw rocks through the windows of the local Catholic church. They stole coins from church sanctuaries where parishioners left contributions in small receptacles for the poor. At school functions, they stole money from coats and purses. Jack crafted a pair of brass knuckles and precipitated a fistfight to try them out. He and his friends set fires. The boys borrowed a rifle one evening to shoot at cans and beer bottles. Jack became bored with these targets and sat on a ledge to shoot at the headlights of cars on a highway below. After Walker and his friends were arrested for a series of burglaries, Walker, as a teenage high school dropout, joined the Navy to escape punishment. In the service, he rose rapidly through the ranks because he was intelligent and easily able to pass the various promotion exams.

During his 21-year naval career, Jack Walker had many sexual experiences with prostitutes. He seemed to be drawn to "bleak harbor hotels, lurid bars, and crude hookers." One of Walker's Navy bosses told Earley: "The problems with John Walker involved moral turpitude. The guy just didn't have any moral standards, as far as I was concerned. He constantly bragged about women, and if a woman looked at him twice, why, he'd be unzipping his britches." A business colleague of Walker described him, years later, as a person who enjoyed involving himself in intrigues.

Walker married, but the marriage was troubled. His wife, Barbara, discovered that he was having many affairs. She described him as moody, continually oscillating from pleasantness to anger and violence. She alleged that Walker intimidated her physically and abused her. When he fell into debt because of failed business ventures, he tried to force her into prostitution to earn money.

Barbara Walker began to suspect her husband's espionage activities in 1967. She found incriminating evidence that he had recklessly left in a tin box in a desk drawer, a box that contained the couple's bonds and other personal items. She found maps, photographs of "dead drops" (locations for secret exchange of information), and even a letter from his KGB contact. Although she warned him that she would report his spying, he did nothing to stop her. Barbara Walker remained silent about it for some time. She later explained that she had always protected her husband to safeguard her children. At some point, all of his children, and a son-in-law, supposedly knew about the espionage as well. He allegedly tried to persuade his daughter to have an abortion when her pregnancy threatened to interfere with his spying. During a custody suit that erupted between his daughter and son-in-law, the son-in-law allegedly threatened to expose the espionage if he lost custody of the child. One of Jack's childhood friends tried to articulate the power Jack had over family and friends: "It was almost hypnotic…I can't explain it, but he was my Svengali. There was just something intriguing about him that drew me to him. He had a certain manipulative power."

Walker loved the fast life; in bars and ports around the world, he enjoyed calling out, "Bartender! I'll have a shot of the scotch that's named after me—Johnny Walker." He was flamboyant. He portrayed himself as a fervent patriot, expressed conservative views, and kept a color photo of then President Ronald Reagan on his wall. He made extravagant boasts about his high-ranking military connections, claiming once that he had keys to the War Room.

In June of 1976, after 19 years of marriage, Barbara Walker divorced her husband and moved to Maine to be as far away from him as possible. Shortly thereafter, Walker retired from the Navy. During his service career he had received two Navy commendation medals, a good conduct medal, the Vietnam Service medal, and the National Defense Service medal.

After retiring, Walker became a private detective and carried such weapons as a cane with a knife concealed within it. Walker was able to purchase office space for his three private detective agencies as well as a houseboat, a camper, two cars, and a single-engine plane that he loved to fly. In a safe deposit box, Walker kept ten 100-ounce silver bars. He told one of his detective employees that the key to his method of operation was to tempt people by playing on their greed. The employee reported that Walker himself "felt basically greedy" and believed that you could get to anyone "through their greed." When his KGB case officer informed Walker that he had been awarded the rank of admiral in the Soviet Navy for his outstanding contributions to world peace through espionage, Walker replied, "Tell them thanks a lot." His reason for spying was to obtain money and what it could buy.

Walker seemed not to be worried that family members knew about the spying. He felt impervious to discovery. In fact, the spy ring itself was a clumsy and bumbling operation, yet it escaped detection for almost two decades. Barbara Walker had warned her husband that she would expose him, but she hoped that he would heed her warning and flee the country. He did not. She finally turned him in during the fall of 1984 when she told the FBI about his espionage. On May 19, 1985, he was tailed by the FBI to a lonely road in a Maryland suburb of Washington. There, Walker made a drop of secret documents intended for his KGB handler and was finally arrested.

After his arrest, Walker seemed unconcerned for his future, stating with open bravado, "I'm a celebrity." He knew what he had to sell, even though the coin this time was different. He agreed to tell the government everything about his espionage activities and to testify against his best friend, Jerry Whitworth, in exchange for a plea bargain for himself and his son. The fourth ring member, his brother Arthur, had already pleaded guilty, been fined $250,000, and been sentenced to three life terms. Whitworth was fined $410,000 and sentenced to 365 years in prison. In exchange for his cooperation, Jack Walker received one life term, as did his son. Michael Walker was released on parole in 2000 at age 37. Jack Walker's expected release date is 2015, when he will be 77 years old.

Psychopaths who commit espionage often betray their country for money, sex, and the thrill of illicit behavior such as conning others, even an entire nation. They are in stark contrast to persons who commit espionage for strongly held beliefs and principles—in other words, those who are ideologues.

People who commit antisocial acts are not necessarily psychopaths. The widely held public notion that the psychopaths among us are crazed killers is also wrong. Psychopaths are people who have severe antisocial impulses. They act on them without regard for the inevitable and devastating consequences these actions may bring to themselves and others. Many psychopaths are not criminals, but they are the predators among us, chronic parasites and exploiters of the people around them. Psychopaths use psychological cues and push emotional buttons to manipulate the vulnerable for their own purposes. They are unable to put themselves in other people's shoes, any more than a snake can feel empathy for its prey.

By Their Acts Ye Shall Know Them

Everyone has antisocial impulses. The vast majority of individuals who take personality tests that measure one's degree of psychopathy do not score zero. Psychiatrically healthy people score within a certain numerical range well above zero but do not rise to the level of a psychopathic personality. In other words, normally functioning people possess some antisocial traits.

Who has not had the wish to take something that belongs to another, or to take harmful advantage of someone for one's own benefit? Good men and women have such impulses but curb them. Bad men and women act them out. The mayhem and personal suffering that psychopaths inflict on society is enormous. Then too, over the course of their lives, psychopaths demand a disproportionate amount of time and financial expenditure, particularly from health care professionals. When they are children, psychopaths are usually delinquent and difficult to manage. As they get older, their predatory behavior usually costs individuals and society both suffering and money. If they become criminal, the costs of incarcerating them are high. So, too, are the costs to society for caring for their deserted and traumatized families.

Not all criminals are psychopaths; in fact, many are not. And not all psychopaths are criminals; in fact, again, many are not. Psychopaths exist at all levels of society, in all walks of life. No profession, however noble, is spared its cadre of them. We know them, if we know them at all, by their acts.

Originally, the term *psychopath* was used in psychiatry to refer to all personality disorders. Later, as we came to understand the spectrum of personality disorders, the definition narrowed. In 1941, in his classic book *The Mask of Sanity*, Dr. Hervey Cleckley gave the psychopathic personality a clinical definition. He described the psychopath as having the traits of guiltlessness, superficial charm, egocentricity (extreme self-centeredness), incapacity for love, an absence of shame or remorse, a lack of psychological insight, and an inability to learn from past experience. *Antisocial personality disorder*, the current official term for psychopathy, was the first personality disorder to be officially recognized within psychiatry and to be included in the earliest version of the American Psychiatric Association's *Diagnostic and Statistical Manual of Mental Disorders*, known to all mental health practitioners as DSM.

DSM-II, published in 1968, changed the term *psychopath* to *sociopath*, and more clearly refined it:

> This term is reserved for individuals who are basically unsocialized and whose behavior pattern brings them repeatedly into conflict with society. They are incapable of significant loyalty to individuals, groups or social values. They are grossly selfish, callous, irresponsible, impulsive and unable to feel guilt or to learn from experience and punishment. Frustration tolerance is low. They tend to blame others or offer plausible rationalizations for their behavior. A mere history of repeated legal or social offenses is not sufficient to justify this diagnosis.

The current version, published in 1994 with text revisions in 2000 (DSM-IV-TR), emphasizes antisocial behavior, more than personality traits and their motivation, in the definition of antisocial personality disorder. The diagnostic criteria for the antisocial personality rely heavily on the research of Dr. Eli Robbins, work that has demonstrated that this disorder is stable and continuous, lasting from childhood through adulthood. This latest version of DSM stresses predisposing childhood factors, such as attention-deficit/hyperactivity disorder and conduct disorder. It also emphasizes criminal behavior over the essential narcissistic features of the disorder. Although the latest DSM also lumps together all delinquents, it does give consideration to the social, economic, and cultural determinants of their delinquency.

Laypersons and some professionals use the term *psychopath* to pejoratively label people who engage in antisocial activities, or simply people that they plainly dislike. Dr. Cleckley's original research demonstrated long ago that the antisocial behavior of common criminals and the antisocial behavior of psychopaths are different. Criminals often have standards that they will not go beyond, or families to whom they will never be disloyal. Although it may seem contradictory, some non-psychopathic criminals have principles and a conscience. An example of this distinction can be made in the case of a career criminal who is surprised in the middle of a robbery and kills two officers to escape capture and imprisonment; he views killing or being killed, which he regrets, as an unavoidable occupational hazard both for himself and the police. The criminal psychopath who kills does so casually, or even for no apparent reason. He feels absolutely no remorse, nor does he give the killing a second thought beyond maneuvering to avoid the consequences.

Psychopaths can be passive or aggressive. Passive psychopaths tend to be parasitic and exploitative of others, whereas aggressive psychopaths commit major crimes. Passive psychopaths (referred to as passive-parasitic, exploitative, or predatory) have frequent scrapes with the law but usually manage to squirm out of serious trouble and punishment. Passive psychopaths commit mostly white-collar crimes. The more aggressive ones, particularly the sexually sadistic, may commit serial sexual murders. Their need for constant stimulation through sexual arousal appears to be a motivating factor in their crimes.

For the most part, however, the average, everyday psychopath among us (and within us) appears to the outside world as a model of normality. As Cleckley wrote,

> There is nothing odd or queer about him, and in every respect he tends to embody the concept of a well-adjusted, happy person.... He looks like the real thing.... More than the average person, he is likely to seem free from minor distortions, peculiarities, and awkwardness so common even among the successful.... Everything about him is likely to suggest desirable and superior human qualities, a robust mental health.

Today, psychiatric clinicians question some of the qualities Cleckley attributed to the psychopath. For example, we no longer agree that psychopaths are charming. Some of them, particularly the aggressive ones, have all the charm of a rattlesnake. Dr. Otto F. Kernberg, a widely respected psychiatrist and psychoanalyst, believes that persons with antisocial personality disorder are basically suffering from a severe type of narcissistic personality disorder. They form only exploitative relationships and lack moral principle. Roughly defined, the psychiatric concept of narcissism refers to a person's sense of self-importance and uniqueness. Narcissism may be healthy or pathological. In the psychopath, it is pathological in the extreme and is malignantly transformed into living, breathing evil.

Pathological Relationships and the Emptiness Within

As noted above, the psychopath typically manifests pathological self-importance, or narcissism, displayed as excessive self-centeredness. Other characteristic traits are grandiosity (displayed as nonsexual exhibitionism), recklessness, overambitiousness, an attitude of superiority, overdependency on admiration, and, alternating with these characteristics, bouts of insecurity and emotional shallowness. The reckless grandiosity of psychopaths usually causes them to fail at any enterprise, often spectacularly. Clinicians sometimes quip that psychopaths "snatch defeat from the jaws of victory," and that for psychopaths, "nothing succeeds like failure." The two fundamental distinguishing characteristics of psychopaths are the inability to feel ordinary human empathy and affection for others and the perpetrating of repeated antisocial acts.

Why do some people do these terrible things? We now know that empathy has something to do with an anatomical structure, mirror neurons; these have been found in monkey brains and human brains. The cells are located in the brain's motor cortex, where muscle movement and control are initiated. Mirror neuron circuitry allows us to "step into the shoes" of others, to feel their pain. The more empathetic the person, the stronger the person's mirror neuron response. And the weaker the mirror neuron response, the less empathy he or she has. Psychopathic personalities may have a dearth of mirror neurons.

Much of what the world calls evil originates in the pathological self-centeredness of individuals who pursue instant gratification and use others for their self-aggrandizement. Understanding the concept of evil in this way, we can see that by far the greatest evils perpetrated by ordinary people are done to the extent that these people share the personality characteristics of psychopaths. That is to say, the evils are committed in the exploitation of others. For instance, psychopaths can have lustful sex, but for them the experience is devoid of any intimacy or commitment; the partner is essentially an instrument of masturbation. A vibrator or other inanimate object might serve the psychopath just as well. Psychopaths are incapable of falling in love. People are like tissues to be used, generally for unpleasant purposes, and then discarded. Is not this entitled selfishness that destroys the capacity for empathy with other human beings the heart of evil?

For psychopaths, the world is a giant dispensing machine from which they obtain goodies without giving up any coins. In their relationships they devalue the other person, they are greedy, they appropriate others' property or ideas and feel entitled to do so. They distrust and are unable to depend on others, another part of their stunning incapacity to empathize with, or commit to, other human beings. A patient-victim of a psychopath once described to me that failure of empathy in unforgettable terms. Her cold, distant, scientist father could tell how many cubic centimeters of tears she shed, but he could never understand why she shed them.

I recall a patient who came to me for treatment of his depression. It soon became clear that his depression was secondary to the life problems caused by marked antisocial personality traits. From the first session, he addressed me as "Bob," assuming an easy familiarity, even though I had introduced myself as Dr. Simon. The "Bob sign," as I had discovered from past patients who had addressed me familiarly, was an absolutely unfailing indicator of a short-lived or nonexistent therapy. These persons are unwilling to accept a patient status, this status being, among other things, a deep personal wound. They often leave after a few sessions.

This patient also came late to many sessions, missing others entirely. The patient produced countless excuses for not paying his bill. He constantly referred to others as "scumbags" and "dirtballs," projecting onto others his contempt for antisocial acts that he was clearly guilty of committing himself. His pervasive view of me was that I existed only for his needs, that I was not a person with any needs of my own, and that no matter what he did, I would be there to supply him with positive stroking.

In very short order, I began to feel an intense dislike for the patient, another sure sign that the treatment was going nowhere. Seeing that my attempts to interpret his behavior toward me were met with a quizzical contempt, I asked him directly what he was hoping to gain from treatment. After that session, I never saw him again. Although I must confess that I was relieved, I was left with an unshakable feeling of having been used and depreciated. I had become another failed relationship for him that he could cast on the heap of his other wrecked relations, convinced that all people were worthless "scum." The tragedy is that he was destined to repeat this pattern endlessly and destructively without any reparative insight. Because of his intense self-centeredness and grandiose image of himself, he could not tolerate any insights without feeling the threat of psychological disintegration. His antisocial acts were driven by the need to exploit and depreciate others to maintain a grandiose, powerful view of himself.

The master spy Jack Walker's exploitation of others is described by author Pete Earley:

> John A. Walker, Jr., had an uncanny skill to see the fragilities of those around him. He was able to identify flaws in their personalities and, like a chameleon, he became whatever he needed to become, whatever they wanted him to be, in order to take advantage of them, manipulate them, and profit from their weaknesses. This was not done by chance. It was calculated, precise.

Although psychopaths can detect the foibles of others readily and exploit them, they lack psychological insight into their own vulnerabilities. For instance, their devaluation of everyone else as a defense against the enormous envy that they feel toward others creates a blind spot in their interaction with the world. It often happens that while the psychopath is busy conning his or her victims, he or she is easily gulled by another predator.

Psychopaths experience chronic feelings of emptiness and of personal isolation. They have *stimulus hunger*, a need for constant stimulation, perhaps to dispel their diffuse sense of the meaninglessness of life. Some find this state unbearable and kill themselves. But what keeps the vast majority of them from doing so? Dr. Kernberg describes the motivation of the most common type of psychopath, the passive-parasitic type:

> [He or she finds] gratification of receptive-dependent needs—food, objects, money, sex, privileges—and the symbolic power exerted over others, by extracting such gratifications from them. To get the needed supplies while ignoring others as persons and protecting oneself from revengeful punishment is the meaning of life. To eat, to defecate, to sleep, to have sex, to feel secure, to take revenge, to feel powerful, to be excited, all without being discovered by the surrounding dangerous though anonymous world—this constitutes a sort of adaptation to life,

even if it is the adaptation of a wolf disguised to live among the sheep, with the real danger coming from other wolves, similarly disguised, against whom the protective "sheepishness" has been erected.

The conflict that psychopaths experience is not that of the normal person, between the push of internal impulses and the pull of conscience, but the conflict between their own impulses and the rest of society. Unable to self-reflect, unable to feel sadness about lost opportunities or relationships, stuck in a pattern of deep mood swings, psychopaths exhibit a value system that is more like that of a child than that of an adult. What they admire are outward things—beauty, wealth, power, adoration by others—and what they discount (and despise) are hard-won abilities, achievements, acceptance of responsibility, and loyalty to ideals. The psychopath is a study of the triumph of style over substance. As Jack Walker stated, "Everyone is corrupt... everyone has a scam." Therefore, psychopaths have no conscience to trouble them and prevent them from such usual psychopathic activities as lying, cheating, stealing, forging, swindling, and prostitution (among the crimes of the passive-exploitation, parasitic type of psychopath), or from assault, armed robbery, and murder (among the crimes of the aggressive psychopath). Earley summed up his impressions of Walker in this way:

> Most of the criminals whom I have met as a journalist seem to have had some moral code of conduct, however twisted and slim, beyond which they could not trespass without traces of guilt and occasional remorse. John didn't. He was totally without principle. There was no right or wrong, no morality or immorality, in his eyes. There were only his wants, his own needs, whatever those might be at the moment. In John's world, only fools believed that they were their brothers' keepers. . . . John could say to me, with all seriousness, during one of our last sessions together, "I have lived every fantasy that I have ever had. I've done everything I wanted to do. And the real mistake I made in life was letting myself be surrounded by weak people."

Largely because psychopaths lack any moral center, and because they also project their own desires onto others, they are unable to imagine moral, ethical qualities in others. At Walker's sentencing hearing, Judge Harvey said to the defendant, "One is seized with an overwhelming feeling of revulsion that a human being could ever be as unprincipled as you." Walker said nothing to the judge at that time, but later told Earley, "I figured Harvey would grandstand for the press. Fuck 'em."

Here again is the fundamental difference between normal human beings and psychopaths. As Kernberg puts it, "The antisocial personality's reality is the normal person's nightmare; the normal person's reality is the nightmare of the psychopath." For example, most people would find spying against their country to be utterly repugnant and could not imagine doing so. In contrast, the psychopath who spies finds commitment to another person, to family, and to country ridiculous, and cannot imagine making or keeping such commitments.

After his conviction in 1995, Aldrich Ames, the CIA agent turned KGB spy, responded to a CNN interviewer who asked why he had committed his crimes, "You might as well ask why a middle-aged man with no criminal record would put a bag over his head and rob a bank." And he added, "At the time that I handed over the names and compromised so many CIA agents in the Soviet Union…I had come to the conclusion that the loss of these sources to the United States government, or to the West as well, would not compromise significant national defense, political, diplomatic interests…. And I would say that this belief of the noninjurious nature of what I was doing…permitted me to do what I did for much more personal reasons. The reasons that I did what I did were personal, banal, and amounted really to kind of greed and folly…. It was a matter of pursuing an intensely personal agenda, of trying to make some money that I felt I needed very badly, and in a sense that I felt at the time, one of terrible desperation."

While Robert Hanssen felt he was keeping his commitments to his wife and family, he stockpiled pornographic images on his computer and dallied with a stripper, giving her expensive presents, including a Mercedes, a computer, and a sapphire necklace. He expressed contempt not only for his FBI associates but also for his KGB handlers, believing he was too smart and too sophisticated to be caught, except by a betrayal.

The Psychopaths Among Us

At one time, people thought there were few psychopaths among us, but now that estimate has to be revised upward. Moreover, society is beginning to recognize that psychopaths, more than people with any other mental disorder, threaten the safety, security, and serenity of our world. The history of humankind is replete with the incredible destruction inflicted by nations upon one another. What is less readily visible is the harm done to individuals, to families, and to society by antisocial behavior. And it is important, finally, to understand that the antisocial tendencies that emerge in psychopaths are harbored by every human being.

A national comorbidity survey found that 5.8% of males and 1.2% of females showed evidence of lifetime risk for psychopathy. Antisocial personality disorder is most commonly diagnosed in the 26- to 40-year-old age group; in those older than 40, the incidence diminishes. Approximately 20% of prison inmates are psychopaths, and they are responsible for more than 50% of violent crimes. In maximum-security prison populations, 75% or more of the inmates may have the disorder.

The combination of minimal brain dysfunction, attention-deficit/hyperactivity disorder, and conduct disorder, which contributes to antisocial personality disorder, is more common in boys than in girls. Another part of the difference can be traced to socialization and acculturation norms: girls are taught to control overt expression of anger, more so than boys. Onset of antisocial symptoms typically occurs for boys at age 7, though for girls the symptoms show up (albeit in less severe form) at around age 13. The age difference at onset may be related to the biological differences between the sexes.

Other studies show that antisocial boys are more likely to come from large families in which their interaction with other deprived, aggressive boys fosters the development of antisocial behavior. When the family shows a predominance of girls, such antisocial behavior in the boys is inhibited. Antisocial girls come from families that tend to be more troubled than those of antisocial boys, but both male and female siblings from extremely troubled families are at great risk for developing antisocial personality disorders.

The causes of antisocial personality disorder cannot be ascribed to social class, cultural conflict, membership in a deviant subgroup (such as a gang), keeping bad company, residing in a high-crime neighborhood, or even brain damage. Important factors in the development of the disorder are maternal deprivation during the child's first 5 years, which leads to insufficient nurturing and socialization, and having an antisocial or alcoholic father, even if he is not in residence. Other studies, however, show that adequate discipline can decrease the risk in children whose parents are antisocial. More moderate correlations between adult antisocial behavior and certain other childhood factors have been found. These factors include early-onset conduct disorder (before age 10 years) with or without accompanying hyperactivity, attention-deficit/hyperactivity disorder, and mild signs of neurologic deficit. Emerging evidence indicates that the brains of psychopaths do not process feelings and emotions properly. Neuroimaging studies show that psychopaths use different areas of their brain in regulating emotion than do normally functioning individuals. Twin and adoption studies also indicate a possible genetic factor. The most plausible model for causation involves many factors, with a combination of genetic, developmental, and environmental factors all interacting to produce an antisocial personality.

But I must again emphasize that the tendency toward antisocial behavior is present in everyone, to varying degrees, and in every vocation—including that of world leaders. A classic set of experiments by Dr. Stanley Milgram has dramatically demonstrated this point. In Milgram's study, subjects were brought into a setting that looked like a learning laboratory. They were asked to administer what they were told were mild electrical shocks to other subjects (who were actually Milgram's colleagues) when they did not come up with the correct answers to questions being put. As the experiment progressed, the subjects were asked to administer more and more severe punishment, even though the people being shocked were objecting and voicing their pain. Although the subjects often expressed disapproval of what they were being asked to do, the majority of them complied with the commands of the experimenter and continued to deliver the shocks, even when the selector button read "Danger: Severe Shock."

Milgram wrote that the study revealed the "sheer strength of obedient tendencies manifested in this situation." The subjects followed the instructions of the experimenter, even though the experimenter had no authority to enforce the command to shock the victim. The subject was free to walk away at any time, but most did not. The study demonstrated that ordinary, decent people would knuckle under and unquestioningly obey authority to severely harm another person. But it further demonstrated that ordinary people, under the sanction of "authority," could clearly manifest sadistic behavior that in any other context would be dubbed antisocial.

The social context that permits or suppresses those antisocial tendencies present in all humans is an important factor in the actual emergence of antisocial behavior. In a retrospective study, the background and personality development of a group of German SS officers were investigated. These men had participated in the mass murders at Nazi concentration camps. The investigators wanted to know about their behavior before and after they started such work. They found that the SS men had invariably displayed severe personality disorder symptoms from early childhood. The researchers theorized that it was these disorders that allowed the men to commit murder in the concentration camps, so long as their SS training and the command structure of the concentration camps sanctioned such behavior. It was possible to learn this because after the SS men were captured, they reverted back to their prior non-antisocial personality functioning, both during and after imprisonment. Among the SS officers, the tendency toward antisocial behavior was present to a greater degree and surfaced in a socially facilitating situation.

Doctor, Lawyer, Entrepreneur

More than 150 years ago, Gogol wrote a description of the psychopath Nozdryov in his book *Dead Souls*. His prediction that the Nozdryovs of the world would not die out was quite correct. Psychopaths, particularly the passive predator types, continue to exist at every socioeconomic and cultural level of our society. "Corporate" psychopaths regularly perpetrate spectacular scandals on Wall Street. In fact, if one wants to study psychopaths, one should go to Wall Street. Sometimes it is hard to tell the successful person from the psychopath. For example, entrepreneurs regularly manipulate other people, but this manipulation is goal-oriented, aimed at establishing a lucrative business. The psychopath's manipulation is different. It becomes the means of providing instant gratification of his or her needs, rather than a way of dealing with the reality at hand, or it may be the sheer pleasure in perpetrating a scam—conning people and making them appear foolish. The entrepreneur's life is productive, whereas the psychopath's may only seem productive for a while, but will inevitably become self-destructive. For example, the psychopath's need to express a hostile impulse or to get even, no matter what the personal cost may be, frequently derails him or her from any long-term attempt to achieve positive goals.

The medical profession, like all others, contains its share of psychopaths. Some run afoul of state licensing boards and lose their licenses;

some slip by with only recurrent disciplinary actions and fines. Most get in trouble by exploiting their patients, by providing substandard care, and, frequently, by perpetrating Medicare/Medicaid scams.

The following portrait of a psychopathic psychiatrist is fictional but draws on a number of real cases for its antisocial characteristics and behaviors:

> Dr. Williams is 42 years old, divorced from his third wife, and under indictment for Medicare fraud. He is a bright man with a good deal of personal charm. He has practiced psychiatry for more than 10 years.
>
> As the indictment proceeds through the courts, a dossier is assembled on him from many disparate sources, some legal, some professional, some personal. Dr. Williams's marriages have never lasted more than 2 years. He is not permitted to see the two children from his first marriage because of his ex-wife's allegations that he physically and sexually abused the children. His second and third marriages were to former patients. Both women now give him a wide berth, seeking at all costs to avoid further involvement with him.
>
> As he will tell anyone who asks, Dr. Williams became a physician to make money. Medical school was relatively easy for him, despite skipping classes to go drinking, because he cheated on most of the exams. On occasion, he broke into departmental offices the night before examinations to steal copies of them. The medical school disciplined him for drunkenness three times but graduated him in the bottom third of his class. As a specialty, he chose psychiatry because it could be done alone and without the scrutiny of colleagues. In an unguarded moment, he remarked to a colleague that he thought most psychiatric patients were hopeless leeches who never grew up. He obtained patients easily because of his charm, but had little real interest in them unless they were sexually or financially attractive. He dragged out the treatment process for wealthy patients—2- or 3-hour sessions, keeping less monied patients waiting—and sometimes sexually exploited the attractive ones. In a spectacular series of cases that made the front page of the local paper for weeks, he was alleged to have sexually exploited several of his female patients. The cases were settled out of court.
>
> Healthier patients saw through Dr. Williams's superficial charm, for soon after initiating treatment they felt the bite of his barely concealed supercilious attitude toward them. They soon left treatment. Patients with low self-esteem would stay and would tolerate his behavior (he sometimes even yawned or fell asleep while a patient was relating a personal tragedy), blaming themselves for being uninteresting. Many of these patients were later exploited by Dr. Williams for sex, money, or both. He followed no particular rational treatment method. He viewed patients as inferior beings who deserved what they got in life.

His contempt facilitated the suicides of two of his more depressed patients, but he managed to avoid censure or inquiry into his conduct.

In fact, Dr. Williams was incapable of understanding the inner life of his patients. He could not comprehend his patients' conflicts, defenses, or the psychological significance of their developmental history. He had no empathy for their personal struggles. To Dr. Williams, the patients were merely projections of his inner needs—objects to be manipulated for his own gratification. If they could not provide him with praise, admiration, sex, or money, he had no use for them.

This meant that he had no concept of treatment boundaries. Where he as a doctor began and the patient ended was a mystery to Dr. Williams. And, having no concept of this boundary, he would touch his patients as he pleased, even after some of them indignantly complained and asked him to stop. His appointment schedule was a shambles, his patients frequently irate. Were it not for his long-suffering secretary—a former patient to whom he paid a paltry salary— he would not have been able to manage his practice at all.

The more agonized the patient's story, the more boring he found it. His eyes would glaze over as his mind wandered into hedonistic fantasies. He would be unable to sit still for very long or to listen to patients without intruding and inflicting on them stories of his own life, which he offered as uplifting homilies. His stories had a grandiose, fantastic quality that emphasized his accomplishments and the great personal difficulties he had had to overcome to make those achievements. They were all lies, though ones that the doctor half believed. Equally important, they enthralled some patients, who were able to escape confronting their personal difficulties while listening to Dr. Williams' tales. More often sooner than later, these patients would have to be seen by other psychiatrists because they had been left untreated for so long that they were seriously regressed and in the midst of acute crises.

Dr. Williams continued to receive referrals because of two personal characteristics. One was his quick wit, which passed for high intelligence, and his great personal charm. However, those few colleagues who came to know him found that the charm ran thin. His contempt was hard for him to disguise if he felt envious of a colleague. There were stories that he had seduced the wife of one colleague and the fiancée of another, both of whom he envied. Referrals also came from other mental health professionals because he was the author of some articles on sexual dysfunction that produced a brief flurry of interest. It was later learned, however, that these were plagiarized from the work of other people and that a number of cases in which he reported treating patients for sexual dysfunction were wholly fabricated.

Dr. Williams had no friends and few acquaintances outside of his practice. When he was forced to spend time alone in his apartment, he would feel unsettled and have a creeping sense of internal void, a consuming nothingness, a deadness within himself. To escape these feelings, he drank or took tranquilizers until, intoxicated, he fell asleep. He was rarely actually depressed or anxious except at those times when he ran afoul of the law or his profession. One such time was when he was sued for sexual exploitation of a hospital patient.

Although the sexual misconduct case was settled out of court, it was only the tip of the iceberg. Dr. Williams was a serial exploiter of female patients, a predator who gradually seduced low-esteem patients by manipulating them from his position of professional power. These women were told that having sex with their psychiatrist was an accepted form of treatment. To gain control of some of these women, he would oversedate them, or even addict them to medication. His sexual activities with patients were perverse, involving sadomasochistic practices. He would soon tire of one woman and unceremoniously dump her for another. In some of these instances, the rejected patients would attempt suicide; a few, successfully. Other psychiatrists would be called in to pick up the emotional pieces of the survivors.

Dr. Williams also exploited patients by involving them in business deals. He would either intrude himself into the patient's business life when he saw a lucrative opportunity, or he would extract money from patients by involving them in his own poorly thought-out business ventures. Patients invariably lost money, and when they did, he would contemptuously discharge them from his "care." He manipulated less wealthy patients by getting them to do menial tasks for him, such as cleaning his office, collecting his mail, and getting his lunch.

The lawsuits, ethical complaints, and disciplinary actions by professional bodies mounted, but Dr. Williams never suffered a single pang of remorse or guilt for any of the patients he had harmed, particularly not for those he had sent to an early grave. Eventually, to make a quick buck, he got involved in a Medicare scam and, after the scam was discovered, was indicted. Knowing he would be convicted, he gave up his license to practice medicine in exchange for a deal that permitted him to stay out of jail and to have only a 6-month suspended sentence. He then moved to another state, which had no licensing requirements for psychotherapists, and set up a new practice.

Criminal Psychopaths

Criminal behavior, or *adult antisocial behavior*, as it is referred to by psychiatrists, encompasses a wide spectrum of conduct and describes normally functioning people engaged in making a dishonest living, perhaps out of necessity; those who are driven to criminal behavior out of guilt in order to be caught and punished; and those who are brain damaged, either by birth or by drugs. Narcotics, alcohol, and other drugs that strongly affect the brain are contributing more and more to the rising tide of antisocial behavior. Dr. Dorothy Otnow Lewis, a psychiatric expert on criminal behavior, points out that we need to distinguish criminals with antisocial personality disorder—the psychopaths—from individuals whose criminal behavior is a result of their psychosis, below-average intelligence, or brain damage. Because a large proportion of the criminal population has these latter disorders, it follows that those with antisocial personalities represent only one segment of the criminal population.

At the far end of the criminal spectrum are those referred to as serial sexual killers. Many are sadistic, sexual psychopaths. They must be distinguished from unfeeling, predatory individuals with sexual perversions who run afoul of the law but are not psychopaths. A lethal mixture exists when powerful sexual and aggressive impulses are combined within an antisocial personality. Arthur J. Shawcross's murder sprees terrorized New York's North Country, where he killed 11 women, most of them prostitutes. At Shawcross's trial, Dr. Park Elliot Dietz, a forensic psychiatrist, reported that he had examined the killer and determined him to have an antisocial personality disorder. Dr. Otnow Lewis, who also testified in the trial, said Shawcross had multiple personality disorder. She also diagnosed brain damage, seizure disorder, and posttraumatic stress disorder secondary to the patient's Vietnam War experiences and severe early childhood abuse.

In *The Misbegotten Son: A Serial Killer and His Victims,* Jack Olsen gives a detailed account of Shawcross's progression from birth to serial killer. As a child, he was very troubled; he displayed a triad of behaviors that some psychiatrists believe precedes homicidal behavior: fire-setting, cruelty to animals, and bed-wetting. Shawcross also bullied classmates, insulted teachers, and roamed the woods of New York's North Country with fantasied friends. He was ridiculed by other children, even though he shared his toys and money with them. In school, he achieved top grades and excelled in sports. By doing so, he confounded the psychiatrists who began to examine him regularly after the second grade.

While serving in the armed forces in Vietnam, Shawcross wrote home letters about his gruesome battlefield experiences. Upon his return to Watertown, New York, he committed a series of arsons and burglaries. Shawcross was arrested and convicted and served 2 years in prison, after which he was paroled in the care of his parents. He then strangled a boy and a girl. After he was caught, Shawcross was able to plea-bargain the offenses down to a single count of manslaughter, for which he was sent to prison.

Incarcerated, he continued to be a mystery. At Greenhaven, a maximum security prison in Stormville, New York, a psychiatrist described him as a dangerous schizophrenic pedophile who also suffered from intermittent explosive personality disorder. Several psychiatrists could not agree as to whether he would ever respond to treatment. After having served 14 years and 6 months of an indeterminate sentence, Shawcross managed to persuade a parole board to give him an early release. Olsen cites the report of a psychiatrist who examined Shawcross for that parole hearing; the report states that the strangler was "neat, clean, quiet, cooperative, alert," with "positive attitude," "no evidence of any perceptual disorder," "no delusions, no morbid preoccupations, memory intact," "intelligence good, good reality contact, denies suicidal or homicidal ideation," "not depressed, not elated, mood stable," and "not emotionally ill at present." It is not unusual for sadistic murderers to appear quite normal or even to be model prisoners while they are within the confines and structure of an institution.

Shawcross attempted to settle in one community after another in upstate New York but was invariably run out of town. Unbeknownst to the Rochester police, Shawcross was smuggled into that large city and soon began stalking prostitutes, generally troubled, diminutive women. Their nude, mutilated, sexually assaulted bodies were found in icy streams and swamps. One prostitute survived her encounter with Shawcross by playing dead so he could achieve a pseudonecrophilic orgasm. Shawcross did perform sexual acts upon some of his victims after they were dead. At his trial, the psychiatrists once again could not agree on an exact diagnosis for Shawcross. However, he was convicted and sentenced to life imprisonment without the possibility of parole.

Necrophilic sexual psychopaths derive sexual gratification only when they can have complete command of a woman's body without the woman present. The total sense of power acts as an aphrodisiac but also dispels fears of inadequacy with women. Sexual fantasies involving sleeping women are common among men. In medieval times, demons or spirits called the *incubus* and the *succubus* were thought to have sexual intercourse with sleeping women and men. The necrophilic psychopath pursues a much distorted and debased version of this common fantasy.

The Lady Next Door

Shawcross was widely reviled as a serial killer and was the object of a massive manhunt. By contrast, Virginia McGinnis operated almost without interference during a criminal career in which at least four people who were near her died. The story began to unfold in the wake of the death of Deana Hubbard Wild, a 20-year-old woman who had been a house guest of McGinnis and her husband. The McGinnises had driven Wild to a 400-foot cliff along Big Sur, California, for a sightseeing trip, and, according to the McGinnises, while their backs were turned, Wild had fallen from the cliff "without a sound." Wild's distraught mother, who lived in Louisville, Kentucky, asked a tax attorney to look into her daughter's death because she needed help in collecting the daughter's burial insurance. The attorney, Steven Keeney, was amazed to discover that Virginia McGinnis had purchased a life insurance policy on Wild one day before the "accident," and that the beneficiary was McGinnis's imprisoned son.

Suspecting foul play, Keeney investigated further, as detailed in David Heilbroner's book *Death Benefit*. Keeney learned that both of McGinnis's sons had been previously charged with murder, and that they had both been in and out of prison. Moreover, he discovered that three of McGinnis's relatives had fared badly under the care of this woman, who called herself a practical nurse. Her 3-year-old daughter was found hanged in a barn. McGinnis claimed it had been an accident. Her husband died suddenly one evening while she was nursing him, and so had her own mother. Further inquiry uncovered a series of thefts, fires, and poisonings from which she had reaped the insurance benefits.

A pattern of antisocial behavior dated back to her childhood. Keeney compiled a 600-page report on her life and crimes. The child of a people-hating dairy farmer, McGinnis was abused in her early years. Ill fed, she lived in filth and smelled of cow manure and kerosene. She had no friends. She became a bully and a juvenile delinquent. She flashed polished paste diamonds to her classmates, then stole their lunches. Like Arthur Shawcross, McGinnis displayed the prehomicidal triad of behaviors: fire-setting, cruelty to animals, and bed-wetting. Brought to trial for Wild's murder, McGinnis was portrayed by the prosecution as a remorseless killer who beat the system repeatedly in collecting money from the insurance policies of her victims. Evidence was produced about her remorseless, treacherous, sexually promiscuous, glamour-loving behaviors. After watching her for 2 months, the jury dubbed her the "ice lady."

The jury did so, writes Heilbroner, because "outwardly she still appeared so *normal*, the lady next door who efficiently did away with her house guest and who had left a wake of fires and bizarre deaths. In the hours when she drove Deana up to Big Sur, making small talk, smiling like a loving friend, she had countless opportunities to turn around. Instead, she was intent on betrayal." This description brings to mind Cleckley's classic depiction of the psychopath's "mask of sanity." Indeed, the forensic psychiatric expert consulted by Keeney suggested that Virginia McGinnis was a psychopath. She received a life sentence without possibility of parole. Heilbroner concludes:

> Keeney knew that [this] wasn't the abstract evil he had studied in the seminary. This evil had a human face and a human heart. It lived next door, smiled as it passed you on the street, and called you neighbor. This evil was woven into the fabric of the human soul. Aragon [the prosecutor] is right, Keeney thought, we are all "of the same fabric."

To this conclusion I can only add that the warp and woof of that fabric is different for the bad men and women who do what good men and women only dream of doing. The good boy wishes to trade his bratty brother for a cold soda on a summer day but does not do so. The bad woman does not hesitate to "trade" an innocent woman's life for the proceeds of an insurance policy. All human beings wish to do the forbidden. Fortunately, the majority of humankind is able to resist these antisocial impulses. And, unfortunately, as the examples in this chapter have shown, psychopaths will be with us forever. We cannot escape the possibility that at some time in the future, a particularly virulent psychopath may become evil incarnate and leave all of humankind for dead.

Are Psychopaths Treatable?

Despite valiant efforts, the treatment of antisocial personalities by mental health professionals has been an abysmal failure. The shortest chapter in a psychiatric textbook is usually the one on the treatment of psychopaths. Psychopaths fear intimacy. They cannot accept criticism, though it might be constructive, or accept authority figures. They resent anyone who attempts to thwart their behavior, even though such thwarting might be in their best interest. Often the victim of inconsistent parenting and of a chaotic family environment, the psychopathic person cannot trust the therapist enough to establish a treatment alliance between them.

Robert E. Hare, Ph.D., a prominent researcher and expert on psychopaths, does not recommend treatment. He advises: "Don't waste your time. Nothing you can do can make a difference at all." Furthermore, Dr. Hare suggests that psychotherapy for psychopaths is an oxymoron. "What do you treat? They have no subjective distress, they don't have low self-esteem, they are not dissatisfied with their behavior. Do you treat personality traits that they don't want to change?" In fact, a number of studies have found that psychotherapy is likely to make psychopaths worse.

One of the great psychological paradoxes that forensic psychiatrists uncover in some psychopathic criminals is the presence of a sadistic, punitive conscience. Not having had appropriate models for behavior in their childhoods, many never mature past the eye-for-an-eye, harsh, primitive conscience of the child. If their own conscience struck them down, its punishment would be awful. To escape that possibility, these psychopaths reject all moral standards and ideals. Thus it becomes extraordinarily difficult for them to face the emotional pain of their own punitive consciences.

In the course of my forensic practice, I once examined a 38-year-old man in jail who was accused of murdering a friend in the course of an argument. I was seeing him at the request of defense counsel to determine his competency to stand trial. He had experienced a brief psychotic episode in jail, so his competency was in doubt. This man had a long history of antisocial behavior. A number of psychiatrists in the past had made the diagnosis of antisocial personality disorder, which clearly was correct. I spent many hours examining this articulate man and found no evidence of psychosis. I believed he was quite capable of understanding the charges against him and assisting counsel in his own defense.

I was struck, however, by a strong moralistic streak that he expressed openly. He went out of his way to harshly condemn other prisoners, particularly those charged with child abuse or wife beating. As a younger man, he had wanted to be a preacher. My sense of this prisoner was that he was burdened by a rigid, lashing conscience that was constantly threatening him with destruction. He was driven to commit antisocial acts as a means of expiating his burden of guilt. He subconsciously saw to it that he was caught and punished. As it happened, he was released shortly after I examined him when another person confessed to the crime. Soon after, he hanged himself. I had the distinct impression that his sadistic conscience viciously raged at him because of the "undeserved" good fortune of his release, which, he concluded, demanded his death.

Psychiatrists who work in a noncriminal setting are not ordinarily sought out for treatment by the psychopath unless the psychopath is in the midst of a legal crisis or some other sort of trouble. In difficult situations, the psychopath pressures the psychiatrist to remedy his situation, not himself. Medications are of little use with the psychopath and are likely to be abused. When a psychopath becomes depressed or anxious, however, medications may help these symptoms. If he or she is incarcerated and unable to act out, painful symptoms of anxiety, depression, or even psychosis may emerge that are more amenable to treatment.

Memberships in altruistic organizations such as the Guardian Angels or self-help groups such as Alcoholics Anonymous or Narcotics Anonymous may redirect a psychopath's antisocial impulses into productive channels. For a few psychopaths, some improvement in their condition comes with age. Although re-arrest levels are high for criminal psychopaths, a decrease in the rate of recidivism does occur with increasing age. However, the psychopathic personality traits and the propensity toward violence continue unabated.

This finding gives little support to the theory that antisocial personality disorder is the result of delayed maturation. The notion that psychopaths are merely developmentally arrested children is badly flawed. Children who go through normal stages of development have a vastly different growing-up experience than do children who become psychopaths. On a sweltering summer day, the aforementioned normal, thirsty 10-year-old who thinks he would gladly exchange his baby brother for a cold soda is expressing a normal impulse toward immediate gratification. But he does not make the swap. He knows full well that he must do no such thing.

The child who grows up in an environment rife with child abuse, parental separation or loss, and many of the other deprivational factors mentioned above cannot be said to have had a developmentally normal childhood with merely arrested development as a consequence. These are the children who go on to delinquent behaviors such as cruelty to animals, fire setting, truancy, running away from home, and forcing others into sexual activity. Some who engage in these activities have precursors of antisocial personality disorder such as attention-deficit/hyperactivity disorder accompanying conduct disorder. These disturbed children should be distinguished from other children with attention-deficit/hyperactivity disorder or conduct disorder, who may act impulsively but display age-appropriate empathy, relatedness to others, and conscience.

4

Why Do They Rape?
The Inner Life of Rapists

A sudden blow: the great wings beating still
Above the staggering girl.

—William Butler Yeats

Vicious attacks on women along the beaches of San Diego began in the spring. In the wee hours of one morning, while a couple was sitting on the beach, a lone male gunman with a nylon stocking over his head robbed them and raped the woman. On the Fourth of July, a man of similar description raped a woman at another beach. Two weeks later, at another beach, the gunman approached two young girls, ages 13 and 14, and ordered them to tie up their somewhat older male consort. After this, he repeatedly raped the girls. During the assaults, the attacker asked one of the crying girls to become more sexually involved in the act. He asked the other if she was a virgin, and when she said yes, the rapist said he would change that soon.

The police had very little to go on and no definite leads. They staked out decoy teams, but the rapist eluded them. Police officials trying to understand his pattern noted that he would generally force the female to tie up the male and to create the appearance of a robbery, with the rape almost incidental to it. They thought this method had a fundamental psychological purpose: taking pleasure in terrorizing his victims.

In the early hours of another summer morning, two men and a woman, all in their twenties, went for a swim at Torrey Pines State

55

Beach, near San Diego. Although they had heard about a rapist, they did not let the stories deter them from their fun. As they emerged from the water, they were accosted by a man wearing a nylon stocking to conceal his face, dressed in dark clothes, and carrying a pistol. He ordered the woman to tie up the men. When she hesitated, he rammed the pistol against her head. As she began to cry, the attacker handed her his heavy-duty flashlight so he could tie up the second man himself. The man being tied up lunged at the attacker and was shot in the chest. During the scuffle that ensued, the second man was shot in the abdomen. The attacker also received a bullet wound and a bite before running off. The three victims made their way to a convenience store and called for help.

A few hours later, a man and his wife arrived at the emergency room of a university hospital in San Diego, seeking help. The man's hand was injured, he told the emergency room doctors, when he was jumped by some men after his car had broken down. He was treated but was also investigated. When sand was found on his clothes, the investigators became suspicious. Next, they turned to the bite marks on his back and ear: those were found to match the teeth of one of the male victims of the dawn rape attempt, who was still undergoing surgery at a nearby hospital. The final piece of evidence sealing the case was the heavy-duty flashlight that the female victim had brought to the convenience store. On it was engraved the name of the man with the injured hand, Henry Hubbard. He was the last man the police would have suspected as the predawn rapist: a 30-year-old, model police officer with numerous commendations.

As the case readied for trial, facts came out about Hubbard. A few years earlier, he had starred in a local television documentary, *The Making of a Cop*. Hubbard had even once played baseball in the San Diego Padres minor league system. Fellow police officers who worked with him were shocked to learn that he had been the vicious rapist responsible for attacking not only the three people on the Torrey Pines Beach but also the victims in the earlier incidents. To his fellow officers, he had always seemed "normal."

However, a psychological evaluation revealed that Hubbard's father had regularly humiliated and abused him. On weekends, the father would slip into drunken rages and hit the boy and his mother, sometimes while brandishing a gun. During the week, the father was a sober, respected school administrator and teacher, but as the week ended, he became a monster. Hubbard, too, followed this Dr. Jekyll and Mr. Hyde behavior pattern. In his model police officer character, he was very kind and caring toward women, whereas as a rapist he turned cruel and vicious, lacking any sense of compassion or empathy. To Hubbard's friends and fellow officers, the scariest aspect of the entire affair was his ability to function in an apparently normal way in society by day, yet become a violent rapist at night. He pleaded either guilty or no contest to numerous counts of kidnapping, robbery, rape, and attempted murder and received a prison sentence of 56 years.

Rape: New Definitions, New Terror

During the past decade in the United States, rape has increased four times as fast as the overall crime rate. In 2005, there were 191,670 reported victims of rape, attempted rape, or sexual assault; these figures do not include victims age 12 or younger. There were also rapes of young boys and men. The definition of rape is also shifting and expanding as our understanding of this crime increases. Basically, rape is considered a penetration offense. The FBI defines *rape* as "carnal knowledge of a female forcibly and against her will." This is the definition that the FBI was still using in 2005, the most recent year for which figures are available, in compiling its Uniform Crime Reports. As written, the definition is controversial, because carnal knowledge refers to penile-vaginal intercourse only. In the FBI definition, the only exception to that notion is homosexual rape. However, the rape of men is not always perpetrated by homosexuals. This is just one of the reasons some states are revising the old definition of rape.

Newer statutes define rape as nonconsensual penetration of an adult or adolescent obtained by physical force, by threat of bodily harm, or when the victim is incapable of providing consent because of mental illness, mental retardation, or intoxication. These redefinitions go beyond penile-vaginal intercourse to include oral and anal sodomy, as well as penetration by fingers or objects other than the penis. They progress beyond the previous definitions to expand our understanding of the methods that are used to gain compliance. Furthermore, the sex of the offender in this definition is not specified. The emphasis is placed on the perpetrator's violent acts rather than on what the victim experiences. In such reformed statutes, female-female, female-male, marital, and acquaintance rape are recognized. Even with this greatly revised definition, there are still problems with the way the statutes delineate the concepts of force and consent.

The FBI Crime Classification Manual (1992) lists 13 different categories or types of rape, including stranger rape, acquaintance rape, date rape, multiple or group rape, and marital rape. There are many categories in which the attacker is known to the victim; perhaps that person is a coworker, a fellow student, a relative, a neighbor or friend of the family. Almost two-thirds of all rape victims know their assailants. The figures on acquaintance rape are likely to be incorrect because this category of rape is underreported. The victim's embarrassment about the crime is a significant factor in underreporting.

Serial Rapists

Those who rape three times or more, like Henry Hubbard, are known as *serial rapists*. These are not brooding loners, as popular understanding would have it, but are often articulate, highly intelligent men who hold jobs, have wives or girlfriends, and generally get along easily with others. The majority of serial rapists were sexually abused as children. Because rapists are extremely likely to repeat their crimes, the category really represents the difficulty that the authorities have in catching rapists—a process that usually takes a long time. In other words, the serial rapist category contains intelligent, cunning men who know how to cover their tracks. To ensure their continued "success," serial rapists work to protect their identity. Their methods of operation vary with their age and experience. For instance, they may improve their techniques with information gleaned from reading newspaper accounts of similar crimes, by watching expert panels on television, even by attending courses on criminal justice and psychology. Serial rapists also become more proficient over time and are able to learn from their mistakes.

Nonetheless, each rapist displays certain characteristics and ritual approaches to the crime—and in the expression of these, he invariably leaves his "signature" at the crime scene, and on the victim. For example, Henry Hubbard's signature was to force the rape victim to first tie up the man who was with her. These ritualized behaviors provide the authorities with important clues about the rapist's fantasy life and motivation. Law enforcement officers are then able to work backward: from the *what*—the behavior—they can deduce the *why*—the fantasy and motivation—in order to eventually discover and apprehend the *who*.

Acquaintance Rape

Although girls are generally raised to be wary of strangers, they often do not expect to fear their friends. An assault by a monstrous psychopath lurking in the shadows may account for only one out of five rapes. It is the boy in math class, the guy in the adjoining office, or the friend of the brother who is more likely to be that girl's or woman's rapist. Familiarity with this person causes the potential victim to let down her guard, so that, after the event, the victim may even wonder if she was really raped. Unfortunately, both men and women have been socialized to think that male aggression leads to female sexual arousal. That may have been a motivating factor in Henry Hubbard's demand that the victim become more sexually involved. In this scenario, a woman's *no* is really a *yes*. Stereotypical thinking confounds the category of acquaintance rape for both perpetrator and victim. Was James Bond a rapist, or was he merely forceful, and were the many women he encountered simply compliant?

Date rape is only one kind of acquaintance rape. The public tends to believe that acquaintance rapes arise from dating situations that are sexually ambiguous. Some do. But in the most accurate rape study, the National Women's Study, 20% of rapists were described as friends. Husbands committed 16% of rapes, boyfriends committed 14%, and 9% were ascribed to non-relatives such as handymen, coworkers, and neighbors. The acquaintance factor reduces the likelihood that a woman will be able to successfully fend off a sexual assault, particularly after the perpetrator gains entrance into the home.

In a study funded by the National Institute of Mental Health (NIMH), researchers found that the behavior of women attacked by acquaintances differed in two basic ways from the behavior of women attacked by strangers. Only 11% of acquaintance-rape victims screamed for help, compared with more than 21% of stranger-rape victims; and only half as many acquaintance-rape victims ran away, compared with stranger-rape victims. The study further showed that almost 20% of women from both groups physically struggled against their assailant—a fact that shows acquaintance rape is not just the result of a misunderstanding between amorous partners.

The principal investigator of the NIMH study notes that 20 years of research has shown that screaming and running more often lead to foiling a rape than struggling does. Despite these findings, the vagaries of assailant, victim, and situation are such that no stock prescription for avoiding rape can be given. Experts in acquaintance rape suggest certain preventive measures, such as following one's instincts about danger, using alcohol only moderately, avoiding men who drink heavily, running if attacked (no matter what the state of one's undress), and always reporting attempted or completed rapes.

Spousal Rape

Spousal rape was officially recognized by the law in 1982, when, for the first time, a Florida man was pronounced guilty of raping his wife while she was living with him. All 50 states now have laws against marital rape. A majority of states, however, to avoid wandering into the thicket of tangled marital relationships, place added legal burdens on women who accuse their spouses of rape.

Group Rape

The FBI defines *group rape* as that committed by three or more offenders. If there are only two in the group, each is considered an individual rapist. In the group, dynamics such as contagious behavior and the defusing of responsibility are common. In highly defined groups such as gangs, the subculture may foster gang rape. Twenty percent of all rapes are group or "multiple" rapes. Perhaps the most notorious gang rape was that of the Central Park jogger, which occurred in 1989. In addition to raping the victim, a gang of youths bludgeoned her, beat her senseless, and left her for dead. She was discovered and taken to a hospital. Her attackers were eventually put on trial and convicted.

Rape of Males

The rape of males is significantly underreported. According to the Department of Justice, an estimated 123,000 men were the victims of rape attempts between 1973 and 1982—attempts in which the rapists were heterosexuals, homosexuals, or bisexuals. In 1994, 4,890 males ages 12 and over were raped.

Statutory Rape

Statutory rape means that the female victim is under the age of consent, usually defined as under 16 years of age, and that the male perpetrator is over that age. Women have also been accused of statutory rape: Jean-Michelle Whitiak, a 24-year-old swimming instructor, pleaded guilty to one count of statutory rape, admitting that for the previous 3 years she had had an affair with a 14-year-old boy. Women commit approximately 20% of the sex abuse against boys.

Rape: Statistics, Demographics, and Motivation

There is a plethora of statistics about the crime of rape. The figures can shed light on many different aspects of the crime, the criminals, and the victims. It is estimated that 1,871 women are raped in this country every day, one every 1.3 minutes. The National Women's Study estimated that 683,000 adult women are raped each year. In 2005, 93,934 forcible rapes were reported. The group at highest risk is women between the ages of 16 and 24. The statistics show that about 70% of rape victims are unmarried. Many are quite young: almost one-fifth of the victims are between the ages of 12 and 15. Even so, women of all ages are at risk. One out of every four women will be raped at some point during her lifetime, but only 16% will report the assault to the police, and less than 5% of the accused offenders will go to jail. Nearly half—48%—of all rape cases are dismissed before trial. Of convicted rapists, 21% are released on probation, whereas an additional 24% are sentenced to a local jail, in which they spend only an average of 11 months before again being released. Since the first publication, in 1992, of these release figures, convicted rapists have been receiving much longer prison sentences.

Rapists tend to be older than most other criminals; most of them are between the ages of 25 and 44. The rape is rarely the rapist's first sexual experience. Various studies show that anywhere from one-third to two-thirds of rapists have been married. This research suggests that the individual's marital status or presumed ability to have consensual sexual relationships is not directly related to whether or not the person commits the crime of rape. Although the figures show that 51% of rapists are white, 42% black, and 6% have other racial backgrounds, these percentages must be viewed with the understanding that rape is so underreported that the attacker's race may not be properly reflected in the statistics.

Power, rather than sex, is the major motivation for rape. This assertion is partially borne out by FBI statistics showing that 71% of arrested rapists have prior criminal records and that their prior crimes tend to be assault, robbery, and homicide. Further evidence for this contention comes from the fact that rape frequently occurs during the commission of another crime. In 20% of single-offender rapes, and in 62% of multiple-offender rapes, the rapists are under age 21. In 30% of all rapes, a weapon is used; 25% of the weapons are handguns, 44% are knives. Rape may result in the unintended death of the victim through excessive violence, or she may be intentionally killed to eliminate a witness to the crime. When convicted rapists are released from prison or from probation, 52% of them will be rearrested within 3 years.

Reported rapes occur close to home, often *in* the home. Many take place in the victim's neighborhood, on a street or in a parking lot. One-third occur in the victim's home. Reported rapes happen more often in June, July, and August than in other months, and are more likely to take place on the weekends than during the week. Interestingly, the clustering of reported rapes on the weekends is more common for black victims than for white victims, and for the victims of group rape rather than for the victims of single-perpetrator rape. Rape, as with most other crimes against the person, is highly race-specific: 78% of white victims are raped by white men; 70% of black women are raped by black men. Rapes occur mostly at night, generally between the hours of 8:00 p.m. and 2:00 a.m. Group rape occurs more frequently than single-perpetrator rape during those hours.

Aside from the physical consequences for the victims, which often are considerable, the psychological consequences are frighteningly severe. Many women who are raped experience posttraumatic stress disorder symptoms, develop depression, and consider suicide. About half of the victims experience sexual difficulties in their own relationships within 15 to 30 months following the rape.

The Inner Life of Rapists

The brain is the *potential rape* organ. In human beings, most sexual acts have their origin in fantasy. Among rapists—in contrast to what happens with the sexual fantasies of "normal" people—the fantasies of control, domination, humiliation, pain, injury, and violence are acted out.

Rape is a crime of violence. Most rapists have the precise purpose of humiliating and harming the victim. The rapist finds sexual pleasure in the victim's pain and fear. The victim's sexual compliance may even increase the intensity of the rapist's aggression. The expressed aggression may then further stimulate the rapist's sexual arousal, in a spiraling cycle of violence.

No single psychological profile provides the answer to why people rape. Rapist typologies overlap and are constantly undergoing modification as new data accumulate. Not all rapists fit in these categories so neatly. It is important not to mistake the lens of classification for the real object: the uniquely individual psychology of each rapist. Even there, we can only view the rapist "through a glass darkly." Yet being able to identify various groups of rapists by means of their characteristics, behaviors, motivations, and backgrounds can assist in helping to apprehend rapists. Classification also provides information for judicial decision making, law enforcement, treatment of rapists, and rape prevention.

Psychiatric studies have identified the following four basic profiles of rapists, each based on their motivations:

- *Compensatory:* sexual behavior is an expression of sexual fantasies.
- *Exploitative:* sexual behavior is an impulsive, predatory act.
- *Angry:* sexual behavior is an expression of anger and rage.
- *Sadistic:* sexual behavior is an expression of sexually aggressive fantasies.

Based on their degrees of aggressive motivation, rapists can be further classified into *instrumental* and *expressive* types. In the instrumental type, the rapist's aim is primarily sexual. Aggression is used for the purpose of forcing compliance from the victim. In the expressive type, the aim is primarily aggressive. The aggression is intended to harm the victim. Instrumental rapists are the compensatory and exploitative types, whereas the expressives are the displaced anger and sadistic types. The classifications are further refined by adding the qualities of *high or low impulse* to each group. The rapist's high or low impulsivity rating is derived from his or her behavior in nonoffense areas such as work, relationships, promiscuity, changes in residence, finances, and other life situations.

As noted above, less than 5% of all accusations of rape or attempted rape result in arrest and convictions. Therefore, rapists who are jailed (and studied) do not represent a random sample of all rapists, and the profiles may not encompass all the varieties of rapists.

Again, the prevalence of acquaintance rape is vastly underreported. A rapist who confounds classification in this group of offenders, perhaps a professional, and who does not rape other men's wives or daughters, but who does rape his own wife or girlfriend, is not likely to become involved with the legal system. Mental health experts do argue, however, that even such a man is describable as a rapist within the categories outlined just above, with their chilling mixture of expressed aggression and sexual fantasies.

Moreover, statistics and psychological profiles gathered from interviews with convicted rapists in prison are significant enough that an incontestable fact can be understood from them: rapists themselves were often the victims of horrendous childhood abuse and of pathological families. Someday we may find that specific kinds of child abuse predispose the victims to become adults who rape. No such specific set of factors has yet been found, nor do most abused children turn into rapists in their later lives. But one thing is abundantly clear: the most consistent element in rape of all kinds is an absence of empathy, the absence of an ability by the attacker to put himself or herself in the victim's place. This can be traced back to the victimization of rapists as children, a victimization that results in their own emotional paralysis. Abused children who become rapists are those who grow up feeling martyred, vengeful, and entitled to abuse others as they were once abused. In these individuals, compassion is dead, and the world is a jungle in which they must hurt or exploit others to survive.

Every Man a Rapist at Heart?

The plain facts are that most criminal rapists are ordinary folks who generally live ordinary lives but are driven by their personal emotional demons to commit the crime of rape. Many rapists, like Henry Hubbard, hold down good jobs at which they are proficient. Many are married and have children. Just as important, most of these individuals are rarely out of touch with reality; psychiatrists define the state of being out of touch with reality as psychosis. Thus, rapists do not appear to be very different from the rest of us. In fact, they give the lie to the artificial separation of "us" and "them" that so often characterizes our discussions of law-abiding citizens and criminals.

Rape fantasies are common. Research has consistently demonstrated that some "normal" men, who have no history of sexually aggressive behavior, are aroused by rape stimuli that involve adults. In a study of 94 men's erotic fantasies during masturbation or intercourse, 33% fantasized about raping women. In a survey of college men, 35% indicated that they would rape, if they could be assured of not getting caught. But rape fantasies are not exclusively confined to the mental domain of men. Women undergoing intensive psychotherapy occasionally reveal fantasies that involve raping men or other women. Among female patients with multiple personality disorder, a male alter-personality may come forward that harbors intense rape fantasies. Moreover, controlled aggression plays a role in normal sexual relations—it can add playfulness, creativity, variety, and additional gusto to consensual sex. Some evolutionary psychologists have even found that the psychological profiles of rapists are practically indistinguishable from those of non-rapists, leading them to take the hugely controversial position that the proclivity to rape is an evolved behavioral adaptation that is universally present in normal human males. These researchers conclude that under certain appropriate, reproductive risk-benefit conditions, any normal man is likely to commit rape. An immediate caveat must be added to this contention: the presence or frequency of conscious or unconscious rape fantasies does not make every man a rapist, nor does it make every woman a willing victim. Fantasy, however powerful, cannot come close to the actual rape experience of degradation and violence.

Most of those who imagine sexual sadism confine themselves to fantasy and never engage in a sexually sadistic act, much less in a sexually sadistic crime. Even among the group that do act out their fantasies, most sadistic behavior is limited to lawful or quasi-lawful behavior with consenting or paid partners. It is only a small group of sexual sadists who act out their fantasies at the expense of an unwilling partner. Unfortunately, it is an even smaller group that comprises those who are apprehended and criminally charged with rape.

The question still remains: Are all men rapists at heart? I think not. I know of no scientific research that would support such a conclusion. The enormous psychological differences among the billions of men on this earth alone would preclude such a sweeping generalization. Everyone must contend with the base, the foul, the ugly within themselves, but not every man's dark side harbors a rapist. Bad men do what good men dream, but not every man dreams about doing all the things that bad men do.

The Compensatory Rapist

Rape is a crime of aggression. The rapes of infirm 80- and 90-year-old women are examples of pure hate and aggression. In instrumental aggression, the amount of force used does not go beyond that which is necessary to coerce the victim's compliance. If the victim is injured, that is usually accidental. If the victim resists, the instrumental rapist does not usually become angry in response. Sometimes, if the victim becomes aggressive, or screams and fights back, the rapist may stop and flee. The compensatory rapist—a subcategory of the instrumental rapist—exhibits behaviors that emanate both from sexual arousal and from compensatory ideas about himself or herself.

The compensatory rapist's rape is usually planned or premeditated. His sexual behavior toward the victim is driven by elaborate sexual fantasies. These may involve having a Hollywood-style romantic sexual relationship, fending off homosexual fears, and the indulging of passive sexual wishes by putting himself in the shoes of the victim, to give just a few examples. The sexual behavior of the rapist may also serve nonsexual purposes, such as attempts to deal with deflations in self-worth, reverse a passive lifestyle, compensate for fears and inadequacies arising from child abuse, or defend against a threatening emotional or mental collapse. Such rapists fantasize about, or live out, a variety of sexual perversions, including voyeurism, exhibitionism, cross-dressing, fetishism, the making of obscene telephone calls, and bizarre masturbatory practices. High sexual arousal may lead to loss of control and to distortion of reality. For example, the rapist may expect the victim to respond sexually and accept a "date" after the assault.

The compensatory rapist is more likely than other rapists to give the victim his name and address, or to allow himself in other ways to be identified. He is more likely than other rapists to fondle, caress, engage in foreplay, and perform cunnilingus on the victim. He may ask to look at the victim naked, ask her to kiss him, or engage her in conversation that intends to reassure her—and himself. Premature ejaculation is common. In summary, the compensatory rapist attempts to make up for severe feelings of male inadequacy and failure.

The following example depicts a typical compensatory rapist:

> Mike, a 27-year-old married man with two children, a daughter age 8 and a son age 6, was apprehended shortly after raping a woman and giving her his telephone number. When his psychiatric history was

taken, it provided a classic illustration of the development and behavior patterns of a compensatory rapist. During the previous 6 years, Mike had been engaging in frequent episodes of exhibiting himself, voyeurism, and the wearing of women's underwear. On the day of the rape, he had first exposed himself in his car to a woman who was just getting off a bus. He had previously watched this woman get off the bus at the same time for a number of days. She was tall, well-dressed, and attractive. He experienced intense sexual fantasies of domination toward her. In his fantasy, she began by strenuously resisting him but was overcome by his sexual prowess and the desire it aroused in her.

This day, he stopped the car and opened the door to expose himself, fully naked. She reacted with surprise and fear. He interpreted this reaction as sexual arousal on her part. Stimulated, he drove on but circled back and forced the woman into the car at knifepoint, then demanded that she remove her clothes. She resisted, but complied after he threatened to cut her throat. He fondled her breasts and forced her to perform oral sex. He then attempted oral-vaginal contact but was unable to complete the act because she was wearing a tampon. He ripped out the tampon and flung it in her face. She cried uncontrollably. After he made many attempts to reassure her, saying "I will not hurt you," her crying subsided. Now she was frozen with fear. He attempted intercourse but ejaculated prematurely after the first penetration. Interpreting her paralysis as quiet acquiescence and a sign of sexual arousal, he gave her his telephone number and dropped her off at the original bus stop.

In his childhood, Mike's family consisted of an abusive, alcoholic father, a passive, compliant mother, and three older sisters. The father was frequently in drunken rages. In such states, he would beat Mike for minor infractions and berate him as a "loser." Mike felt terrorized by the father, yet longed for a loving relationship with him. As the youngest of four siblings, and the only boy, he also was subject to secondary abuse: one of the sisters, who had been sexually abused by the father, in turn sexually abused Mike by performing enemas on him. He witnessed the physical abuse of his mother and heard brutal sexual encounters between his parents. From his adjacent bedroom, he would hear his mother crying and whimpering. At other times, he heard her and his father laughing together in bed. He imagined his father hurting his mother and her sexually enjoying it. Unconsciously, Mike identified with his mother as a means of obtaining the yearned-for love from his father.

As an adolescent, Mike was involved in the vandalizing of cars and homes. He was ignored by his peers. Shy, he did not date, but he began engaging in peeping-tom activities and masturbating while dressed in women's clothing. He spent long periods of time alone, fantasizing about women undressed and how he would dominate them.

In these fantasies, he felt very powerful. In his scenes, the women did anything that he requested, but if they refused, he forced them to comply with his wishes. After their initial resistance, the women would experience erotic ecstasies and become his sex slaves forever. These fantasies of sexual dominance allowed him to compensate for his feelings of alienation and male inadequacy and to fend off his father's scathing definition of him as a loser.

In school, Mike performed poorly. He was unable to concentrate and left formal education at age 16. He held a succession of menial jobs and then joined the military, where he completed 4 years of service but had numerous disciplinary actions brought against him. He had a brief, superficial courtship with a woman—his first—and asked her to marry him. As the wedding date approached, his exhibitionistic activities escalated. For instance, he would display himself from the window of his apartment or from the taxi he drove. The marriage proved turbulent. His wife drank excessively and berated him for his many real and imagined inadequacies. After receiving emotional bashings from his wife, he felt deflated and depressed. He then would perform exhibitionistic and masturbatory activities in women's clothes. His relationship with his daughter was distant, and he spent little time with her. It was after a particularly hateful, withering verbal attack from his wife that he raped the woman who stepped off the bus.

Mike's rape was typical of the compensatory rapist, an acting out of his lifelong fantasy of dominance over women as a means of compensating for his personal limitations and inadequacies. His grandiose fantasy of himself as a compelling sexual object led him to misinterpret the victim's startled reaction to him as sexual arousal. His passive-dependent sexual wishes toward his father and his feminine sexual identification with his mother were projected onto the victim, whom he saw as enjoying his sexual assault. In this acting-out, he psychologically compensated for feelings of fear, sexual doubts, loneliness, abandonment, passive homosexual desires, and his general life failures. Despite knowing that he assaulted and raped the victim, he was so distanced from reality by his fantasy that he gave the victim his phone number, enabling him to be identified and arrested.

The Exploitative Rapist

The exploitative rapist's sexual behavior takes the form of an impulsive, predatory act. It has far less psychological meaning to the offender and is less a part of his fantasy life than for the compensatory rapist. Exploitative rape is driven by situation and opportunity, rather than by conscious fantasy. The rapist, a man on the prowl for someone to exploit, intends to force the victim to submit. He is not concerned with the arousal or welfare of the victim, or with forming a relationship with her. He may not be sexually aroused as the incident begins, but the situation itself may trigger his arousal. Low-impulse exploiters display sexual behavior in response to a threatened macho self-image. High-impulse exploiters are usually antisocial personalities—psychopaths.

The following example depicts a high-impulse exploitative rapist:

> Joe, a 34-year-old engineer, regularly patronizes a bar, where he frequently meets and sexually exploits women. At age 24, he was dishonorably discharged from the army with a diagnosis of antisocial personality disorder. Joe has had numerous scrapes with the law, especially for repeatedly writing bad checks. At the bar, Joe meets Lisa, a 20-year-old secretary. In talking with her, he discovers that she has an alcohol problem. Lisa confides that she loses her memory of events when she drinks. Joe reassures her and orders another round of drinks. Eventually, they go to his apartment. Joe presses some more drinks on Lisa. When he attempts to have sex with her, she refuses. Joe grabs a baseball bat and threatens to kill her if she does not submit. Paralyzed with fear, she submits. Joe forcibly performs sexual intercourse. Eventually, Lisa falls asleep. The next morning, she awakens on the couch with no memory of the rape. Joe tells her they had a wonderful time together, listening to music, before she fell asleep.

The Sadistic Rapist

Sexual sadism was named after the Marquis de Sade, who wrote vividly about sexual acts of domination, degradation, and violence. The sexual sadist becomes sexually excited in response to another person's suffering. All rapists cause their victims to suffer, but only sexual sadists intentionally inflict psychological and physical suffering to enhance their own sexual arousal. During their sexual assaults, all too often they perform acts of extreme cruelty.

For rapists who employ excessive aggression, the arousing sexual aspect of the assault is intimately linked to hurting or humiliating the victim. Such aggressive behavior is usually poorly controlled, reaching peaks of brutality and violence before subsiding. The offender's aggressive behavior goes far beyond what might be necessary to obtain the victim's compliance for a sexual purpose. For instance, the sadistic rapist is verbally abusive, sometimes shouting obscenities at the victim. Compliant behavior by the victim may arouse more aggression from the attacker or may provoke cold, calculating, viciously demeaning behavior as a means of expressing his power and control.

The sexually sadistic rapist aims at abusing, hurting, humiliating, or killing the victim through the use of a large variety of implements and behaviors: knives, sticks, cigarettes, bottles, restraints, blindfolds, pinches, spankings, paddlings, whippings, beatings, electrical shocks, strangulation, mutilation, and an almost infinite variety of other tortures. If the sadistic behavior is less severe, the aggression may take the form of inserting foreign objects into the vagina and other practices that may be strange but do not cause substantial physical injury. The sadist's violence is usually directed at body parts having sexual significance: the breasts, buttocks, mouth, anus, and genitalia.

The following example represents a sadistic rapist:

At a party, Sam, a 26-year-old, straight-A graduate student in mathematics, meets an undergraduate woman. During the party he spikes her drink with a tranquilizing drug, then escorts her out of the party and to his apartment. Although she is partially awake, she is unable to resist his advances. He becomes sexually aroused. He has prepared a "rape kit," for this attack has been carefully planned. He ties her arms and legs to the four points of the bed, and shaves her vaginal hair. Then, hooking up to her genitals an electrical device that he has designed for such an occasion, he gives her electrical shocks until her screams bring someone knocking on his outer door. He sends the knocker away. He inserts a soda bottle into the victim's vagina and anus. With a pocket knife, he carves Xs and Os into her abdomen, and with a cigarette he burns her breasts. When she screams, he punches her in the mouth, drawing blood. "Blood turns me on!" he shouts, "Blood turns me on!" He becomes sexually excited and, in a frenzy, performs vaginal and anal intercourse, and then forces her to perform oral sex. Later, Sam falls asleep. His victim is able to escape and to call the police.

Sam is the third of four sons born to a family in which the parents divorced when he was 3 years old. Both parents physically abused him. His father locked him in a closet for hours. Although he kicked and screamed, these actions brought no response from his parents. His mother was seductive and sexually abusive, taking baths with him and masturbating him. When he became sexually excited, she would laugh at him. He found it difficult to get along with his brothers or with other children and frequently got into fights. He did well in school but had few friends. He began to peep on his female neighbors and make obscene phone calls. As an adolescent, he was arrested for setting fires and for cruelty to animals. On one occasion he was apprehended with blood all over his hands and clothes, which was discovered to have come from a cat whose abdomen he had slit open before hanging it in a tree. He had also tortured other animals with a cattle prod, then killed them. During these actions, he masturbated.

Sam's frequent bed-wetting caused him to be the butt of his brothers' jokes. His mother's bathing of him continued until he was 14. During these baths, she would wash his private parts and tell him sexual jokes. On several social and family occasions during his adolescence, she humiliated him by revealing the fact that she still bathed him.

Sam developed fantasies of sexually dominating and hurting women, particularly by using knives and electric shocks. He imagined using naked women as dart boards, carving out board games on their abdomens. Baroque in detail, these fantasies were accompanied by masturbation. He spent a great deal of time each day intensely elaborating his sadistic fantasies.

In college, Sam had a few dates but quickly acquired the reputation of being an "animal" because he slapped and punched his dates if they refused his sexual advances. He once stuffed a date into the trunk of his car and, after she became hysterical, sexually forced himself on her.

In such ways, Sam redirected the hatred he felt toward his mother against other women. In his childhood years, his mother forced him to experience inappropriate sexual stimulation, coupled with humiliation. The sexual and aggressive overstimulation that Sam experienced found its first outwardly harmful expression in wetting his bed, setting fires, and torturing animals. This triad of behaviors has been associated with the violent behaviors of some individuals in later life. Hostility, hatred, and sexual pleasure continued to be combined in his mind and coalesced into compelling fantasies. Later, by acting out his detailed, sexually aggressive fantasies, he found sexual excitement in physically hurting women.

The Displaced-Anger Rapist

Sam was a sexually sadistic rapist, and although he felt much hatred, he was not considered a displaced-anger rapist. The distinction is an important one. For the displaced-anger rapist, sexual behavior is an expression of anger and rage. The victim is the displaced object for the rapist's aggression. Usually, the rapist's anger originates in early relationships that were abusive and depriving. There is no erotic aspect to his aggressive acts because the pervasive feelings he has are of contempt and hate. His abuse is more likely to be verbal rather than physical. His hatred of women, however, may be expressed through actions that run the gamut from verbal abuse to murder. Although sexual feelings or fantasies may trigger the aggressive behavior, the sexual assault itself is frequently devoid of sexual meaning. A sexual attack on a victim may occur directly on the heels of a real or perceived insult to him, or a rejection of him by a female figure that is significant in his life.

Whereas sexual sadists direct their attacks at sexual parts of the body, the anger rapist's violence is not so ritually fixated or directed, as in the following example:

> Tom is a 27-year-old store manager. His marriage of 3 years has been extremely stormy from the beginning. He was physically abused as a child by his alcoholic mother. He had numerous hospitalizations for traumatic head injuries from the abuse. Occasionally, he was knocked unconscious. As an adolescent, he was frequently involved in fights. His coworkers at the store were afraid of his temper.
>
> On this particular day, Tom comes home early from work to find his wife in bed with a neighbor. Tom threatens to kill them both and storms out of the house. He then breaks into the home of a 78-year-old woman a few houses down the street and rapes her. Tom is immediately apprehended.

Everyone's Ultimate Nightmare

Rape has devastating physical and psychological consequences for its victims. Short of homicide, rape is the ultimate violation. It is an invasion of a person's innermost, private space. It is not only an orifice that has been invaded, it is the self. The psychological damage that follows this loss of autonomy and control may be severe and permanent. Some rapists use the blitz attack, first stunning and overpowering their victims, then forcing themselves on them, causing immediate bodily injury. Other rapists use a surprise attack, for example, waking a woman who was previously sleeping. The most insidious rape approach is a con, wherein a man passes himself off as a policeman or repairman to place himself in a position to rape the woman. Each of these approaches produces a different pattern of psychological damage in the victim.

As many as 80% of rape victims develop posttraumatic stress disorder (PTSD). It is estimated that 1.5 million adult female rape victims suffer from PTSD. Although the disorder severely affects the victim, many experts insist that it is a normal response to a life-threatening event. For the victim, terrifying flashbacks and nightmares of the rape are common, and may persist for a long period. If the rape includes physical injury, the victim's stress disorder may be magnified. If the victim has previously suffered from psychological disorders, he or she will be rendered even more vulnerable to the chronic, emotional consequences of rape trauma.

A few years ago, I evaluated a 22-year-old college senior who had been viciously attacked and raped in her dorm room. Although she had PTSD symptoms, they were surprisingly mild, given the severity of the multiple knife slashes she had received that almost killed her. On further inquiry, I discovered that the brutality of the attack upon her was softened by a profound religious experience she had as she lay on the floor bleeding and in shock. She saw a beautiful white light more intense than anything she had seen before. As she groped toward the light, she experienced overpowering feelings of peace and love. She no longer felt the terrible pain. After being rescued and recovering from her physical injuries, she came to look upon the rape as providing her with a religious experience few other human beings have had: an intimate, life-transforming encounter with God, much like Moses had on Mount Sinai. She became profoundly religious.

Some people want to combat rape by detailing ways in which the rape victim should deal with the attacker. As the profiles in the previous sections have revealed, rapists come in different psychological packages. Therefore, no one method of defense is adequate to the task. Rapists do not wear identifying labels that enable a potential victim to defend herself or himself properly. Resisting robbery is occasionally successful, but often it is not and ends in greater damage to the victim. People are advised not to fight a robber. Should they not fight a rapist? The choice should be the victim's, based on his or her values and the exigencies of the situation. I believe that rape victims should have the option to submit, and that if they do, the law or society should not hold them as an accomplice in their own rape.

Advice on how to deal with a rapist is unreliable because so much of what happens in a particular rape depends on where and when the attack occurs, the type of rapist committing the act, and the psychological and physical strengths and weaknesses of the victim. In some instances, confronting a rapist may burst his fantasy and bring the rape attempt to an end. In other instances, confrontation and resistance by the victim might trigger lethal violence from the rapist. Some rapists are sexually stimulated by resistance, others by expressions of fear. In one instance, a victim was dragged to the roof of her Manhattan apartment building for a rape attempt and was killed while trying to resist the armed intruder. Even women who are trained in martial arts may find that in certain situations it is too dangerous for them to resist a rapist.

Elizabeth Xan Wilson, of Austin, Texas, submitted to a rapist and asked him to wear a condom. In court, she was subjected to a withering cross-examination for having made this request, which the defense insisted was evidence that what had taken place was not rape. Wilson angrily pointed out:

> Rape is the only felony that places the onus on the survivor. If an assailant held you at knife point, asked you for your wallet and you complied, there would be no question that a crime was committed. You would not be asked [in court] if you have consented, you would not be asked if you tried to resist. Only survivors of rape are asked these questions. This [practice] must stop now.

On the stand, Wilson described her ordeal in words that speak volumes about the psychological damage that rape victims sustain:

> It is everyone's ultimate nightmare to confront an unknown, knife-wielding assailant in their home. The terror is indescribable and, unfortunately, never-ending. I am not the same person I was.

How was she different after the rape? She described what many rape victims experience:

> I no longer trust my neighbors or strangers. I have many sleepless nights, bolting upright from the slightest noise, especially when my dog barks. I see men that resemble [the rapist] and I am filled with terror. I awaken many nights at 3 A.M., the hour that my rape began.

She described her self-image, which had been deeply despoiled, as follows:

> I have felt tainted, violated, filthy, and used. I fear that I will never have a healthy relationship with a man if he knows that I have been raped. Who wants damaged goods? This is how I feel, and I don't

know when it will stop, or if it will. I hope it does…. [The rapist] took a part of my life, my soul, my body, and security that will never be replaced or healed.

The law is a blunt instrument, and never more so than in regard to rape cases. If victims want to bring their rapists to justice, they must be prepared to withstand the rigors of an adversarial legal system. They will need a lot of cooperation from medical examiners, police, prosecutors, and grand juries. They will require validation and support from family and friends. And they must have the psychological staying power and the determination to see the case through.

As Ms. Wilson so heartfully articulated, there are many long-term consequences of rape. These include:

- Mistrust and avoidance of men or a hesitation to form relationships
- A variety of sexual problems, which are frequently manifested as sexual disturbances and marital conflicts
- Persistent phobias
- Emotional distress, brought on by events that trigger once more the original trauma
- Heightened anxiety and avoidance of gynecological examinations and procedures
- Suicide or suicide attempts, based on self-blame, guilt, and depression

The emergence of rape crisis centers in the 1970s has been instrumental in the early treatment of rape victims. These centers remain an essential source of the emotional support that enables victims to deal effectively with the psychological traumas caused by rape. Survivors of other experiences that have led to PTSD—such as being in the Vietnam War—have shown that peer support is essential for recovery from the disorder. The interventions of rape crisis centers show similar positive results flowing from their psychological support of rape victims.

There are certain techniques that assist in rape prevention. A male voice or a dog barking in the background on one's answering machine may deter rapists who are hunting for a victim. Contrary to the conventional thinking that designates one's home as the safest place in the world, people must understand that one's own home is an extraordinarily dangerous place in which to encounter a rapist. If a rapist has gained entry, and the inhabitant is alone, it is just the rapist, the inhabitant, and the four walls. When outside the home, individuals should be aware of situations in which they could be abducted. For example, women are advised not to get out of their cars if they are next to a van. When traveling alone and booking hotel rooms, one should be extra vigilant. One can ask for a room above the first floor, a room whose only door leads to an inside hall, a room that has a peephole and chain lock on the door. Once inside the hotel room, one should not answer the door unless the knocker can be definitely identified and is known or expected. Rape crisis prevention centers can provide readers with many other helpful tips.

Rape will continue unabated as long as society and culture empower men at the expense of women. From this perspective, the profiling of rapists deals with only the individual consequences of a male-dominated society, not the fundamental, underlying causes of rape. It is critically important to seek to eliminate rape by challenging societal beliefs and cultural values that promote and condone sexual violence. Every effort must be made to foil attempted rapes by educating potential victims about risks and by teaching realistic strategies for self-defense. We need to reduce the emotional and physical trauma of rape through early, appropriate attention to the individual needs of the rape victim. And, finally, we must prevent recurrences of rape by insisting on the incarceration and treatment of offenders.

5

Stalkers

Forever Yours

If you leave me, I will track you down,
I will kill you.

*—A stalker's prophetic threat
to a woman he later murdered*

Kristin Lardner, a 21-year-old art student in Boston, met Michael Cartier, 22, a nightclub bouncer, in January of 1992. They started dating. On April 16, 1992, they had an argument, and he struck her about the face, knocked her to the ground, kicked her over and over, and told her, "Get up or I'll kill you." By the time she staggered to her feet, he was gone. Two motorists stopped by and assisted her home. She determined never to see him again.

But Lardner had a hard time getting rid of Cartier. Spurned, he called her apartment 10 times a day and showed up at the liquor store where she worked part-time. There, he would be alternately violent and tearful, telling her that he did not know why he always hurt the people he loved. Maybe it was because his mother never loved him. He knew he needed help.

Lardner was now terrified of Cartier. She knew he was on probation, but she did not know why. His probation officer did—it was for attacking a woman with a pair of scissors—and when Lardner complained to the probation officer, she was told to take her complaint to the Brookline District Court. She did, and while she was there she filled out an application for a complaint that charged Cartier with domestic abuse. Now he would be ordered to stay away from her, she thought. She would not have to feel the dread of catching a glimpse of him stalking her or experience the awful panic and terror of a direct confrontation that could turn violent. Inexplicably, the court did not immediately issue a summons for his arrest.

On May 30, 1992, Michael Cartier found Kristin Lardner and shot her in the head and face, killing her in broad daylight. When the police burst into his apartment, they discovered Cartier sprawled on the bed, with a fatal, self-inflicted bullet wound to the head.

After the murder and suicide, the police investigated. They learned that the Brookline District Court had never issued the summons for Cartier's arrest. They found a friend of his who told them that Cartier had spoken to him a few weeks earlier, telling the friend he could not live without Lardner, and vowing that he was going to kill her with a gun he was going to buy. Another friend described Cartier as a man unable to handle rejection, someone who had always been extremely jealous and unpredictable. According to other sources, Cartier had experienced extreme abuse as a child. As a youngster he had shown signs of severe emotional disturbance.

Stalking: An Epidemic Problem

The FBI Classification Manual (1992) defines a stalker as "a predator who stalks or selects a victim based on a specific criterion of the victim." Federal and state laws (all states have enacted anti-stalking laws) define stalking as a crime in which a person "on more than one occasion" engages in "conduct with the intent to cause emotional distress...by placing [another] person in reasonable fear of death or bodily injury," or the "willful, malicious and repeated following and harassing of another person." Plainly and simply, stalking is terrorism directed against an individual in order to obtain contact with and gain control over that individual. In the United States, more than 1 million women and more than 370,000 men are stalked annually.

Despite official classifications, the definition of stalking remains hazy. The term is used very broadly, particularly by law enforcement. For example, the man who cases a woman's home before a sexual assault is often dubbed a stalker. Is the contract killer who follows his victim to determine the best point of attack a stalker? What about the rejected husband or lover who cannot let go? Is the egotistical person who writes a movie star for a date a stalker? Those who are called stalkers present a wide spectrum of behaviors. There is no stalker syndrome, only a common behavioral pathway to the victim for a broad variety of motives. Stalking is frequently precipitated by a rejection or the onset of a mental illness. The stalkers most often examined by psychiatrists are those with the delusional belief that they have a special relationship with a stranger, who is then pursued.

In most cases, the stalking victim is a woman and the stalker is a man, but there are cases in which women stalk men or stalk other women. Men stalk other men, and they stalk children; and children stalk other children. Stalkers may be straight or gay. They are not hit men or professional kidnappers; for one thing, those criminals tend to work in groups. Many stalkers are loners who have abnormal mental and emotional fixations on a specific individual.

Stalking and Intimate Partner Violence

The statistics on stalking and intimate partner violence are chilling. Each year, 4.8 million women experience intimate partner–related physical assaults and rapes. Men are the victims of about 2.4 million intimate partner–related physical assaults. Studies reveal that 76% of intimate partner murder victims were stalked by their intimate partner; 67% were physically abused by their intimate partner; 89% of murder victims who were physically abused were stalked in the 12 months before the killing; and of the 79% of abused victims who reported stalking to the police, more than half were murdered by their stalkers. Although intimate partner stalking does not necessarily result in physical violence, the psychological violence is severely damaging and long-lasting.

Domestic violence is a frequent backdrop for stalking. The stalking usually begins when the abuse victim leaves or when the abuser is forced to leave by the authorities. About 30% of women who suffer physical injury by spousal abuse are eventually killed by their partners. The FBI estimates that one in four women who are murdered are killed by husbands or partners. Doctors are told that every physician in America, regardless of specialty or where his or her practice is conducted, has seen a battered women in his or her office in the last 2 weeks.

Battered spouses often find it very difficult to leave an abusive partner. Victims stay for many reasons: first and foremost, there is the real threat of further harm or even death if they attempt to leave. Abused women are used to hearing the very real threat, "If you leave me, I'll kill you." Also, they may feel ashamed, they may feel grateful when the abuse stops and bend over backward not to reexperience the terror of abuse, or they may have nowhere to go or no means of financial support. In between the violent episodes, the spouse may be loving, kind, a good provider, and an esteemed citizen. Victims often are bewildered when the abuser apologizes for the progressive violence but then blames the abused person for the incidents.

Stalking is often an invisible crime until violence breaks out. One study showed that the time from the beginning of stalking to the occurrence of violence was 5 years. Until the violence reaches such a level that the victim has to go to the police or to the hospital, the victim usually does not talk about being stalked. Most stalking victims suffer in silence. The act of stalking plays on a victim's deepest fears of being hunted, harmed, and killed. Common symptoms include anxiety, insomnia, social dysfunction, and depression. Kristin Lardner must have experienced such feelings. Even reporting stalking to the authorities does not always bring protection; 54% of women who reported stalking to the police were killed by their stalkers. This was Kristin Lardner's fate.

Stalkers are motivated by myriad reasons. In cases where celebrities are stalked, mentally disordered people desperately seek contact in the search for identity, love, power, and relief from their personal problems. Some stalkers even seek contact with total strangers to redress perceived or real grievances or wrongs. Statistics reveal that of all the victims of stalkers, 38% are ordinary people, mostly women; 17% are high-profile celebrities; and 32% are lesser-known celebrities. Of the remainder, 11% are corporate executives stalked by current or former employees, and 2% are people such as supervisors stalked by disgruntled subordinates and psychotherapists stalked by current or former patients.

Stalking has always existed. It is rooted in the ancient concept that women are chattel or property. By wielding power over a man or woman, the stalker is asserting that he or she will be part of the victim's life whether the victim likes it or not. In the past, stalkers were brought up on charges of criminal trespass or not prosecuted at all. The residue of this old way of looking at stalking can be seen in the common but erroneously held belief among men that women somehow entice their stalkers. In fact, however, 90% of stalkers suffer from mental disorders, and the remaining 10% are very upset or angry persons.

Today, stalking is recognized as a major social problem, with an estimated 200,000 stalkers on the loose in the United States. Some experts assert that this figure is apocryphal and that nobody knows how many people are stalked. One out of every 20 women, at some time during her life, will be stalked by a former boyfriend, an ex-husband, or a stranger. Statistics show that 77% of women stalked and 64% of men stalked know their stalker. Most of the targets of stalkers are single or divorced women between the ages of 20 and 45. The stalking may begin in a benign fashion, perhaps with a compliment, but can escalate into a pattern of surveillance, obscene language, harassment, threats of bodily harm, and actual physical injury or murder.

Stalking occurs at all socioeconomic levels. Proof that education and professional stature are no bar to stalking comes from the case of then 63-year-old Sol Wachtler, the former chief judge of the State of New York. After Joy Silverman ended a relationship with Wachtler, he conducted a 13-month campaign to threaten and terrorize her. Wachtler was arrested when he demanded that Silverman pay him $20,000 or he would kidnap her 14-year-old daughter. He received a 15-month federal prison sentence and was fined $30,000 for stalking and threatening Silverman and her daughter. Before the court, Wachtler explained his bizarre, 2-year harassment as the result of a "sick and aberrational" attempt to create a situation that would recapture the woman's need for him.

Stalker Typology

The Celebrity Stalker

In our mass-entertainment culture, some entertainers may enjoy an audience of 100 million people or more. These large audiences, coupled with our fascination with the personal lives of entertainers, sports stars, and other celebrities, have produced some inevitable consequences. Out of 100 million viewers, some will feel that the entertainer is speaking, singing, or performing directly to or for them. Others will develop the notion that their own destinies are inextricably intertwined with that of the media star. Some will write love letters. Others will write hate letters or letters that say they are being tormented or abused from afar by the entertainer. Still others will have deviant sexual thoughts. Considering that scantily clad entertainers enter the bedrooms of millions of viewers, many of whom may themselves be in various stages of undress, it is not difficult to understand that this situation will stimulate some viewers to act in aberrant ways.

One of them was Teddy Soto, an admirer of Christina Applegate, who played the "teenage sexpot" character of Kelly Bundy on Fox television's show *Married...With Children.* Soto was noticed hanging around the security gate of Columbia Pictures television studios, where the sitcom was taped. He was recognized as a man who had previously been arrested after being spotted near Applegate's home. When he steadfastly refused to leave the security gate at the studio, the guards arrested him.

Soto may have had trouble distinguishing between the actress Christina Applegate and the Kelly Bundy character she played. Applegate has been emphatic in telling people that privately she is the antithesis of the Kelly Bundy character, who on television wears extremely tight skirts and tops that reveal cleavage. Soto is an example of how tenacious some people will be in their attempt to contact media stars about whom they have developed an obsession—or a delusion.

Only a small minority of stalkers are disgruntled fans. The vast majority of stalkers of public figures are mentally ill. They tend to be media addicts who are highly self-absorbed loners. Some of them delude themselves into thinking that they have a special relationship with a famous person. Others believe that they can become celebrities themselves by their association with a famous person—even if it means killing that person. Mark David Chapman, who stalked and killed John Lennon, was one of these. He described himself as a "nobody" who "didn't know how to handle being a nobody." Chapman said he struck out in anger "to become something he wasn't, to become somebody." Margaret Ray, a 41-year-old stalker, reportedly believed she was actually a specific somebody, the wife of David Letterman, and she repeatedly broke into the talk-show host's home.

Forensic psychiatrist Park Elliot Dietz has researched the subject of celebrity stalkers and has found that celebrities who are perceived as "nice" attract more pursuers than do those celebrities with a less friendly image. The obsessed fan generally pursues the nonthreatening, "girl-next-door" types, not the actresses who project strong personalities, such as Elizabeth Taylor or Joan Collins. The friendly, outgoing image of actress Rebecca Schaeffer, who starred in the television series *My Sister Sam,* attracted the attention of a man named Robert John Bardo. He sent her a fan letter. She did what most actors and actresses have been urged to do in such instances: she sent him in return a picture of herself with a brief thank-you note. In this case, it was a mistake because Bardo misread this as a real interest in him, and he stalked and killed Schaeffer. Almost always, a confrontation between the stalker and the person who is the object of his or her intense fantasy is ineffective in deterring the stalker, no matter what the celebrity's intent. Such contact will likely reinforce the stalker's unshakable belief that a love relationship exists between him or her and the celebrity. The only way for a person being stalked to help himself or herself is to enforce complete separation from the stalker.

People in love think constantly about their loved ones. What is she or he doing now? I wish I could see her this very moment, at work, at play. What is he thinking about? Is he thinking of me? Even reasonably healthy people "mind stalk" those to whom they are attracted. People harbor subconscious wishes to merge with others that derive from the earliest stages of human development. But aberration can occur. I once examined a short, skinny man with a hawklike appearance, who repeatedly stalked and injured his ex-wife. When I asked him why he did this, he chillingly said: "Before we married, I loved her. Once we married, she was mine. And since I'm no good, she became worthless. She is me. I can't let her go." So it is no wonder that stalkers reflect the entire spectrum of psychopathology, from the moonstruck adolescent to the delusional psychotic. The difference between the healthy and the nonhealthy is that the latter are driven by internal psychological needs to actually pursue their object of interest, whether or not that person wants to be pursued. Stalkers cannot confine their obsessions or delusions within their heads; they must act them out. Bad men do what good men dream.

Many stalkers are men who have been rejected by women. Most stalkers are mentally ill loners without meaningful lives of their own. But there is some psychological distance between a vengeful ex-spouse and an obsessed celebrity stalker. In the following pages, I look into some of the psychological profiles of stalkers, but I need to warn the reader in advance that the categories into which stalkers are placed are not as neat or as all-encompassing as those for rapists or for other criminals described in other chapters. The lines separating categories of stalkers must not be seen as hard and fast.

The Immature Romantic Stalker

Let us begin with that moonstruck adolescent. It is not unusual for an adolescent to become infatuated and romantically preoccupied with some person. Indeed, the relationship may be totally one-sided and exist only from afar because the idealized person of the adolescent's ardor may be unaware of this interest. The young romantic sits outside the person's house, hides in the bushes, follows his or her car to steal a glimpse, or telephones and hangs up just to hear the voice of the person. Boys are acculturated through television and movies to persistently pursue the woman of their desire. Unlike adult stalkers, adolescents usually do not make threats. In developmentally normal adolescents, these pursuit behaviors usually cease as the person matures. Most people have gone through this phase. In some adults, however, the behavior may continue and become fixed—and that, of course, can cause problems.

The Dependent, Rejection-Sensitive Stalker

Generally, the dependent, rejection-sensitive stalker is a person who is extremely sensitive to being rejected and at the same time is extremely dependent on the person with whom he or she has a "love" relationship. This jilted lover gathers intelligence on the person who has rejected him or her and attempts contact through incessant phone calls, e-mails, letters, gifts, and visits. Some rejected lovers badger the victim's friends, coworkers, or relatives for information. Others go further, reading the victim's personal mail, breaking into his or her house, checking the computer, listening to the answering machine, even watching the person sleep. The most vicious of this category of stalkers applies every means of harassment and of psychological terror he or she can dream up. Some of the more harsh tactics include pouring weed killer on a lawn, taping gun cartridges to a car window, leaving threatening notes scrawled in nail polish, destroying property, sabotaging cars, killing the victim's pets, and threatening the victim's children.

Many of the men in this category hide their dependency feelings behind a hypermasculine, macho image and are chronically abusive toward women. They attempt to cover their deepest fear—that the woman will leave them for another man—by saying, in effect, "If I can't have her, nobody else will." Michael Cartier, the Boston nightclub bouncer, had been overheard saying words to that effect, and in many ways Cartier fit the profile of a dependent, rejection-sensitive stalker.

Many such stalkers sustained significant losses in their childhoods, either through the death of a parent or through psychological and physical abuse or parental neglect. Stalkers usually have an impairment of attachment, reflecting childhood disturbances in their relationships. They are unable to grieve normally, let go, and find other relationships. Often, the abandonment rage is a defense against feeling intolerable hurt and humiliation from childhood rejections that get tacked onto the current loss.

Cartier was reported as having been abused as a child, although the abuse was denied by his mother, who insists that he was born troubled. As evidence, she cites early behavior in which he took bottles away from his baby stepsister and lit matches behind a gas stove. At age 5 or 6, the mother reported, Cartier ripped the legs of his pet rabbit right out of their sockets. By age 7, he was in a state-supported residential treatment center for troubled children. At 12, Cartier graduated to a treatment center for disturbed adolescents. He dropped out of high school because he was facing about 20 criminal charges that he had accumulated in various Massachusetts jurisdictions. He expressed his extreme bitterness toward his mother in his wish to get a tattoo depicting her hanging from a tree with animals ripping at her body. At age 18, Cartier asked his stepsister if she wanted him to kill their mother. He had beaten several women before Kristin Lardner, and, as he had with her, would then break into tears and ask for their help, citing his belief that his mother had never loved him.

The Borderline Personality Stalker

The label *borderline* is an attempt to convey the notion of the thin line walked by the individual between relative normality on the one side, and, on the other side, serious problems in being able to correctly differentiate reality from fantasy. It is from this group that most celebrity stalkers come.

Borderline individuals have unstable but intense personal relationships that alternate between extremes of overidealization and devaluation. They can change from adoration to hate in a heartbeat when the person being idealized does something—or is perceived to have done something—that pricks the balloon of perfection.

In psychiatry, the mechanism of imbuing a person with either all good or all bad characteristics is known as *splitting*: the good and the bad representations exist simultaneously but are kept apart from each other through a failure of cohesive integration; they are split. The borderline stalker does this to the idealized person, but he or she also splits his or her own self-image. Most normal people are able to integrate the good and bad perceptions and feelings they have about themselves and about others into a realistic whole. Borderline individuals cannot. They also tend to be impulsive, to be emotionally unstable, and to shift moods rapidly for periods that may last from a few hours to a few days. Depression is a common complication of borderline personality disorder. Such depression further influences the borderline individual's behavior. For instance, it magnifies inappropriate, intense anger and an inability to control one's temper. The utter hatred vented by individuals with borderline personality disorder can be withering. Their sense of self can be so fragile that the slightest insult or criticism can produce in them intense feelings of rejection, abandonment, and shame. And when rejected, the borderline individual may discharge his or her hatred in attempts to destroy the victim's career, reputation, family, friends, and, in some instances, the victim's life.

Rejected borderline individuals often threaten suicide. They exhibit marked disturbances in self-image, sexual orientation, career choice, types of friends, and value system. They experience chronic feelings of emptiness or boredom, and often make frantic efforts to avoid real or imagined abandonment. Borderline individuals tend to project their disavowed, unacceptable thoughts and feelings onto others, whom they then try to control. This is a common underlying psychological mechanism observed in borderline stalkers. Impairments in reality testing and the blurring of boundaries between themselves and others facilitate this process. Such was the situation in the movie *Fatal Attraction*, with its classic borderline female stalker.

Borderline patients are typically difficult to treat. One minute the therapist may be revered like a god. In the next moment, if the borderline patient feels provoked or rejected, the therapist can be attacked with a venomous, eviscerating hate that cuts to the soul. Recently, I was asked to evaluate a couple experiencing marital problems. The husband had borderline personality disorder. The wife experienced depression secondary to the marital discord. In a separate interview, the husband described his wife adoringly but, without blinking an eye, went on in the next breath to make astonishingly degrading, depreciating comments about her. He was totally oblivious to the utterly contradictory views he held of his wife. The simultaneously held split images that stood in such sharp contrast were mind-jolting to me. When I interviewed his wife, she told me that she could tolerate her husband's irresponsible spending, even his affairs with other women, but she could no longer withstand his bouts of virulent hate directed at her.

As with the rejection-sensitive stalker, the borderline individual is often found to have experienced physical or sexual abuse as a child. In general, the categories of rejection-sensitive and borderline have many overlapping characteristics. Among celebrity stalkers, however, there appears to be a troubled combination of low self-esteem and an over-idealized view of their victims. One wants to say to them—as some who wish to help them do—"get a life," because they do not seem to have lives independent of the celebrity they are stalking. In fact, obtaining a life is exactly what they are doing by stalking a celebrity. In fastening their lives to a well-known figure, celebrity stalkers attempt to achieve meaning. Overidealization, however, is a fragile thing, and one that easily and quickly can turn to murderous anger and hate.

All of the characteristics that psychiatrically define a borderline personality disorder seemed to be on display in an interview that Larry King conducted with Mark David Chapman, the assassin of John Lennon. As a youngster, Chapman idolized John Lennon. When Chapman insisted that the man who shot Lennon was not the man he had become after some years in treatment and confinement, King asked him who he had been at the time of the murder:

> CHAPMAN: On December 8, 1980, Mark David Chapman was a very confused person. He was literally living inside a paperback novel, J. D. Salinger's book *The Catcher in the Rye.* He was vacillating between suicide, between catching the first taxi home back to Hawaii, between killing, as you said, an icon.

At the time, Chapman went on, Lennon was "an album cover to me. He didn't exist, even when I met him earlier that day when he signed the album for me—which he did very graciously." Chapman believed that he was unable to "register" that Lennon, or Lennon's son, whom he also met that day, were human beings: "I just saw him as a two-dimensional celebrity with no real feelings." King asked him why he had wanted to shoot the "album cover":

CHAPMAN: Mark David Chapman at that point was a walking shell who didn't ever learn how to let out his feelings of anger, of rage, of disappointment. Mark David Chapman was a failure in his own mind…. He tried to be a somebody through his years but as he progressively got worse—and I believe I was schizophrenic at the time, no one can tell me I wasn't, although I was responsible—Mark David Chapman struck out at something he perceived to be phony, something he was angry at, to become something he wasn't, to become somebody.

Chapman told King that before he stalked and killed Lennon he had gone to art galleries and had his picture taken with other celebrities: "I felt important while I was with them. And then, after, you disintegrate again."

The love and hate that seem to have alternated in Chapman toward Lennon were similar to what Robert John Bardo apparently felt toward the actress Rebecca Schaeffer. At Bardo's trial, forensic psychiatrist Park Elliot Dietz explained on the witness stand the mechanism of good-bad splitting that is so often seen in borderline individuals. Dr. Dietz said that Bardo's love and hate existed simultaneously in his mind and that he could switch between love and hate "in an instant." That was why, Dr. Dietz testified, Bardo could love and adore Schaeffer at the same time that he was plotting to kill her. In his opinion, it was a sudden switch that occurred in Bardo's brain during his second visit to Schaeffer's doorstep that led to the fatal shooting.

The Erotomanic Stalker

A person who suffers from erotomania has the entrenched delusion that he or she is ardently loved by some other person. This delusion usually involves idealized romantic love and spiritual union, rather than simple sexual attraction. The one loved is usually of higher status than the adorer, a famous personage or a superior at work, although it can also be a complete stranger. Approximately 25% of delusional stalkers have stalked others before switching (often after a job reassignment) to the current victim. Margaret Ray, arrested repeatedly for stalking David Letterman, previously had stalked Yul Brynner. The erotomanic individual makes persistent efforts to contact the one about whom he or she has delusions through the telephone, by letter, by e-mails, through visits, through the sending of gifts. Whatever obstacles are put in the erotomanic individual's path are viewed as tests of the ardor of their love.

Studies show that people who write love letters to a delusionally loved person, even if the letters make no threats, are nonetheless prone to violence because of their abnormal craving for contact with the loved person. Research reveals that threatening letters sent to Hollywood celebrities were not associated with approaching them. Nor were the threatening letters sent to members of the U.S. Congress. Disorganized letters (that is, those showing evidence of psychotic thinking) also were less often associated with approaches to famous persons. People who wrote 10 to 14 letters had a 66% likelihood of approaching the celebrity. Those who wrote fewer or more letters were less likely to approach.

Interestingly, there is a dichotomy between the gender groups of erotomanic stalkers. In clinical practice, psychiatrists see mostly female erotomanics, whereas in forensic practice, they tend to encounter more males. Males more than females tend to run afoul of the law in their pursuit of delusionally loved persons or in some misguided effort to rescue them from an imagined danger.

Under current standards of diagnosis, those suffering from erotomania are classified as having a delusional disorder that is distinct from schizophrenia or mood disorders. Erotomania can exist across a whole spectrum of psychiatric disorders. Only 25% of stalkers are pure erotomanics; the other 75% have a second psychiatric disorder such as schizophrenia, borderline personality disorder, or a mood disorder. The symptoms persist, studies show, for an average of 10 to 12 years and are not as uncommon as once thought. Apart from the delusion and its consequences, erotomanic individuals do not display odd or bizarre behavior and may not intend any harm to their victims. In fact, they generally do not understand that their victims are being harmed by their stalking; on the contrary, they believe the victims are enjoying the attention.

During a preshow warm-up of the game show *Wheel of Fortune*, a man in battle fatigues and dog tags jumped out of the audience and screamed to letter-turner Vanna White that her boyfriend was dangerous and associated with the Mafia, but that he was there to protect her. Security guards escorted him from the studio, but he returned again and again. Court papers later revealed that he had been calling the show's production office and stating that he wanted to marry Ms. White.

Margaret Ray insisted that she was already David Letterman's wife. She broke into his home for the seventh time 3 days after being released from serving a 9-month sentence for trespassing on his property. For her, as for the battle-dressed admirer of Vanna White, arrests and imprisonments were merely obstacles to be overcome, opportunities to demonstrate the strength of their love.

John Thomas Smetek, later described as a 39-year-old drifter from Texas, walked up to a repertory theater where actress Justine Bateman was appearing in a play. Business card in hand, he pushed past patrons waiting in line and presented the card to a ticket taker. A love note to Bateman was written on its back, and with it Smetek delivered a verbal ultimatum: he was going to kill himself with a .22-caliber pistol. Eventually, Smetek was talked into surrendering. He was charged with two felonies and a misdemeanor, but he explained to the authorities that he had done all of this so that Justine Bateman would know how much he still cared about her. He claimed to have had an affair with her 7 years earlier. Authorities determined that he had been stalking her since March. At that time, he had bluffed his way onto the set of her television series, *Family Ties*, and twice managed to come face to face with her before disappearing. At the theater the night before the suicide threat, he had also come near her, shouting "I love you" to her as she left a rehearsal.

"I love you 6 trillion times," John Hinckley, Jr., wrote to the object of his unrequited ardor, actress Jodie Foster, just a few days before he set out to assassinate President Ronald Reagan. "Goodbye," he wrote to her. "Don't you maybe like me just a little bit?" He was trying to impress her with what he was about to do, although he did not spell it out. "You know a few things about me, dear sweetheart, like my obsession with fantasy; but what the rabble don't yet understand is that fantasies can become reality in my world."

The Schizophrenic Stalker

Schizophrenic individuals experience illogical, bizarre, and delusional disturbances in their thinking. They also exhibit many other disturbances in their perceptions, emotions, sense of self, volition, and relationship to the outside world. Schizophrenic individuals often have hallucinations, mainly auditory and visual. Their emotions are flat; their sense of self is fragmented. Withdrawn and self-absorbed, they often exhibit unusual or bizarre mannerisms but are usually loners who try to avoid all contact with other people.

Most schizophrenic stalkers do not wish to make contact with their victims. But some are driven to make contact because their own bizarre delusions convince them that they are tormented by their victims or that they have been somehow ordained, fated, or commanded to contact their victims. It is such schizophrenic individuals who are compelled to pursue their victims, driven, as it were, to seek relief by contact with them. When stalking is a symptom of chronic schizophrenia, this behavior may become intractable. Some schizophrenic individuals are psychologically fused with their victims, hopelessly unable to discern where they stop and the other person begins. Thus, killing the victim is tantamount to committing suicide.

Michael Perry, who had escaped from a mental institution, stalked singer-actress Olivia Newton-John. He wrote her two letters saying that he wanted to get in touch with her to prove to himself that she was real and not just a "Disneyland mirror image." Reportedly, he believed that Olivia Newton-John was responsible for dead bodies that were rising through the floor of his house and that her eyes changed colors as signals to him. He compiled a death-list of 10 names that included Supreme Court Justice Sandra Day O'Connor. He killed five persons, including his father and mother, whose eyes he shot out. Two weeks after those murders, he was in a hotel room in Washington, D.C., near the Supreme Court building. There were seven television sets in the room, all of them tuned to static and with eyes drawn on the screens with a marker. Fortunately, he was arrested before killing any more people on his death list.

Individuals like Perry can be extremely dangerous because of their persecutory or messianic delusions about specific individuals. But the majority of schizophrenic individuals who have delusional beliefs are too disorganized and self-absorbed to be capable of planning and carrying out a reasonably competent, sustained stalking.

As an aside, let me point out that some serial murderers, particularly serial sexual murderers, are stalkers, in that they often track their victims. Richard Ramirez, a California serial killer, was dubbed by the media as the "Night Stalker," but there was no discernible pattern in his killings and so could not be said to have stalked anyone. Most serial killers who stalk are not interested in the socioeconomic status of their victims or in their specific personalities, and so do not really fit into this chapter about stalkers. Serial murderers who stalked, such as Ted Bundy and Edmund Kemper, are discussed in Chapter 11.

The Cyberstalker

The Internet provides the stalker with another avenue by which to arrive at a person's doorstep. The stalker can obtain private information to facilitate pursuit of the victim as well as to communicate with the victim for the purposes of harassment and threats. Cyberstalking statistics show that between January 1, 2000, and December 2001, 83% of cyberstalking victims were women and 64% of the harassers were men. When the victims were asked where they first encountered the abuser or stalker, the top three locations were e-mail (39%), chat room (15%), and message board/forum (11%).

Most cases were resolved after reports were made to the stalker's Internet service provider. Prosecutors are increasingly prosecuting cyberstalking crimes. Cyberstalking is just another example of how far stalkers will go to harass and frighten their victims.

Prevention and Protection

Preventive Measures

Stalking is psychological terrorism. Inflicting terror on the victim often is intended, but it is also sometimes an unintended consequence of the stalker's obsession. No matter where the victim goes, he or she is at risk. It is difficult to appreciate the intensity of fear felt by victims for their lives. The horror is so intense and constant that it often defies our understanding and taxes our ability to empathize with the victim. The stalking victim gradually becomes a captive of the stalker. As the terrorism escalates, the victim's life becomes a prison. Friends may fall away for fear of becoming entangled and stalked themselves. The victim scurries from the protective cover of home to work and back, much as a prisoner is shuttled from cell to cell. Frequently, the workplace is no refuge from the stalker. Some victims are too terrified to leave home. They live in solitary confinement, peering out at the world from behind blinds. Sometimes, if help cannot be obtained, the only release is death—at the hands of the stalker. Such was the fate of Kristin Lardner, who was gunned down in broad daylight by Michael Cartier.

If the stalker shows up repeatedly at the victim's place of work, the victim may lose his or her job. Friends may have to do the victim's shopping. E-mail contacts can be endless and visually threatening. The telephone may ring incessantly. One victim's home was buzzed by a stalker in a small plane. Other victims have lost pets, cars, homes, and have had defamatory material spread about them (e.g., the victim has AIDS) at work, school, or on the Internet. Some victims of stalkers have had to move away from their homes, their towns, even out of the country. As an extreme measure, a few stalking victims change their identities. Andrea Evans, who had a starring role on ABC's *One Life to Live*, a series taped in New York City, felt forced by a Russian immigrant stalker to give up her job and her city. He sent her letters with threats written in blood, and despite his frequent hospitalizations, he continued to disrupt her life for some time. Eventually, her career in shambles, Ms. Evans left New York for an undisclosed location.

Actress Theresa Saldana's stalker, Arthur Jackson, came all the way from Scotland to see her, then stabbed her 10 times and left her for dead. Imprisoned in California, he frequently indicated in letters that he intended to finish the job of killing her when he was released. For the new threats, he received additional jail time. Jackson has been described by psychiatrists as a very dangerous, paranoid psychotic. He said that he wanted to kill Saldana so they could be united after death. Upon his release in the U.S., he was returned to Great Britain to stand trial for another violent offense, and in 2004 was reported to be in a mental institution there. Arthur Jackson is a classic example of a stalker who is "forever yours."

All states and the District of Columbia, recognizing the magnitude of the stalking problem, have passed anti-stalking laws. Victims can also obtain restraining orders to try to stay out of the clutches of stalkers, but these orders have had inconsistent success. Restraining orders are not effective against desperate people who have nothing to lose. To obtain such an order, the victim must go to court, itself a difficult process. Then, once the protective or restraining order is in hand, the victim must deal with the possibility that it may further inflame a determined stalker, perhaps pushing him or her over the edge into violence. Experts now suggest that the victim who obtains a protective order should also attempt to have criminal charges pressed. The combination may get the stalker off the streets and into jail, preventing immediate physical harm to the victim.

A federal task force has recommended that stalking be considered a felony offense. A number of states have already taken this step, codifying stalking as an offense punishable by up to 5 years in prison. The most effective laws concerning stalking are those that define the offense broadly, stating, for instance, that it means willful, malicious conduct that involves repeated harassment. Under such a definition, any word, gesture, or action that is intended to diminish a person's safety, security, or privacy will meet the definition of stalking and give the authorities reason to charge the stalker. In some states, however, the anti-stalking law is hampered by stipulations that an arrest warrant can be obtained only if the stalker has also made a "credible" threat against the victim, such as causing the victim to fear death or bodily harm. Unfortunately, this makes it necessary for the victim to prove violence directed against him or her even before that violence takes place. Moreover, threats are not highly correlated with actual violence.

Protecting Yourself

Laws aside, the reality is that stalking victims are and must be responsible for their own safety. Here are some techniques to decrease the risk of being psychologically or physically harmed by stalkers:

- Take the stalker seriously.
- Inform family and friends about the stalker.
- Improve home security with deadbolts and outside lights.
- Establish workplace security.
- Have coworkers screen your calls.
- Obtain witnesses to any stalking.
- Vary your driving routes.
- Do not get out of your car when next to a van.
- Limit the time you spend walking.
- Unobtrusively take pictures of the stalker.
- Make a record of the stalker's patterns.
- Use telephone caller identification devices.
- Do not respond to the stalker's calls, e-mails, letters, or invitations to meet.
- Remain in public places, and try not to travel alone.
- Maintain a continuing relationship with the police.
- Call police immediately if you are physically threatened by the stalker.
- Consider obtaining a restraining or protective order.
- Couple the protective order with the pressing of criminal charges whenever possible.
- Obtain legal counsel.

No one wants to move and take up a new identity. Total protection is too expensive and restrictive. But careless disregard can be fatal. A balance must be struck between the freedom of one's lifestyle and adequate security. With the enactment of laws making stalking a felony and public understanding of the dimensions of the problem, help for stalking victims and potential victims has arrived. Police everywhere are now listening seriously to women who complain of being harassed and stalked. Law enforcement agencies are revising their training procedures to take this crime into account. In some cases, arrests are required in cases of domestic violence to prevent the most common form of stalking, which arises from domestic violence. With regard to this particular crime, which is usually directed against women, society finally appears to "get it." Kristin Lardner's death and the violent maimings and deaths of thousands of other stalking victims have galvanized our legislatures and law enforcement agencies to finally face the epidemic of stalking and its related violence.

6

Workplace Violence

Is Your Job a Dead End?

Vengeance is mine; I will repay, saith the Lord.

—Romans 12:18

Gian Luigi Ferri, a 55-year-old mortgage broker, entered the lobby of 101 California Street, a granite and glass skyscraper in downtown San Francisco. He was carrying a black canvas satchel of the sort that attorneys use to hold legal documents. Wearing a dark business suit, he fit in well with the professionally clad attorneys and clients. He took the elevator to the 34th floor of the 48-story building and got off at the law firm of Pettit and Martin. In his bag, rather than legal documents, he carried two legally purchased 9-mm Intratec Tec-9 pistols capable of firing 50 times without having to be reloaded, a .45-caliber semiautomatic pistol, and hundreds of rounds of ammunition. Ferri ambled slowly toward a glass-enclosed conference room. Inside, Jody Jones Sposato, a 30-year-old mother, was the center of a small group of people involved in a deposition for Sposato's sexual discrimination suit against her former employer. With her was her lawyer, 35-year-old Jack Berman, who was advising her while she was being questioned by Sharon O'Roke, also 35, of Pettit and Martin, on behalf of the former employer. The deposition was being recorded by 33-year-old court reporter Deanna Eaves.

Ferri began to spray the conference room with bullets from outside, shattering the glass. Eaves dove under the table but was struck on the

97

right arm. Berman and Sposato were killed outright, and O'Roke received head, chest, and arm wounds. Near the conference room, a legal secretary dialed 911 and then Ferri came face to face with her. She was frozen in fear, but she saw his face. It was blank. He moved on. Attorney Brian Berger yelled at the secretary to run, then he ran to warn another attorney, Allan J. Berk. Ferri shot Berger critically in the arm and chest. Ferri then went in and killed Berk, a prominent labor lawyer, at his desk.

Ferri then went down a stairway to the 33rd floor, fatally wounded law intern David Sutcliffe, and ran into a husband-and-wife pair, attorneys John and Michelle Scully. The gunman pursued them into an empty room. John Scully shielded his wife by taking Ferri's bullets into his own body. As he was dying, he told his wife how to dial for help.

Emergency vehicles arrived and SWAT teams entered the tower. Ferri descended to the 32nd floor, the offices of the Trust Company of the West. There he killed 64-year-old widowed secretary Shirley Mooser and 48-year-old investment manager Donald Merrill, mortally wounded 33-year-old legal secretary Deborah Fogel, and wounded vice-president Vicky Smith and Pettit and Martin attorney Charles Ross, both 41. Then his two Tec-9 pistols overheated and jammed.

He headed down the fire stairs and soon found himself trapped between two teams of police. It was just 15 minutes since he had entered the building. Shoving the third pistol under his chin, Ferri fired a fatal round. The carnage left nine people dead, including Ferri, and six others wounded.

It was later learned that Gian Luigi Ferri had been a client of the Pettit and Martin law firm and that this connection constituted the ostensible reason for his deadly rampage in their offices. A letter found on his body also contained a rant against the U.S. Food and Drug Administration concerning the food additive monosodium glutamate (MSG).

Workplace Violence

I am a psychiatrist. My job can be very dangerous unless I take certain precautions, and I try to take them. How about you? Is your job potentially dangerous, and are you vulnerable at the workplace in some as-yet unexamined way? Most of us spend more time at work than at home or anywhere else. We get to know our fellow workers, but often-times not well enough.

The National Institute of Occupational Safety and Health has iden-tified workplace homicide as a "serious" public health problem. An av-erage of 1.7 million people were victims of violent crime while work-ing or on duty in the United States, according to a report published each year from 1993 through 1999 by the Bureau of Justice Statistics. An estimated 75% of these incidents were simple assaults. An addi-tional 19% were aggravated assaults. For the same period, more than 800 workplace homicides per year occurred. In 2005, assaults and vi-olent acts accounted for 13% of workplace fatalities. Within this cate-gory, 9% were homicides.

Although there are many variations, mass murder in the workplace usually takes one of five forms: 1) a disgruntled employee or former employee kills or injures other employees, 2) an angry spouse or rela-tive stalks employees at work, 3) violence is committed during a crim-inal act such as robbery, 4) violence is committed against people in dangerous jobs, such as law enforcement personnel, and 5) acts of ter-rorism or hate crimes are carried out, such as the terrorist attacks of September 11, 2001, against the World Trade Center in New York and, earlier, the attack by others against Oklahoma City's Alfred P. Murrah Federal Building. Workers, customers, and unlucky bystand-ers are frequently killed or wounded during such outbursts. In any case, the deaths of perpetrators of such violence are usually swift, ei-ther at their own hands or at the hands of law enforcement officials who kill them to prevent more killings. Very few workplace killers walk away from their killing grounds.

On a less overtly violent scale, workplace violence can take the form of sabotage against property or of psychological and sexual ha-rassment of employees. In a survey of 20,314 federal employees, 42% of the women and 15% of the men reported having been sexually ha-rassed. Although more than 90% of the sexual harassment charges filed with the Equal Employment Opportunity Commission (EEOC) have been filed by women, there is an increasing number of charges being filed by men. Moreover, as more women gain power in the workplace, it is likely that the reported sexual harassment of men by women will increase further. Power corrupts, regardless of gender. But it is the workplace mass murders that have caught the public eye. Be-cause most of us work, we feel threatened by this sort of violence even when it is not directed against us. Many people have cause to feel disgruntled because of changes in the workplace due to automation and bad economic conditions. Old-style family and community cohesiveness, no less than employer-employee good relations and loyalty, have gone by the board, with deleterious effects. The availability of rapid-fire, military-style assault weapons has made it possible for a disgruntled person with a private arsenal to kill a lot of people.

The FBI arbitrarily defines *mass murder* as murder involving four or more victims in one location during one event and subdivides the category into classic mass murder and family mass murder. The classic mass murderer was Charles Whitman, the University of Texas "Tower Killer" described later in this chapter. Another example is the killing of 13 students and faculty at Columbine, Colorado, by Eric Harris and Dylan Klebold before they turned their guns on themselves. In 2007, at Virginia Polytechnic Institute and State University in Blacksburg, Virginia, student Seung-Hui Cho killed 32 students and teachers before committing suicide. He became infamous for committing the worst mass shooting by a lone gunman in U.S. history.

Family mass murderers kill four or more family members and may or may not commit suicide themselves. When suicide occurs, it is classified as a murder-suicide. Without suicide, the murder is classified as a family mass murder. On November 9, 1971, John List, an insurance salesman, killed his wife, three children, and mother, then disappeared. His car was found in an airport parking lot. Seventeen years later, a tip was received from a viewer who had seen an age-enhanced clay bust of List on the TV program *America's Most Wanted.* List was arrested in Richmond, Virginia, where he was found to be married and working as an accountant. More recently, in 1999, Mark Barton, a stock market day trader in Atlanta, killed his wife, son, and daughter before going to his former workplace and killing an additional nine people.

There are also *spree murderers* and *serial murderers.* Spree murder is defined as killing at two or more locations with no emotional cooling-off period occurring between the murders. On September 6, 1949, Howard Unruh moved through his neighborhood as he fired his handgun, killing 13 people and wounding 3 others in about 20 minutes. His morbid deed has therefore been classified by the FBI as a spree murder rather than a mass murder. The distinction between the two seems of interest mainly to experts. More recent examples include Martin Bryant of Tasmania, Australia, who in the course of several hours killed 35 people with various automatic weapons in a half-dozen locations in the township of Port Arthur.

The typical mass murderer is as ordinary as many people's next door neighbor, a white male in his late twenties to mid-forties. But he is atypical in that he is frequently a loner who drifts from job to job, existing without close family, neighborhood, or community ties. There are thousands of angry men among us who seek revenge for real or imagined grievances. They also make threats of wreaking violence, but thankfully there are only a few who turn their anger into actual outbreaks of violence. Yet the number of mass murders is mounting. Two or three of them occur each month.

Public perception has it that something snaps and these persons go off and kill the nearest people at hand. That does happen, but the majority of mass murders are planned. Moreover, media coverage of any mass murder is now thought to contribute to the next mass murder— a predictable clustering phenomenon.

Mass murderers tend to have a lethal combination of paranoia (feelings of persecution) and depression. They feel despondent and hopeless while at the same time they blame others for their plight. Their fantasies tend to be straightforward: revenge against the perceived persecutors. They do not entertain the intricate, baroque sexual fantasies of the serial sexual murderer. Nonetheless, they do kill, and, beyond the actual body count, there are many physical and psychological victims of workplace violence. No statistics can capture the immense psychological harm seared into the minds of survivors of this sort of violence. In the Pettit and Martin rampage, John Scully died trying to protect his wife from Ferri's bullets. The Scullys had been married less than a year and were very close. Now his wife must live with the terrifying, agonizing memories of his final moments in the forefront of her mind. Jody Jones Sposato was also killed by Ferri. Her husband Stephen Sposato told a reporter, "They invited me to go to the coroner's office [to identify the body of my wife] and my life was shattered."

Many survivors of workplace violence are scarred by symptoms of posttraumatic stress disorder (PTSD), some for many years afterwards. Terrifying flashbacks that have the clarity of video images, hellish and sweat-drenched nightmares, numbed feelings, and withdrawal from relationships are some of the symptoms that result from life-threatening trauma in the workplace. In fact, a psychological study of 36 employees who were in the building at the time of Ferri's rampage was conducted by a research team from Stanford University School of Medicine. Immediately after the shooting, a wide range of acute stress responses was noted. Reevaluation 7 to 10 months later revealed that one-third of the employees who initially met the criteria for an acute stress disorder had significantly more symptoms of PTSD at follow-up.

Violence against workers has also been charted by occupation, showing that most of the violence is directed at people who interact with the public. The top occupations at risk for a range of physical injuries resulting from violence, as reported by the Bureau of Justice Statistics, are, in descending order, recreational workers, bartenders, cab drivers, retail sales clerks, food service workers, police officers, parking attendants, auto mechanics, security guards, social workers, cashiers, bus drivers, fire fighters, and service station attendants. The rate of injury for the top-ranked category, recreational workers, was 118.5 per 1,000 persons, whereas social workers, ranked much lower, had a rate of 8.5 per 1,000 persons. Many injuries and deaths were associated with robberies and attempted robberies.

As compiled from reports of victims, the following are reasons given by workplace attackers for their violence: irrational behavior, 26%; dissatisfied with service, 19%; interpersonal conflict, 15%; upset at having been disciplined, 12%; criminal behavior, 10%; personal problems, 8%, firings or layoffs, 2%; prejudice, 1%; and unknown causes, 7%. Some of these categories reflect the occasion rather than the reason for underlying rage to explode. Firearms are the weapons of choice used in three-quarters of the deaths. Half the deaths occurred in the southern region of the United States and another quarter in the West.

Types of violence in the workplace have also been studied. In a 1993 survey conducted by the Society for Human Resource Management, 75% of violent incidents were fistfights, 17% were shootings, 7.5% were stabbings, 6% were rapes or other sexual assaults, and less than 1% were explosions. Those who are killed are 3.5 times as likely to be female as male. Homicide is a leading cause of death for women in the workplace. Even though the leading instrument of death on the job is firearms, females were six times more likely than males to die of strangulation. These statistics reflect the fact that women in the workplace are at special risk. Rejection of ardent suitors, or, worse, of workplace harassers, brings with it the increased risk of severe injury or death to the women at the hands of these men. When romances outside the workplace go awry, the rejected male usually knows where the woman is employed and generally has ready access to her workplace. Although the fact has not received much media attention, women who work in retail settings are at high risk of being injured or murdered at their jobs. More women than men work in the retail industry, for instance in convenience stores. Alone and unprotected in such establishments, they are particularly vulnerable and at risk for becoming victims of violence.

Murders at the Post Office

In recent years, certain workplaces have become known as increasingly dangerous locations for workers, patrons, and passers-by because of the killings that have occurred there. The most obvious location, perhaps because of the extensive media coverage, has been the post office. "Going postal" has become a slang phrase for having a psychotic episode and wreaking violence on people in one's current or former workplace. There are 40,000 postal service locations and more than 825,000 postal workers in this country. Dozens of deadly incidents in the past decade have had postal workers or facilities as their focal points. On the same day, May 6, 1993, in two different locations, postal workers lashed out. In Dearborn, Michigan, Larry Jason had been known as a "walking time bomb" who had graphically threatened his supervisors. In San Juan Capistrano, California, Mark Hilburn was fearful of losing his job. Their rampages left four people dead.

On August 10, 1989, John Merlin Taylor, a model post office employee with 27 years of award-winning, exceptional service, went on a rampage in Orange Glen, California, that eventually left four dead, including himself and his wife. In May 1989, mailman Alfred Hunter stole an airplane and strafed the Boston city streets with an AK-47. On August 20, 1986, Patrick Henry Sherrill showed up at work in Edmond, Oklahoma, in full postal uniform but with three handguns in his mailbag. He murdered 14 workers and injured even more before killing himself.

Former workers account for only a small fraction of overall workplace violence, but their rampages can be terrifying. A 35-year-old mail clerk, Joseph Harris, lost his job in the Ridgewood, New Jersey, post office because he threatened a supervisor. Eighteen months later he went to her home and killed her and her fiancée. He then went to the Ridge-wood facility and shot dead two mailmen who had just arrived for work.

On November 13, 1991, 37-year-old ex-Marine Thomas McIlvane found a message from his post office union shop steward on his answering machine, telling him he would not be rehired, that his appeal for reinstatement at a suburban Detroit post office had been turned down. He had been fired for insubordination, cursing a supervisor, fighting with patrons, and for making obscene, threatening remarks to coworkers as well as to supervisors. For months, McIlvane had threatened that if he was not rehired, he would come back and kill. He had been heard voicing the threat that his revenge would make the Edmond, Oklahoma, post office massacre look like Disneyland. His supervisors had described McIlvane as a "ticking time bomb." A former professional kickboxer who also held a black belt in karate, McIlvane had been drummed out of the Marine Corps for deliberately crushing a fellow Marine's car with a tank.

At the post office, a supervisor had requested protection from McIlvane, but the request was turned down. Coworkers established an escape route that they could use if McIlvane turned up. And turn up he did, the morning after the answering machine message, arriving at the Royal Oak Regional Mail Center in Michigan at 8:15 a.m. with a sawed-off Ruger .22-caliber semiautomatic rifle tucked under his raincoat. He killed four supervisors before turning the gun on himself and committing suicide.

Why has the postal service experienced so much violence? No one knows for sure. For one thing, a continuing automation process has been placing great stress on postal employees, who are hard pressed to keep up with the pace of the new equipment. Another major part of the problem seems to come from inadequately careful selection of employees. Lack of tact and management skills among postal supervisors is another contributing factor. Each year, in the postal service, there are 150,000 grievance proceedings and 69,000 disciplinary actions in the army of 825,000 employees. This is a very high index of supervisor-employee difficulties—1 out of every 12 employees is disciplined annually, and 2 out of every 11 file grievances against their supervisors. On the other hand, a report by the Centers for Disease Control and Prevention found post offices have a lower homicide rate than many other industries. Programs aimed at reducing violence in the postal service have led to fewer violent incidents.

In media interviews, an alarmingly large number of postal workers admitted that they strongly identified with the killers in the violent post office events, stating that they themselves harbored similar revenge impulses but did not act on them. In this instance especially, the bad men did what the good ones dreamed about doing. The difference between the two groups depends on many factors—among the significant ones, the degree of depression and paranoia.

Work problems have been common complaints among my patients over the years. I have listened for countless hours to some of my patients' exquisitely detailed fantasies of extreme sadistic torture of their bosses. One of my patients relished her fantasy of beheading the boss's children in front of him, boiling their heads, and then forcing the boss at gunpoint to drink the concoction. As with my other patients who could examine their fantasies, there was very little likelihood that she would act on any of her violent urges. This patient was a very high-functioning, competent executive who was scrupulously law abiding. Perhaps the ability to fantasize and verbalize terrible violence against others helps preempt the need to put violent motives into action.

Not So Ivory Tower

The image of the college campus as a sleepy, peaceful refuge from the world was shattered on August 1, 1966, when Charles Whitman, a 25-year-old architectural engineering student, mounted the 307-foot clock tower atop the University of Texas. Before leaving home for his rampage, Whitman had killed his wife and his mother. Atop the tower, he killed 13 more people by sniper fire and wounded 31 before being killed himself.

Whitman set the pattern for the next 40 years of campus-related killings that seem to have increased the risk of both teachers and students being harmed, as in the actions of Gang Lu, a brilliant but disgruntled astrophysicist at the University of Iowa. During a student-faculty meeting, Lu shot 47-year-old physics professor Christopher K. Goertz twice in the head, killing him instantly. He then whirled and killed 27-year-old Linhua Shan, his perceived rival, who had received a prestigious university award that Lu had coveted. Before Lu was finished, he killed 5 faculty members and seriously wounded another. Then, his mission completed, Lu removed his heavy coat, folded it neatly onto a chair, and fired a .38 slug into his own head.

The cases go on and on, and they involve high schools and grade schools as well as colleges and universities. Inhabitants of Massachusetts, California, Louisiana, a half-dozen other states, and Montreal, Canada have all seen such murders and murder-suicides. Marc Lepine mounted a well-planned aggressive armed assault at the school of engineering (École Polytechnique) at the University of Montreal. Venting his rage principally against women, he killed or injured 14 people with a rifle. After a wounded victim cried out for help, Lepine pulled out his knife and stabbed her repeatedly in the chest until she was dead. He then put the muzzle of the rifle against his head, said "Oh, shit," and shot himself. It was the worst mass murder and hate crime against women in Canadian history. Lepine left a suicide note that said:

> Please note that if I kill myself today 12/06/89 it is not for economic reasons (because I waited until I used up all my financial means, even refusing jobs) but for political reasons. Because I decided to send Ad Patres [meaning gathered to the fathers, or, simply, dead] the feminists who have always ruined my life. For seven years my life has brought me no joy, and, being utterly weary of the world, I have decided to stop those shrews dead in their tracks.

Six months later, Lepine claimed his last victims—Sarto Blais, an engineer who had been at the same school and who could not rid himself of his memories of the killings of his classmates and friends, hanged himself. Then, his parents, themselves seeing no reason to go on living, also committed suicide.

There have been killings at high schools, junior high schools, grade schools. Incredibly, a loaded revolver was discovered at a church preschool in an affluent Virginia neighborhood.

One of the worst cases is the April 16, 2007, killings at Virginia Tech in which a 23-year-old loner from South Korea, Seung-Hui Cho, shot and killed 32 students and faculty, and wounded 17 more, before killing himself. This has been classified as the worst peacetime shooting in United States history. Later investigation revealed that Cho had several times earlier been identified as troubled, but had refused treatment.

Eric Harris and Dylan Klebold, the Columbine High School killers, had planned to set off bombs as well as execute students and faculty with automatic weapons—to kill hundreds and hundreds of people—and be remembered as the most prolific mass murderers of all time.

Fortunately, they did not succeed, but did manage to kill 12 and injure 20 more before placing their guns to their heads.

In all instances in these school shootings, the precise motivations and mental makeup of the shooters remain elusive. There are some clues, however. The U.S. Secret Service developed a profile of 41 school shooters in 37 incidents; they found that the most frequently expressed motive was revenge, and that about three-quarters of the perpetrators had threatened to commit suicide before their attacks. The report described the perpetrators as feeling extremely depressed, with most of them also feeling persecuted and dealing with a significant change in a relationship or a loss in status. These statistics and motivations are consistent with the conclusions reached in other studies of adolescent mass murderers.

Patients Who Kill

Medical facilities such as doctors' offices, emergency rooms, regular wards, nursing homes, and clinics have become increasingly dangerous places for both practitioners and patients because of people intent on murder in such locations. A deranged white supremacist traveled from Maryland to Chicago to shoot to death a plastic surgeon in the doctor's own office. Jonathan Preston Haynes, age 35, told arresting officers that he had gone to Chicago and randomly selected his victim from a phonebook listing for plastic surgeons. He made an appointment with Dr. Martin Sullivan, age 68, then sat quietly in the doctor's waiting room until his name was called. Going into the physician's office, he calmly executed the surgeon, reportedly because Haynes was angry at people "diluting the Aryan beauty by creating ersatz Aryans."

Psychiatrists have long known that the most dangerous time is during the first visit with an unknown patient. According to an American Psychiatric Association Task Force Report, 40% of psychiatrists are assaulted during their careers. Nearly three-fourths of assaults against all physicians occurred during the first meeting of doctor and patient. At that time, the extent of the patient's illness and possible presence of homicidal impulses is unknown to the psychiatrist. The psychiatrist has not had time to develop a working therapeutic relationship that could inhibit dangerous acts. It is quite possible for any mental health professional in such a circumstance to become endangered as the instant object of a disturbed patient's persecutory delusions. While in training, male psychiatrists are often told to wear breakaway, clip-on ties, so that a patient cannot strangle the doctor with his own tie. They are also told to take offices that have separate doors for doctor and patient; otherwise, a doctor who sits with the only door at his or her back may be perceived by the patient as blocking the exit, an avenue the patient might need if he or she fears losing control over violent impulses.

These stratagems are not misplaced. Many mental health professionals have been the victims of workplace violence. One psychiatrist was very seriously maimed by a letter bomb. Others have been killed. Psychiatrist Brian Buss, age 37, was working at a state hospital near Portland, Oregon, when he found it necessary to admit a paranoid psychiatric employee of the hospital to that same hospital for observation and possible treatment. This patient had previously been in a state hospital and expressed fears about having to stay in another such hospital. However, the only alternative, the local community hospital, did not have a psychiatric unit. Buss went into a makeshift seclusion room, alone, to inform the patient that he would soon be transferred to the state hospital where he had been treated a decade ago. The patient became enraged and ordered Buss to leave. When Buss refused, the patient picked up a rod lying on the floor and clubbed him to death. Some time later, when the patient's psychosis had cleared, he was interviewed and made several safety suggestions for the hospital—for instance, that the psychiatrist should never have come into the seclusion room alone and that he should have left the room immediately when the patient had ordered him to do so.

Psychiatrist Michael McCullock, 41, decided to treat a 38-year-old paranoid schizophrenic man with a long history of violence as an outpatient in his private office in Portland, Oregon. He did so despite evidence that the man had made threats to kill a philosophy professor while he had been in college and despite the man's several previous involuntary hospitalizations. The psychotic patient had developed the delusion that Dr. McCullock was torturing him with a brain-stimulating machine and that the only way to stop the torture and pain was to kill the psychiatrist. Barging into Dr. McCullock's office one day and pulling a shotgun from under his raincoat, the patient shot McCullock dead at close range. He then waited calmly for the police. Later, when interviewed, the patient was without remorse. Because of his delusions, the patient believed that he had been justified in killing his psychiatrist.

Similarly, Dr. Wayne Fenton, 53, a prominent psychiatrist, associate director of a division of the National Institute of Mental Health, and an expert on schizophrenia, agreed to do a consultation on a Saturday in his private office with a young man known to be paranoid and psychotic, who was unaccompanied by his parents. Shortly, police were notified by the patient's father that his son had returned from that appointment acting strangely and with blood on his pants and shirt. The police went to the office, found that Dr. Fenton had been murdered. They were soon able to apprehend 19-year-old Vitali Davydov and charge him with the crime.

Today most emergency rooms in hospitals, in addition to handling emergency cases, also function as outpatient clinics, which treat a variety of chronically ill people. In recent years, disgruntled patients who have not found relief for their pain, or who think they have been badly treated, have come back to kill emergency room personnel. That is why most emergency rooms now have security personnel and equipment to detect the presence of firearms.

Doctors may also be the victims of politically motivated attacks, as has been made clear by recent violence against abortion clinics and against doctors who perform abortions. Some antiabortion extremists have become terrorists willing to kill to prevent women from being able to have abortions. Michael F. Griffin, age 32, was found guilty of the first-degree murder of Dr. David Gunn, a physician who performed abortions at Pensacola Women's Medical Services Clinic. Griffin, an antiabortion zealot, shot Dr. Gunn three times as the physician arrived for work during a protest. Antiabortion activist Paul Hill shot and killed Dr. John Britton and his unarmed escort outside The Ladies Center clinic in Pensacola, Florida. John C. Salvi, age 22, opened fire at two abortion clinics in Brookline, Massachusetts, killing two women and wounding five other people. Medical personnel in many abortion clinics are working under a state of siege.

Hospital Killing Grounds

Finally, hospitals and nursing homes have been used as killing grounds by murderers who have access to them and their vulnerable patient-residents. Ex-Marine Donald Swango managed to graduate from Southern Illinois School of Medicine with a medical degree, but his fascination with dying patients was noted. At Ohio State, nurses on the floors that

Swango worked on as a surgical intern noticed more patients dying than usual, and one saw Swango give an injection to a patient who soon sickened. He was cleared by an investigation but resigned and became an EMT in Quincy, Illinois. After paramedics noticed people getting violently ill in the office when he was around, he was arrested in possession of arsenic and other poisons, convicted, and sentenced to five years in prison. After his release, he forged documents to reestablish himself in West Virginia and then, under an alias, in South Dakota. Discovered there, he found his way to Stony Brook in New York State. In every location, patients died for no apparent reason. Only when a former employer in South Dakota called Stony Brook was he exposed and a warning about him sent to all the teaching hospitals in the United States. Swango moved to Zimbabwe, where he killed more people but escaped before being tried. He was on his way to a job in Saudi Arabia when he chose a flight that gave him a layover in Chicago, where he was arrested. He pleaded guilty to three killings of patients, and—nearly 20 years after he began to harm patients and coworkers—received a sentence of life imprisonment without the possibility of parole.

Donald Harvey, a nursing assistant known as the Angel of Death, may have killed as many as 100 victims in healthcare settings. He worked as a nursing assistant in various hospitals. He confessed to killing 15 patients at Marymount Hospital in London, Kentucky, and 15 more at the Cincinnati Veterans Administration Medical Center. While working at Drake Memorial Hospital from 1985 to 1987, when he was arrested, he allegedly killed 21 additional infirm and chronically ill patients.

Harvey at first claimed that he was committing mercy killings, but his real motivation came out later as he told how he obtained great satisfaction from being able to fool "know-it-all" doctors who would assume that their patients had died from natural causes. Psychiatrists described Harvey as a compulsive man who murdered because it gave him a sense of power. He had also killed for revenge after having been homosexually raped. Harvey was not a subtle mercy killer, as his methods of murder also revealed. He thrust a straightened-out coat hanger into the abdomen of a restrained and confused old man, puncturing the man's bowel and causing him to die of peritonitis two days later. For others, he cut off the oxygen supply, suffocated them with plastic bags and pillows, injected syringes full of air, and mixed arsenic and cyanide in patients' food.

Other so-called mercy killings have taken place with some frequency in hospitals, institutions, and nursing homes. Few of these murders have anything to do with compassion and pity for the victim. Most echo Harvey's incentive to kill in order to exercise total power and control over the victim. Motives of nurse-killers or bedside-killers have included the thrill of creating medical emergencies, appearing heroic, enjoying watching patients as they die, and putting patients out of their misery. The most common method of killing is injecting a prescribed drug in amounts that are known to be lethal. Charles Cullen, a nurse, was charged with the murders of at least 40 seriously ill patients. He injected patients with drugs, mainly digoxin, used in cardiac care units, ostensibly to end their suffering. Similarly, Harold Shipman, a British physician, was convicted of killing 15 patients, although a government investigation concluded that he had killed at least 215, making him the most notorious of all medical serial killers.

Patients in nursing homes are sometimes killed by physical abuse. It is my belief that some serial killers work in facilities that take care of the elderly and the very infirm—killers who change jobs frequently and whose crimes are only discovered in the wake of heightened patient mortality rates that are otherwise inexplicable.

It was not until after the death of Dr. David J. Acer, a dentist practicing in Florida, that the workplace violence he allegedly committed was discovered. Dr. Acer had died of acquired immunodeficiency syndrome (AIDS). He had contracted the human immunodeficiency virus (HIV) years earlier but continued to practice dentistry—and did not inform his patients of his condition. The first of his patients to develop AIDS and die was young Kimberly Bergalis. Dr. Acer himself died before he could be questioned about Kimberly's treatment. At least five other patients became infected. It was only possible to test 700 of Dr. Acer's 2,000 patients for HIV. Questions have been raised about whether Dr. Acer might have deliberately infected his patients. His former lover has been quoted as saying that Dr. Acer did do so in an attempt to "prove" that AIDS was not just a disease limited to the population of homosexuals. If Dr. Acer did deliberately transmit the fatal disease to his patients, he would have to be considered a serial murderer. It may be years before the full extent of the damage he allegedly wrought can be tallied. I say *allegedly* because a new scientific study may cast doubt on the original findings that implicated Dr. Acer.

Vigilante Justice in the Courts

As the introductory vignette about Gian Luigi Ferri's murderous assault on the law firm of Pettit and Martin makes clear, lawyers, law firms, and the courts are fast becoming targets of violence. Bad feelings toward lawyers and the court system are today epidemic and are reflected in the current abundance of uncomplimentary jokes about lawyers. Ferri was reported to have laughed himself to tears, a few weeks before the massacre, when told the following joke: "If you were locked into a room with Saddam Hussein, the Ayatollah Khomeini, and a lawyer, and you had a gun with two bullets in it, who would you shoot? The lawyer—twice."

Lawyers are advocates who work within an adversarial system, one that leads directly to the polarization of positions and to the evocation of strong emotions. The courts deal with difficult, contentious, and momentous decisions, sometimes of life and death; stresses on litigants, lawyers, judges, and juries can be extremely high. Letter bombs have been sent to lawyers and judges, injuring some recipients, killing others. Gun-wielding litigants seeking their own immediate brand of justice have killed several lawyers and judges. In one notable rampage, Kenneth Baumrock brought two handguns into a divorce hearing in a Clayton, Missouri, courtroom and killed his wife and wounded four court officials. On the same day in Grand Forks, South Dakota, a similar event occurred in a family court, in which a gunman severely wounded the family court judge.

Lawyers can turn lethal as well. Attorney George Lott began a shooting rampage in a court, killing a defense lawyer and a prosecutor, and injuring two appeals judges. Lott's complaint was that a family court justice had improperly favored his former wife in a child custody hearing. Violent outcomes are not unusual in divorce and custody actions because the litigation process fans intense hatreds.

Death in Familiar Places

Restaurants and financial institutions are increasingly becoming venues for violence as a result of revenge motives acted out in locations where many people are likely to be present. Only a few of the locations have been specifically connected to the perpetrators' grudges against society. In one of the most awful incidents, George Hennard crashed his truck through the front window of Luby's Cafeteria in Killeen, Texas, injuring several customers in his path. Hennard then jumped out of the truck with a gun in his hand and systematically killed 23 lunch customers and employees. Hennard killed mostly women, especially those who had made eye contact with him. He wounded 22 others and then took his own life. It was the nation's worst firearms massacre. Hennard had fired a total of 96 bullets in a few minutes. Of the 136 survivors who were psychologically examined after the rampage, 20% of the men and 36% of the women were found to have posttraumatic stress disorder.

Hennard had no real connection with Luby's Cafeteria, but many other mass killers have targeted restaurants because they once worked in those particular locations or because they believed they had been insulted there. There is a high turnover of employees in the restaurant industry, and often robberies are executed by former employees of a restaurant who are familiar with its operation. In Queens, New York, two men entered a Wendy's restaurant, displayed their guns, took 7 employees, 3 of them known to one perpetrator, into a basement freezer, and shot them in order to rob the eatery of $3,200. Two of the 7 who were shot survived and identified the killers.

Workers at financial institutions are also at risk during robberies. Furthermore, they are targets for disgruntled employees and customers, especially during hard financial times. A disgruntled former employee of the Firemen's Fund, 33-year-old Paul Calden, went to the Island Center Building in Tampa, Florida, killed three of the Fund's supervisors while they were eating lunch, and injured two women. He then drove away and was found later in his car, 12 miles from the site, dead of a self-inflicted gunshot wound. It was learned that he had been dismissed from a job with Firemen's Fund 8 months earlier and that he had been mentally disturbed, troubled by a preoccupation with extraterrestrial contacts.

The General Motors Acceptance Corporation office in Jacksonville, Florida, repossessed a two-year-old Pontiac Grand Am from James Edward Pough, 42, a few months after Pough's wife had left him. He could not pay the debt of $6,394 out of his low hourly laborer's wages. Six months later, Pough walked into the office, killed eight people, wounded four others, then ended his own life with a .38-caliber revolver.

A disgruntled, disabled electrician named Jim H. Forrester drove his Chevrolet Suburban into the office of the State Industrial Insurance System in Las Vegas and went on a shooting rampage through the first floor of the building. In this incident, although no one was killed, about

25 employees later filed claims for stress and for injuries, and many of the 400 employees later received individual and group therapy.

The annals of workplace killers are heavily weighted toward lower-rank former employees, but one of the first such killers to come to the public's attention was a former IBM executive and engineer, Edward Thomas Mann. He had resigned, rather than be fired, after his performance ratings had slipped. Mann charged that he was a victim of racial discrimination. He traded in his white shirt and other appurtenances of IBM life and donned an olive-drab fatigue jacket and ski mask. Then, in pseudocommando style, Mann crashed his bronze Lincoln Continental into the lobby of an IBM office building in Rockville, Maryland. He leaped out of the car with two loaded rifles, a shotgun, and a pistol, using these to kill two people and wound seven more in a long siege, at the end of which he surrendered to police. Two years later, in prison, he hanged himself.

Most perpetrators of workplace violence are white men, but occasionally they are women. In every setting except where women are acutely psychotic, men have a higher incidence of violent behavior. Gail Levine, age 62, was convicted of sabotage against the Pepsi-Cola company by a federal jury in Denver. She had placed a syringe in a Diet Pepsi can during the tampering scare—as delayed vengeance against the company that had fired her husband 18 years earlier. In a rare case of workplace violence perpetrated by a woman, 30-year-old industrial engineer Elizabeth A. Teague attempted to set the Eveready Battery plant in Bennington, Vermont, on fire by detonating several homemade black powder and gasoline bombs. Before the bombs went off, she shot and killed the plant manager and wounded two coworkers at the plant where she had worked. Captured, she complained to the FBI of racial harassment at Eveready, that her home phone had been tapped by the company, and that coworkers had stolen and sold company secrets. Police also found at her home some media accounts that had fueled her vengeful feelings: stories about the Luby's Cafeteria massacre and about Anita Hill's sexual harassment charges against Supreme Court nominee Clarence Thomas.

A Behavioral Profile of the Workplace Killer

There are millions of unhappy workers in the workplace, but only a few of them reach the point of acting out their unhappiness in violence against others. Although the behavioral characteristics of the person who commits workplace mayhem is rather stereotypical, the psychological motivation can be extremely complex and, often, undiscoverable. Typically, the worker is disgruntled and has troubled work relationships, but this is not enough to trigger violence. In general, ordinary occupational unhappiness does not play a significant part in the motivation of workplace violence, although it is often cited as a "cause." Situations, context, genetic makeup, psychological development, physical and mental disorders, cultural and social influences, and many other factors enter into the lethal mix. Even trained professionals are frequently unable to detect a potential murderer. John Merlin Taylor, whose career in the postal service had lasted 27 years, had paranoid ideas about being set up to take a fall. He imagined that he would find money on his route and that this would be used as a way to discipline or fire him. Such a delusion did not, in itself, signal the murderous violence he later wreaked. Taylor gave no warning that he would explode.

Profiling of potential perpetrators of workplace violence is an inexact exercise; it should be viewed as a rough assessment tool that can raise the consciousness of management personnel toward the possible prevention of outbreaks of violence in their workplaces.

The following 10-dimensional behavioral profile (summarized in Table 6–1) characterizes many perpetrators of workplace violence:

TABLE 6–1. A behavioral profile of the workplace killer

1. Disgruntled
2. Disturbed
3. Determined
4. Deviant
5. Distant
6. Dangerous
7. Disrupted relationships
8. Dyscontrol
9. Drugs and alcohol
10. Down and out

---

1. Disgruntled

Virtually all persons who commit workplace violence have major, un-requited grievances against their employers. Often, the employee feels he or she has been "screwed over," used, abused, and discarded like a piece of trash. Frequent absences occur. Usually, disciplinary actions have been taken against the employee in the past. A documented record of escalating labor-management disputes often is found after a violent incident has occurred. Complaints of work stress commonly precede the outbreak of violence. Disgruntled employees or ex-employees whose lives are consumed by pursuing their grievances can turn lethal. For example, James Huberty was described as a bitter man. A 42-year-old unemployed security guard, Huberty lost his job after 13 years of hard work when his employers shut down their plant. He was emotionally cold and had a violent temper; he struck his children and engaged in physical fights with his wife. He was fascinated with weapons, mercenary literature, and army clothing. On July 18, 1984, at 4 p.m., Huberty dressed in camouflage clothing, armed himself, and told his wife, "I'm going hunting humans!" He entered the nearest McDonald's and sprayed the restaurant with an Uzi semiauto-matic weapon and a 12-gauge shotgun. Twenty-one people were killed and 15 were wounded. Huberty was shot through the heart by a SWAT team. A number of mass murderers attack in pseudocom-mando style. Their interest in weapons, mercenary magazines, and the military are often an attempt to cover up deep feelings of inadequacy, as well as to express intense bitterness and hatred toward others and themselves, given that they often also die.

2. Disturbed

Many perpetrators of workplace violence experience some sort of mental disturbance. Some have been diagnosed; others commit their violence and are judged as disordered well after the fact. The patient who killed psychiatrist Wayne S. Fenton was reported to be a paranoid psychotic. Edward Mann, who rammed his car into the IBM offices and was captured after killing two people, was later diagnosed for the first time as suffering from major depression and a delusional disorder. Many workplace killers commit suicide after their rampages and can only be diagnosed in retrospect, and even then without great certainty.

One particular form of mental disorder, *erotomania*, was implicated in a case in California's Silicon Valley. In erotomania, the person feels absolutely convinced that the object of his or her affections feels the same way, even if there is evidence to the contrary. Software engineer Richard Farley met Laura Black, an electrical engineer, at the defense contractor ESL, Inc. When she spurned his advances, he stalked her. Four years after Farley had met Black, he stormed ESL, killed seven employees, and gravely wounded Black. Farley wanted to spill his blood on Laura Black so she would never forget him. From prison, Farley continued to write to Black as she lay in a hospital bed with her survival in doubt. Even though his violence had been acted out, his delusion and disorder continued.

The vast majority of people who are mentally disturbed are no more violent than the population in general. There is no research support for the strong connection the public assumes exists between mental disorder and violence. In fact, a previous history of violence and current alcohol and drug abuse are much more accurate indicators of the risk of violence. Mental disorder represents only a modest risk of violence compared with other risk factors such as male gender, young age, and lower socioeconomic status. Mental disorders, however, can interfere with work performance. A vicious cycle may develop in which declining performance brings managerial criticism, which produces further anger and deterioration in work. The worker's mental disturbance is overlooked, and an opportunity to intervene therapeutically is lost. When mentally disturbed workers are subjected to these downward cyclical stresses, they may be more likely to become violent. Prior brain injuries, posttraumatic stress disorder, depression, mania, substance abuse, personality disorders, chronic pain—any of these, or a combination of them, may, but not necessarily do, form the backdrop for violence. When Texas tower killer Charles Whitman was autopsied, he was found to have had a brain tumor the size of a pecan. The pathologist was uncertain of the role that tumor might have played in Whitman's murderous rampage, but it was learned that Whitman had complained of severe headaches.

3. Determined

Frequently, among survivors of workplace violence, one hears the description of the killer as acting like an automaton—mechanically, coldly, and emotionlessly going about his killing. Gian Luigi Ferri was described as displaying a blank expression while murdering people at the law firm of Pettit and Martin. This observation is counterintuitive, because we would expect peak expressions of strong emotion during the act of killing, such as hate and rage.

It is my impression that many workplace killers commit violence in a mentally-split state. Most workplace killings are planned. Once a plan is hatched, the person is determined to see it through. Perpetrators generally are familiar with weapons, have a military background, and attack the workplace in a pseudocommando fashion. Much like men preparing to go into battle, they are determined and prepare themselves mentally. Part of that preparation is to consciously split off thoughts and feelings that might produce fear or otherwise interfere with the mission.

4. Deviant

The thinking of persons who ultimately explode into violent acts is usually quite different from that of most people. It is odd and extreme. Although such thinking may result from an overt mental disorder, it may also be a manifestation of an eccentric and deviant personality. For instance, the Canadian killer Marc Lepine saw women as the source of all his troubles and wrote that "feminists have always had a talent for enraging me." Low self-esteem and blaming others for one's problems dominate the thoughts of many persons who commit workplace violence. This is deviant thinking, no less so than the thoughts of the white supremacist who killed a plastic surgeon for creating "ersatz Aryans," or Gian Luigi Ferri's invectives against the Food and Drug Administration concerning the food additive MSG. Such individuals often have an arsenal of weapons stashed at home, for defense against the dangers they perceive based on their crank conspiratorial theories.

5. Distant

With a few rare exceptions, workplace killers are loners. Their lack of meaningful contact with other human beings is almost always a symptom of underlying mental and emotional difficulties. Moreover, the scarcity of human contact removes from these loners a potentially critical brake on their aberrant thinking and behavior. People who are regularly in touch with others are more likely to check their thoughts and perceptions with them and to use the feedback to keep themselves within the bounds of normality. Those who are out of touch with people are more likely to become even further out of touch.

6. Dangerous

Like rattlesnakes, people who commit workplace violence usually give warning: they communicate their threats, either overtly or covertly. They do so regularly, over time, escalating the warnings to the point that when the carnage erupts, few who knew them are surprised by it. Potential workplace killers often are fascinated by firearms. Many of them have had military training, or own firearms and are known to be proficient in their use. Some have a history of prior violence that is contained in their criminal or military records. Thomas McIlvane, who killed four fellow postal workers, had been thrown out of the Marine Corps for running over a fellow Marine's car with a tank. The best predictor of future violence is past violence.

7. Disrupted Relationships

Most workplace killers are alienated from their families. Many are divorced. Few have any meaningful relationships. The smoldering rage and hatred resulting from wrecked marital and familial relations can erupt into violence in another arena: the workplace. James Edward Pough's wife walked out of their marriage a few months before his car was repossessed by General Motors Acceptance Corporation. He later went on a rampage against the offices of the financing agency, murdering eight employees and a patron.

8. Dyscontrol

Temper tantrums, violent outbursts, and run-ins with the law are commonly found in the background of some perpetrators of workplace violence. The ex-Marine McIlvane had been disciplined for fighting with postal patrons and for cursing out a supervisor. In such men, the ability to control their violent outbursts is clearly deficient. They seek to resolve conflicts through actions, not through words. And neurological disorders or brain injuries can loosen whatever control they do have. The beginning of loss of control may be signaled by the perpetrator who speaks louder than usual, is easily startled, and becomes increasingly impatient and irritable.

9. Drugs and Alcohol

The use and abuse of drugs and alcohol are well known disinhibitors of violent impulses. Like brain injuries or neurological disorders, they loosen control over violent propensities that the individual may have, leading to outbursts of uncontrollable behavior. Generally, too, people who abuse such substances are found to have underlying personality disorders. Individuals with borderline and antisocial personalities are capable of committing violent acts, and are rendered more so by using drugs and alcohol. Postal worker John Taylor's alcohol consumption was known to have increased before his rampage. It likely fueled his unfounded suspicions that he was going to be set up and made to appear as though he was unlawfully accepting money on his mail route.

A small subset of workplace killings are unplanned. Some individuals, intoxicated on drugs, commit murders outside of work and then go to the workplace and kill again. Ramon Salcido stayed out much of one night drinking and taking drugs. Early the next morning, he took his daughters, ages 1, 2, and 4, to a county dump and cut their throats. Somehow, the youngest child survived. Salcido then drove to his in-laws' house, where he killed his mother-in-law and her two children. He returned home and killed his wife. Salcido then drove to the winery in Sonoma, California, where he worked. There he killed one employee and wounded another.

10. Down and Out

Employees who turn violent in the workplace are at the end of their emotional, personal, and financial ropes. Consumed with rage, they feel they have nothing to lose by going on a rampage. They see this as a final opportunity to turn the tables on coworkers and superiors who had once appeared to them invulnerable and to force these tormentors to experience vulnerability. Most workplace killers are in their thirties or forties and have failed to meet their occupational goals. Also, over the course of their working years they have accumulated personal and job setbacks to the point that they feel they are at a dead end. Joseph Wesbecker, described in the next section, fit this description. It takes time, augmented by bad experiences, to make a workplace killer.

Three Life and Death Histories

In the backgrounds of Gian Luigi Ferri, Joseph Wesbecker, and Patrick Henry Sherrill, many of the behavioral aspects of the workplace killer listed in Table 6–1 can be observed.

When Ferri's carnage at Pettit and Martin was over, his ex-wife could not believe that her former husband could have been the perpetrator because "the man I married hated violence." Nor could one of Ferri's former assistants at his failed mortgage company, who said, "You don't expect that from someone you know, no matter how lonely and sad and miserable he is."

Ferri immigrated to the United States in 1964. He studied biology and psychology at the University of California at Santa Cruz, from which he received a bachelor's degree. Thereafter, he worked as a mental health counselor for the Marin County Department of Health and Human Services. He married and divorced quickly. After his divorce, Ferri did volunteer work for the televangelist Reverend Terry Cole-Whittaker, a former Mrs. California. He adopted her slogan, "Prosperity, Your Divine Right," but prosperity did not shine on him. He was involved in a failed Midwestern trailer park venture and got legal counsel from Pettit and Martin. Not satisfied with their work, he eventually turned to another law firm and won a million-dollar settlement.

Ferri tried other ventures, all of which went under. He slid into financial decline. At work in his own firm, he displayed an explosive temper. His former assistant later noted that Ferri did not know such basic things as the procedure for verifying bank deposits. Ferri found himself unable to pay the rent on his one-bedroom apartment, where he lived alone. He received a notice that gave him 2 weeks to pay the money he owed or be evicted.

Although he had won a million dollars in his lawsuit, Ferri continued to harbor resentment against the legal system. It was that resentment that he focused on Pettit and Martin. When his rampage was over, a four-page letter was found on his body. Part of it said, "I spent the last 13 years trying to find legal recourse and to get back on my feet, only to find a wall of silence and corruption from the legal community." He also blamed the food additive MSG for having nearly killed him on three occasions. Later, a videotape was found that showed him, weeks before the carnage, taking target practice in the Mojave desert.

Joseph Wesbecker, unlike Ferri, had been previously known as a violent person. When the emotionally disabled employee showed up unexpectedly at the Standard Gravure Corporation in Louisville, Kentucky, his recent history of violent tendencies and mental disturbances was well known to management. For the past 13 months he had been considered disabled and was on disability pay at 60% of his annual salary.

Wesbecker had begun working for Standard Gravure 20 years earlier. In the company, which prints Sunday supplements and inserts for newspapers, he had been very well liked by coworkers. However, his "nice-guy" image had begun to change with the onset of emotional problems and a divorce. Coworkers became worried when he began to read *Soldier of Fortune* magazine and when he let them know he had ordered through the mail an Uzi semiautomatic weapon.

Wesbecker went to management and requested a less demanding position because of his mental and emotional troubles. He became very agitated because he had been assigned to work on equipment that caused him extreme stress. Wesbecker believed that fumes from a chemical used in the printing plant were causing his physical ailments. A doctor's report supported the request, and although Standard Gravure rejected it, the company did put him on disability. Wesbecker felt that the employer had inflicted a gross injustice upon him, considering his long years of service. Coworkers noted that his emotional problems seemed to get worse after that happened. Wesbecker clashed with management and openly complained to his union and to coworkers that he was being treated unfairly. Union officials learned from him that he was bitter toward the owner and CEO of Standard Gravure, as well as toward certain supervisors in the pressroom. He was worried that his disability benefits would end and that he would be left with nothing.

Wesbecker tried to commit suicide three times, and was, in the opinion of coworkers, becoming more paranoid each day. He was taking the antidepressant medication Prozac (fluoxetine). During the year he was on disability, Wesbecker made threats that he would get even with Standard Gravure. So it was no surprise to some coworkers when one morning he entered the plant carrying an AK-47 semiautomatic assault rifle, two MAC 11 semiautomatic pistols, a 9-mm semiautomatic pistol, and a .38-caliber revolver with assorted ammunition and began shooting. Within a few minutes, he had killed 8 people, wounded 14 others, and taken his own life. In the lawsuit that followed, a jury found that Prozac did not cause the violence.

Patrick Henry Sherrill was a 44-year-old part-time mailman in Edmond, Oklahoma. He had held his job for only 16 months, and during that time he had been suspended twice, once for failing to deliver mail and being rude to patrons, and a second time for spraying a dog with Mace. Coworkers thought him a total incompetent, unable to even find the local Wal-Mart. In fact, he was a strange and lonely man. He had no personal ties. He had never married. After his mother died, he had lived practically as a recluse in her house. As though to underscore his solitariness, he rode around Edmond, alone, on a bicycle built for two. He was viewed by coworkers as a very angry, surly person, whose best mood still revealed a dark sullenness. Neighbors reported him to the police for peeking in their windows and for spying on them with a telescope. Later on, a friend from his high school days would recall that Sherrill had confided to him a deep fear of becoming mentally ill, as his father had done in middle age. Sherrill was also overly sensitive about his premature baldness. He had a shooting range in his home. His interests were limited to the military, pornography, and his ham-radio hobby.

An ex-Marine, Sherrill was an expert marksman, with an excellent record as a member of the local National Guard marksmanship team. He boasted of having been in Vietnam, although in actuality he had never left Camp Lejeune, North Carolina during his tour of duty. He had received an honorable discharge from the Marines. Sherrill spent the next 20 years drifting from job to job, never spending more than 9 or 10 months at any of them, before being hired at the Edmond post office. At home he kept military uniforms, marksmanship medals, *Soldier of Fortune* magazines, and a pamphlet entitled, "Dying: The Greatest Adventure of My Life—A Family Doctor Tells His Story."

On the day that Sherrill was rebuked at the post office for poor performance, he left in a rage. The next morning at 6:30 A.M., he clocked in, then drew out of his mailbag two .45-caliber automatic pistols and 100 rounds of ammunition that he had signed out from the National Guard's armory. Within 15 minutes, he had shot to death 14 postal workers and injured 6 others before killing himself.

Workplace Violence: Causes or Triggers?

The availability of sophisticated, rapid-firing guns has been suggested as one major cause of workplace violence because these weapons permit the killing of large numbers of people in a short period of time, as occurred at Columbine and Virginia Tech. However, practiced marksmen such as Gang Lu can kill people as quickly and efficiently with single-shot weapons as George Hennard did with his semiautomatics at Luby's Cafeteria. Forensic psychiatrist Park Elliot Dietz believes that the problem is not guns but movies that "star" guns. His message is that guns do not kill but television and movies do. Mass murderers, he believes, take their inspiration from the mass media. Unlike serial killers, who elaborate their own deviant fantasies and carry them out, mass murderers do not have much imagination. In the instance of workplace killers, life imitates entertainment.

Before going on his rampage, Gang Lu left a typed statement for the media to find and print. It read, in part,

> My favorite movies include *No Way Out, Die Hard, Indiana Jones,* and Clint Eastwood's movies where a single cowboy fights against a group of incorporated bad guys who pick on little guys at their will or cover up each other's ass. I believe in the right of people to own firearms.... Even today, privately owned guns are the only practical way for individuals/minority to protect themselves against the oppression from the evil organizations/majority who actually control the government and legal system. Private guns make every person equal.... They also make it possible for an individual to fight against a conspired/incorporated organization such as Mafia or Dirty University officials.

Violent movies and television programs may contribute to the violence potential of certain children. The reality of murder scenes—the terrible carnage, the awful suffering, the hideous aftermath for survivors and families of victims—is not and cannot be realistically portrayed by the entertainment media. Thus, a vital feedback mechanism to inhibit aggression is absent in dramatizations of violent acts. Individuals particularly at risk of being overly influenced by media representations of violence are those who have been abused physically and psychologically. They have felt helpless, terrorized, and angry as a result of their abuse. By identifying with the perpetrators of violence, they are able to temporarily ease their sense of terrifying vulnerability. They replay such depictions over and over because they have been traumatized. After chronic exposure to violent programs, identification with violent protagonists can become an entrenched defense against their own chronic fears and feelings of helplessness. Because all children must deal in varying degrees with feelings of fear, power-lessness, and dependency, no child is really immune from the adverse influences of violence as portrayed in the media.

More than 2,000 studies of the popular media and violent acts show a correlation, if not an absolute causal linkage, between television violence and aggression. I have no doubt that what we put into our minds strongly influences what comes out. But exclusive focus on popular media as the cause of upsurging violence in America ignores other important factors. Changing parenting styles that permit children to watch violent programs, the great increase in divorce rates that produce more single-parent households, escalating drug and alcohol use, the availability of guns, the collapse of urban communities, child abuse, and domestic violence—to name just a few—are other important contributors to violence.

Stanton E. Samenow, a clinical psychologist and the author of *Inside the Criminal Mind*, holds that television never made a criminal out of anyone. He thinks that emotional violence is rooted in the American tradition of personal liberty and individualism. It is this ethic that gives to a small group of people with deviant worldviews the freedom to violently act out their visions. Samenow cites the observation that these individuals are incapable of recognizing they are the agents of their own problems. They are unable to understand what Shakespeare's Brutus was told in *Julius Caesar*: "The fault, dear Brutus, is not in our stars, but in ourselves, that we are underlings."

Robert K. Ressler, former FBI agent and head of the consulting firm Forensic Behavioral Services, observes that 40 years ago, when people reached their boiling point, they had a nervous breakdown. Today, the aggrieved individual may pick up a weapon and "get even."

On a different scale, I have treated patients who have destroyed multiple relationships because of an inability to tolerate their feelings of self-hate without projecting them onto others. It is very difficult for many of these patients to hold such feelings long enough to be able to examine them in therapy.

Unfortunately, the tendency to direct violence toward others is being facilitated by the availability of firepower capable of carrying out such actions on a mass scale. Roger Depue, former head of the FBI's Behavioral Science Unit, notes that for years many commentators have been telling the public that the problems of individuals are caused by society. This, in effect, produces for certain individuals an excuse and a rationale for attacking society. Some perpetrators are quite open in stating that they want to strike back and to hurt as many people as they can, no matter who those people are. John Douglas, the former Unit Chief of the FBI's Behavioral Science Investigative Support Unit, states that violent individuals, having failed in their lives, take their own lives after a murderous incident (or have others kill them) because they cannot face the likelihood of being convicted and going to jail—of failing again.

Forensic psychiatrist Park Elliot Dietz has learned through interviews that killing does not exorcise the killer's psychological demons. He states that "those who kill out of paranoia are shocked to learn that killing does not relieve their symptoms." He believes wider circulation given to this notion may deter potential copycat killers.

Studies show that individuals who have been laid off, rather than fired, display a six to seven times higher level of violence against others, which is defined as inflicting harm requiring medical attention or producing loss of functioning for one or more days. The same six- to sevenfold increase also shows up in the consumption of alcohol after being laid off. The statistics are about the same for women as for men.

Work, Love, and Hate

Over a century ago, Freud observed that work and love give essential meaning to our lives. Satisfying work provides stability, direction, security, a sense of achievement and self-worth, a feeling of belonging, camaraderie, and, of course, a source of income. Although many people love their work, many others, more accurately, love work, though not necessarily their own jobs. When someone loses a job, it can be a severe blow to the psyche. For most individuals, losing a job is a traumatic event, but one that they eventually accept and resolve by going forward. For a small minority, the loss of a job can be a death sentence.

Some people's entire identity and sense of worth are inextricably tied up with their jobs. The term *workaholic* is often used to describe people who live to work, rather than work to live. It is such people who are hit hardest by the loss of a job. It becomes a significant failure in life rather than a traumatic but survivable event, one that may be beyond the individual's control. People who live to work can become totally devastated by the loss of their job. They can become psychologically ill, possibly because so much emphasis has been placed on work that relationships and resources that could sustain them through a crisis have not been developed. If there are other negative factors operating in their lives—divorce, financial difficulties, health problems, the lack of personal support, or failures in other venues—the loss of a job combined with other setbacks can further destabilize them mentally.

Particularly if the loss of the job is seen as abusive or unfair, some manifestation of rage, embitterment, and a desire for revenge may begin to surface in the individual. When companies treat their employees as disposable machine parts, this attitude may contribute to a discharged worker's feelings of bitterness. Automation itself, which replaces human beings with machines, also engenders feelings of worthlessness in people who are displaced. These factors combined with corporate downsizing, increased stress at work, and the heightened competition for fewer available jobs all promote anger and violence, particularly in susceptible individuals. And among people who have recently been laid off, as we have seen, alcohol and other drugs can lower resistance to acting out violently. In the past, dedicated workers enjoyed job security and the esteem of their employers. These circumstances are rapidly vanishing, and workplace violence may be one unintended result.

For some people, the loss of a job may be a blow that reverberates with some hidden vulnerability rooted in their past. It may trigger an overwhelming rage that seems out of proportion to the immediate loss they have experienced. Such persons look into the abyss and consider violence. "I'll show you that you can't do this to me and get away with it," they think; they conceive violence as a way of restoring their self-esteem. As their vengeful, bitter, envious thoughts continue spiraling downward, they may think, "I can make the life of others a failure, and at the same time nullify my pain and failure, by snuffing out their lives. Why should other people go on having what they want and enjoying themselves, when I can't?" They then decide that if they are going to die—and most decide that they will not survive their rampages—they will not die alone. Some killers may kill familiar coworkers for "companionship."

These individuals may also contemplate the notion that after they are done, the media will report what has happened to millions upon millions of people throughout the world. Their name will become a household word for a few minutes. Even a few moments of notoriety are acceptable, so long as their personal psychodrama hits the world stage. They may decide to leave a suicide note so that the world will understand their "just cause." Whereas most people die quietly and unnoticed, perpetrators of workplace violence will leave this world in a blaze of horror, even though killing innocent people is the last, and the most pathetic, refuge of the defeated. And so, psychologically armored, they gather their weapons and go to wreak vengeance on the world and on themselves. In most incidents, these individuals appear to be calmly going about their gruesome task. And although these perpetrators may be in a seeming dissociated mental state, their methodical, calculated, cold-blooded killing spree is usually the result of deliberate, covert planning.

If workplace violence often is a staged suicide using the murders as a prop, there are plenty of disgruntled and disordered employees who commit suicide without killing anyone else. Some work-related suicides do take place on the job, but most—as in police suicides—take place outside the workplace and principally at home, even though the acts are clearly interwoven with the suicide victim's work. Policemen see the unabated dark side of life, often developing psychological disorders such as major depression and posttraumatic stress disorder, which can sometimes prove fatal.

When a troubled worker displaces his or her violence to a non-work setting, that is known as "silent workplace violence." More often than not, this silent violence does not emerge as suicide, but is directed into physical and psychological abuse of the worker's family.

Preventing the Unpredictable: Listening for the Snake's Rattle

In the wake of one of these terrible incidents of workplace violence, people often say that the supervisors should have known it was going to occur because warning signs were clearly present. It is true that there usually are warning signs displayed. As with rattlesnakes, most people who commit workplace violence emit sounds of warning and distress before they strike. But the predictive "signal" for violence is often of low fidelity, and it is further degraded by the background noise of undecipherable motivational and situational factors that lead to garbled messages and error. For example, John Taylor, the mailman who thought he was being "set up," told managers about his fear, but he was not reassured by their denials. Taylor's paranoia was a clear signal that he was in mental trouble, but by itself it was not enough to warn that he was at high risk for violence. He displayed other signals to friends: some knew or suspected that he was drinking more alcohol in the weeks before the event than he had done before. Alcohol abuse is also a warning sign, for excess drinking can spark a mental disorder or be a symptom of a developing mental crisis. There was also a third signal that few knew about: Taylor was having trouble at home with an unemployed 22-year-old stepson. These signals of potential violence were all important; yet none of them, alone or together, including Taylor's growing paranoia, could be said to have predicted the killings, even in hindsight. It is likely, though, that psychiatric examination of Taylor before the incident might have provided an opportunity for intervention and treatment, thereby possibly preventing the outbreak of violence.

The following are some guidelines for the prevention of workplace violence by employees or former employees:

- Conduct an initial screening of job applicants to exclude violent or seriously dysfunctional people. Those who are potentially violent usually have prior histories of making threats or acting in a violent manner.
- Foster a supportive work environment.
- Make conflict resolution possible by promoting team-building and negotiation skills.
- Post a clear, written policy against sexual or any other form of harassment.
- Provide fair and reasonable grievance and review procedures.
- Both management and other employees should identify, as early as possible, those persons who may be at risk for violence. Most potential perpetrators make threats before they explode. Every such threat must be taken seriously and must be seen as a reason for intervention. Part of the process must be to allow the person making the threats to fully ventilate his or her feelings to a mental health professional. That professional must be willing to listen in a non-judgmental way to the person's *full* story in order to effectively diffuse potential violence.
- Provide effective and appropriate intervention-prevention programs, consisting of many factors including evaluation and treatment support.

- Establish a workplace violence aftermath debriefing program for all employees and their families within 12 hours of an incident. Provide aftercare for employees who have been psychologically traumatized by workplace violence.
- Identify and assess workplace stressors with measures to reduce employee job stress.
- Identify abusive managers with written policies for counseling, discipline, transfer, or termination.
- Educate employees to recognize violent tendencies in themselves and other employees, to seek help, or to report threatening comments and behaviors.
- Create a central office for reporting threatening behaviors.
- Provide appropriate and supportive out-placement programs for former employees.

The clustering of workplace violence in other places throughout the country may follow a mass murder in the workplace. Knowledge that there is a clustering phenomenon can be used as an early prevention alert to heighten security and to institute other preventative measures.

The notion that mental health professionals can predict violence is a myth. Psychiatrists have long known that they cannot predict violence with any great degree of accuracy. The clinical prediction of violence is accurate less than 50% of the time. Simply flipping a coin would increase accuracy to 50-50. One of the reasons that psychiatrists and other mental health professionals have such a low predictive rate is that they overpredict violence out of concern for their patients as well as endangered third parties. They are able to achieve better predictive rates when the base rate of violence in the underlying group is well known; for example, we can make accurate predictions in 25% to 30% of cases in disturbed psychiatric inpatients. Actuarial assessment attempts to predict reasonably accurate risk probabilities of violence for specific populations, for example, the likelihood of new violence by a previously violent offender when considering him or her for parole.

The forensic psychiatrist has an even harder job in conducting assessments of potential violence for the courts, especially because the evaluation must address a person's *dangerousness*—a legal term of art that is very vaguely defined by the courts and has little clinical meaning. The courts want to know if the person in question is going to act violently at some point in the future. Psychiatrists, however, cannot predict dangerousness, although the courts insist that we do so. The United States Supreme Court has held that if jurors must make decisions about dangerousness, certainly psychiatrists are in an even better position to do so. Psychiatrists can assess the risk of violence, as well as manage violence. They can assess the risk of violence based on the evaluation of certain risk factors—for example, those listed in Table 6–2. The assessment of violence risk factors is a here-and-now evaluation. Violence risk assessment is a process, not an event, meaning that a potentially violent person should usually be assessed more than once. That is why the use of the term *imminent* violence is a fiction; it presumes a predictive capacity that does not exist. Mental health professionals cannot reliably predict when or even whether violence will occur. The purpose of clinical violence assessment is to inform treatment and management of the *potentially* violent individual; it is a lot like weather forecasting: pretty good for the moment but not so good for the longer term. And, as with weather forecasts, the assessments of potential violence must be frequently updated to be of value.

In assessing violence risk factors, psychiatrists especially look for the presence of mental disorders. However, the connection between mental disorders and violence is murky. More violent crimes are committed by people who are not identified as mentally ill than by those who have been so diagnosed. So many factors enter into the making of a violent episode that credible analysis of predisposing factors is a daunting, if not inherently impossible, task. The most reliable risk factor for future violence is past violence. Threats made against specific individuals are another serious risk factor. The combination of a history of past violence and present threats is an ominous sign that heightens the risk of violence dramatically. Coworkers who after a violent event say that people should have seen it coming because of previously uttered threats could actually help prevent some of this violence. Management and workers need to learn how to identify such expressed warnings and take action to diffuse the potential for violence.

Threats must be taken seriously. However, forcefully confronting the disgruntled employee may increase his or her humiliation and rage. Counterthreats can also cause an escalation in the risk of violence. Engaging the employee in a fair and reasonable grievance procedure is often the best way to productively harness and diffuse work-

---

TABLE 6–2.   **Factors to consider in psychiatric assessment of violence risk**

- Specific person threatened[a]
- Past violent acts[a]
- Individual-specific violence risk factors (triggers)
- Motive
- Therapeutic alliance (ongoing patient)
- Other relationships
- Psychiatric diagnosis (major psychiatric disorders and personality disorders)
- Control of anger
- Situational status
- Employment status
- Epidemiological data (age, sex, race, socioeconomic group, marital status, violence base-rates)
- Availability of lethal means
- Available victim
- Violent feelings or impulses, acceptable or unacceptable
- Specific plan
- Childhood abuse (or witnessing spouse abuse)
- Alcohol abuse
- Drug abuse
- Mental competency
- History of impulsive behavior
- Central nervous system disorder
- Low intelligence

---

[a]When a specific person is threatened and past violence has occurred, a high risk rating for violence is achieved.

Source.   Adapted from Simon and Tardiff 2008.

place anger. A referral for evaluation and possible treatment should always be considered because disgruntled employees may have depression or some other psychiatric disorder. Some potentially violent employees may refuse referral to a mental health professional, considering it another insult.

Except when violence is random, it is usually the interactive result of a specific individual and a specific situation. If that trigger situation never occurs, some potentially violent people are able to keep their violence from exploding. Almost everyone can become violent, given the right circumstances. Moreover, the violence may be appropriate if, for example, one's life or the life of another person is threatened. It is clear in retrospect that the repossession of James Pough's red Pontiac Grand Am became a specific trigger for his violence against General Motors Acceptance Corporation, although the deeper psychological meaning that the car had for him will never be known.

Is Your Job A Dead End?

Have you or your coworkers ever given any thought to what you can do to assess the risk of a potentially dead-end job? If the evidence mounts that you are heading for emotional trouble, will you seek help? Do you know where to go to get it? Have you ever considered violence as a possible (though illusory) solution to problems, as some of the workers who "went postal" said they had? Equally important, are you able to identify and to help coworkers who seem dangerously distressed and headed for violence? Or will you do as most people have done, deny and ignore plain signals of trouble that are invariably present before violence breaks out? Violence in the workplace is everyone's concern. The prevention of violence begins with the worker's recognition that his or her place of employment can be a dangerous place and that he or she, in concert with enlightened management, must take prudent precautions.

7

Multiple Personality and Crime

A Real Whodunit

Though a good deal is too strange to be believed,
nothing is too strange to have happened.

— *Thomas Hardy*

An unusual witness took the stand at a rape trial in Oshkosh, Wisconsin. A 27-year-old woman testified that Sarah was "the name of the body" she inhabited. It was also the given name of the rape victim. Sarah had no memory of having met the man on trial for raping her, 29-year-old grocery bagger Mark Peterson, but testified that she had been told about the rape by her other 6 personalities and 15 personality fragments who also inhabited her body. They said it was the naïve and fun-loving Jennifer who had had sex with Peterson. He had violated "the body."

Wisconsin law states that it is a crime for anyone to have sexual intercourse with a mentally ill person, if that person does not understand the consequences of his or her conduct and if the accused knows of the impaired mental condition. At the trial, Peterson maintained that sex with Sarah had been consensual and that therefore no rape had taken place.

Sarah had been diagnosed with multiple personality disorder (MPD). She testified that when another personality takes over, she has no control of what happens. However, she had learned in psychotherapy how to call up and speak with some of the other personalities. The prosecutor asked Sarah to summon them, one at a time. She bowed her head. Her eyes closed. Within a few seconds, her facial expression and voice changed. Moments later, the judge swore in another personality, "Franny."

The maternal one who takes care of the child personalities, Franny testified that she had been sitting with friends in the park when approached by Peterson, who asked her out. Two days later, Franny "bumped Sarah to a dark place" and accompanied Peterson to a local cafe, where she told him about the other personalities. On the way, Peterson asked Franny if he could speak with the naïve 20-year-old, "Jennifer," who loves dancing to rock and roll.

At the trial, the prosecutor requested that Jennifer take Franny's place on the stand. Once again the eyes closed, and a few moments later Jennifer appeared and waved to the jury. She, too, was sworn in. Jennifer testified in a high-pitched voice that Peterson had driven her to a park and "poked a hole in me with this thing.... I put my arms around him and said it was nice. Mark [then] said, 'Time to pull out. I don't want you pregnant.'" The prosecutor asked Jennifer if she knew what "pregnant" meant. She replied, "Yes. A guy puts his finger on your belly button, and a baby comes out."

"Emily" was summoned. The 6-year-old personality testified that she was "peeking" and saw Peterson "wiggling his butt" as he lay on top of Jennifer. Leslie, a jokester personality, wanted to tell the court a joke but suppressed the urge when reminded of the seriousness of the proceedings. Leslie—also sworn in separately, as Emily had been— told the court that she had found semen in Jennifer's shorts later on during the morning after the sexual intercourse.

Franny, recalled to the stand, described how she had become angry when Emily and Jennifer had told her what had occurred: "I trusted that man, and he did harm to the body," Franny said. When they told Sarah, she had begun to shake.

Further testimony came from Sarah's downstairs neighbors, a couple who had been with her on the day that the Franny personality had met Mark Peterson. The couple had explained to Peterson that Franny's real name was Sarah and that Sarah suffered from a mental illness. Peterson had nonetheless asked her out to dinner, and when she declined, he had obtained her phone number by other means. Two days later, at an early hour in the morning, Peterson had shown up at

Franny's door and asked her out for coffee. She had accepted. At that point, the husband of the neighbor couple had again reminded Peterson of Sarah's vulnerability and her mental illness. Mark and Sarah went off for coffee and all that followed.

The neighbor also testified that he had been present when Sarah was being told by Franny and Emily about the sexual intercourse with Peterson. It was after this that Sarah had become outraged and reported the incident to the police, who had taken her to the hospital, where she was examined for signs of rape. After deliberation, the jury found Mark Peterson guilty of second-degree sexual assault. Jurors disagreed as to whether the woman had MPD. However, in the police report signed by Mr. Peterson, his admission that he knew of other personalities led to his conviction. On appeal, a circuit judge ordered a new trial. The district attorney decided not to put the woman through a second trial that could cause her condition to deteriorate.

Multiple Personality Disorder: A Primer

People with classic MPD generally have two or more fully developed personalities, although sometimes they may have only one completely developed personality and other fragments or personality states. These personalities each contain unique memories, patterns of behavior, and ways of relating to other people. Some of the various personalities may not know of the others' existence. Very few people with MPD have only two personalities. Most have between 6 and 12. In recently reported cases, about half have more than 10 personalities. A few have 50 to 100. Doubtful claims of hundreds, even more than a thousand alternate personalities have been made by some persons.

The transition from one personality to another is spontaneous. Usually it takes place within a few seconds, as with Sarah, but it can happen gradually, over hours or days. Staring, rapid blinking, and changes in the patient's usual facial appearance may accompany the transition. Stress or psychologically meaningful cues in the environment often trigger the switching of personalities. Transitions also occur when conflicts break out between personalities or in response to a plan previously agreed to by the various personalities. Hypnosis or drug-assisted interviews can facilitate personality switching.

When MPD patients seek help, the personality that presents for treatment usually has little or no knowledge of the others. The various personalities may be friends, companions, or enemies. They may be aware of each other, or not. Whatever the style, only one personality at a time interacts with the outside world, though others may be listening in and possibly influencing what is happening. Six-year-old Emily, for example, testified that she had been "peeking" as Sarah was raped. Each personality may report being of a different age, race, gender, or from a different family than the others, and behave according to those differences. Emily, clearly a 6-year-old, had the sexual awareness of a young child, not that of the adult in whose body she was housed.

Some MPD patients may recognize that they have lost periods of time, develop amnesia about these times, or are subject to confusion for brief or even extended periods. These patients typically report awakening in strange places. Someone whom they met as one personality may hail them as a friend when another personality is in charge. The latter will be baffled by someone who seems to be a complete stranger. Some personalities who are unaware of losing time subconsciously fill in amnesic gaps with fabricated memories (*confabulation*), or have access to the memories of the other personalities, which they report as if these were their own. If asked about the memory lapses, some MPD patients will admit them, but very few will openly volunteer such information, fearful of being viewed as "crazy" or of being called a liar.

Individual personalities of MPD patients may be quite different from each other in behavior, beliefs, styles of problem solving, and responses to perceived or real attacks. A quiet, "old maid" personality may alternate with a promiscuous, loud, brassy, bar-hopping, devil-may-care personality. A childlike personality may flee in terror from an attacker, whereas another personality might passively submit to the same attacker, or a third might launch a vicious counterattack. One of my male MPD patients with a dozen personalities found eight different books lying around his house, all being read at one time. The topics varied greatly, from science, weight lifting, cooking, art, comics, cars, and baseball to Zen Buddhism, none of which interested him in the least.

Several of the personalities may function reasonably well in the patient's workplace or in interactions with other people. These "functional" personalities may alternate with others that function poorly or that even appear to have a specific mental disorder. Among the more common disorders represented in these patients are mood disorder, anxiety disorder, and the maladaptive personality traits that indicate personality disorder. When such disordered personalities are present, it is often difficult for the therapist to determine whether each of these is a separate psychiatric disorder or if they are just different facets of one patient's MPD. Sarah, for instance, was receiving medications for severe anxiety and depression, even though some of her personalities were neither anxious nor depressed.

The personalities may be so different that the eyeglass prescription for one may not fit another of the patient's personalities, probably reflecting different stress levels. Similarly, the different personalities in one body may have different responses to the same medication, different brain wave patterns, IQ scores, and handwriting. Distinct differences also exist in preferences for foods, friends, types of entertainment, and other interests.

The personalities are sometimes aware of one another and may talk with one another. Sarah had heard voices "babbling" in her head since she had been 4 years old. Other MPD patients wake up at night and hear multiple-party conversations going on inside their heads. Usually, if someone reports conversations with dissociated parts of themselves, these may be taken as indicators of a psychotic state. Not so for MPD patients. They are not considered to be psychotic. Their dissociated experiences are different from the delusional and hallucinatory experiences reported by people with other mental disorders, such as schizophrenia. Particularly in forensic settings, reports of dissociated conversations often contribute to the misdiagnosis of MPD patients as malingering psychopaths or schizophrenics. The confusion is made more likely because many of the behaviors observed or reported seem psychotic or seem to be evidence of severe lying: amnesia, the use of different names, reports of finding surprising things in one's possession, self-mutilation, and suicide attempts. These behaviors make more sense when seen as part of an MPD patient's illness but are often mistaken as symptoms of other disorders.

Most of the personalities are given distinct proper names, usually different from the person's first name and often from the last name as well. The name is usually announced to the person the first time the personality "comes out" and may reflect the kind of abuse that the personality has experienced, or the sort of function it performs. "Floozie" may be the name given to a disavowed immoral, sexual personality, whereas "Abigail" may denote a morally strict, priggish personality. Some personalities do not have a proper name and are called strictly by their function: "protector," "organizer," or "executioner."

Personalities are organized by the function they serve for the person. There are usually two camps: protective personalities and destructive personalities. When the destructive personalities take control, they may engage in self-mutilation, attempt to complete (or actually succeed in completing) suicide, abuse children, or commit assault, rape, or even murder. Destructive personalities harbor anger, guilt, and hatred that they direct at the host personality. "Ginger," one of Sarah's personalities, was an alcoholic who drank and drove, an activity surely intent on "harming the body." Sarah's male personality, known as "Shadow," took on the pain of her childhood and was rageful and violent. At times, he lacerated Sarah's arms by crashing them through windows. "Patty" and "Justin," also destructive personalities of Sarah's, would put out cigarettes in her hands. For most of us, our minds are occupied by one person. As much empathy as we can muster for another person, we cannot experience his or her feelings. But MPD patients feel like they are experiencing someone else's feelings when in contact with an alternate personality. It would be very disconcerting to have a number of persons inhabiting our minds as do MPD patients—particularly persons who hate us.

It is when destructive personalities erupt into the real world that persons with MPD may commit violent crimes. More women than men have MPD, but incarcerated males have a higher incidence of MPD than is generally reported in the psychiatric literature. Males with MPD appear to be at a greater risk for external violence than do females with MPD.

The murderous rage and hatred that is often manifested by the destructive personalities is directly traceable to the extraordinary physical and sexual abuse that most people with MPD have experienced in their childhoods. Some of the destructive alternate personalities repeat the hatred, assault, and rape that the MPD patient experienced in childhood. Often, the heinous crimes they commit are directly reflective of the abuse they themselves once received. The protector personalities are also formed in reaction to this child abuse. They protect the host by encapsulating painful memories and thereby permit the host personality to function in society.

In fact, many MPD patients are quite functional, hold down responsible jobs, maintain stable relationships, and find some enjoyment in life. But, all too often, the more disturbed among MPD patients live in chaos, the result of various alternative personalities, many of them destructive, taking over the host personality and plunging it into disaster characterized by frequent hospitalizations, attempted suicides, and, rarely, terrifying crimes.

Sowing the Winds of Child Abuse

In 97% of cases of MPD, psychiatrists have found that the patients experienced severe child abuse before they had reached age 6 or 7. Usually after the age of 7, children develop psychological means of managing traumatic experiences other than by dissociation.

Before going into the specifics of the MPD sufferer's abuse, I want to stress the magnitude and seriousness of the problem of child abuse in general. In the United States and elsewhere in the world, the staggering statistics of child abuse are exposing the darkest side of humankind. In 2005, 3.3 million referrals alleging 6 million cases of child maltreatment were reported to child protective services agencies. Neglect was the most common form of child maltreatment. Of the 6 million cases, 63% were classified as neglect; 17% physical abuse; 9% sexual abuse; and 7% emotional maltreatment. Because of the underreporting of child abuse, the actual number of child maltreatment cases is much higher.

This rate reflects only the reported cases; many more instances of child abuse go unreported. Some experts believe that the actual rate of abuse is at least twice as high and that 3 million cases annually represents only the tip of the iceberg. For example, 10% to 15% of all "childhood accident" cases treated in emergency rooms are actually the direct result of physical abuse. Although estimates vary, in 1993 the National Committee for Prevention of Child Abuse reported 1,299 confirmed child deaths from mistreatment that ran the gamut from neglect to physical injury and sexual abuse. Some experts put the actual death toll at 5,000 a year. These fatalities result from the following causes: abuse, 55%; neglect, 40%; and both, 5%. Much violence is curtailed by societal restraints. However, when the front door closes at home, violence may break out within the family. For many abused children, home is the most dangerous place to be. Children may unwittingly precipitate violence by just being children, or they may stir up latent problems and violence in the parents. Often the messenger is harmed.

The country has been slow to awaken to the horrors of child abuse. However, the death of 6-year-old Lisa Steinberg at the hands of her adoptive parents became indelibly etched in the minds of Americans. As millions of spectators watched on television, Hedda Nussbaum accused her common-law husband, disbarred lawyer and cocaine addict Joel Steinberg, of striking Lisa with fatal blows. Pounded into unconsciousness, Lisa was left lying on the floor of the couple's middle-class, Greenwich Village apartment for 12 hours. While Steinberg went out to dinner, she remained unconscious, with water and undigested food from a recent meal oozing out of the side of her mouth. Nussbaum was unable to find the psychological strength to do anything about the situation. When Steinberg returned, Nussbaum informed him that Lisa could not be revived. Steinberg insisted that he and Hedda freebase cocaine before calling for help. Steinberg reportedly tortured Lisa and Hedda Nussbaum for years. In court, Steinberg received a sentence of 8 to 25 years for manslaughter. The charges against Nussbaum were dropped as the result of a successful battered-woman syndrome defense. Steinberg was released in June 2004 after serving 17 years of his sentence.

Then there was Susan Smith, who drowned her children by strapping them into safety seats in her car and driving it into a lake. She first received national attention by reporting that a passing carjacker had abducted the children. Smith went on television, tearfully begged for the return of the children. She showed home videos of them and herself, looking for all the world like a devoted mother gamboling on the floor with her two happy toddlers. Friends described her as a loving mother. Later, she confessed to killing the children. She let it be known that because she was severely depressed she had intended to kill herself along with them, but at the last minute had changed her mind and let the children go alone to their watery deaths. She received a life sentence for the murder of her two sons. During the trial, the dark underside of a small southern town was exposed—the lies, the adultery, the incest, and the human failures.

There is little in the psychiatric literature or in the experience of most forensic psychiatrists to indicate that mothers kill their children in a cold-hearted, calculating manner. Most often, the killings are formed in a state of fear, panic, dissociation, depression, or psychosis. Susan Smith was sexually abused as an adolescent, but it is unlikely that she would have developed MPD at that age. Instead, she had a history of deep depression and had attempted suicide twice as a teenager. No psychiatric diagnosis can explain everything about this unfathomable human tragedy. Perhaps F. Scott Fitzgerald came closest to the truth about such situations in *The Crack-Up*: "In a real dark night of the soul, it is always three o'clock in the morning." Every parent, except for the few saints among us, has now and then caught a terrifying glimpse of that darkness.

Incestuous abuse accounts for a large proportion of all child abuse. Its true dimensions are unknown, but by extrapolating from a 1986 landmark study—itself skewed toward underreporting—an estimated 60,000 per million, or 6%, of women in the United States may have been abused by close blood relatives (including stepparents) before they reached the age of 18. In 75% of cases, the incest abuse victim is a daughter and the perpetrator is her father. Therefore, as many as 45,000 per million women may have been incestuously exploited by their own fathers.

Male incest survivors have been underestimated, and, until recently, their plight has been denied and ignored. One such survivor was Dr. Richard Berendzen, who made national headlines when he resigned as president of American University in Washington, D.C., after having been caught making bizarre, obscene phone calls to women about having sex with children. His own sexual abuse at the hands of his mother was later described in his book, *Come Here: A Man Overcomes the Tragic Aftermath of Childhood Sexual Abuse*. At least 20% of sexual abuse against boys is directly perpetrated by women. It has been estimated that approximately 5% of women are pedophiles; that is, they have sexual desires directed toward children. Other perpetrators include babysitters, mentally disturbed mothers, mothers who enable men to abuse their sons, teachers, mentors, neighbors, and family friends.

Almost all parents at one time or another experience angry or violent feelings toward their children, but most do not act them out in an abusive manner. Similarly, some parents experience sexual feelings toward their children. Many do not act them out. Others do. Child abuse, more than any other destructive act, reflects the theme and title of this book: that bad men (and women) do what good men (and women) only (occasionally) dream.

Reaping the Whirlwind of Child Abuse

Children of abuse become future abusers. This does not occur in every instance, of course, because there are many who are determined never to repeat the abuse of their own childhoods. Surprisingly, studies show that 70% to 90% of abused children do not abuse their children as parents. But the fact is that the vast majority of abusers were themselves abused as children. What is it that perpetuates the cycle of abuse? Abused children model their behavior after that of the abusing parent by means of a psychological mechanism called *identification with the aggressor*. By becoming like the abusing parent, the child seeks to transform his or her helpless and terrifying dependency on an unloving parent or caretaker into power over others who take on the dreaded position of victim. This process of identification is facilitated by the child's perception that he or she is blameworthy and that the parent is always right. Many abused children internalize the identification with the abusing parent and direct it at themselves. This often results in physical complaints (somatization), depression, self-mutilation, or destructive lifestyles. One of my patients who had been severely abused as a 9-year-old child did not develop MPD, but later blamed himself for everything that went wrong with his life—an orgy of negative omnipotence. Instead of feeling anger at others when it was clearly appropriate to do so, he turned the anger on himself, flagellating himself, as it were, with merciless blame. Although he was aware of his persecutory side, he was unaware of carrying around within himself the abusive parent. Long-term psychotherapy enabled him to gain control of his self-inflicted abuse.

The wind is sown with abuse of children, and the whirlwind is reaped when those former children abuse the next generation. The cycle of sowing and reaping the child abuse whirlwind seems endless and full of despair. For the abused child, the consequences can be enormous, depending on the type, severity, and frequency of abuse. These consequences affect every important aspect of a person's life—physical health, psychological health, and basic life choices of career, marriage, and lifestyle. Childhood abuse and neglect increase the likelihood of that person's arrest as a juvenile by 53%, as an adult by 38%, and for a violent crime by 38%. As adults, females tend to remain victims of abuse, whereas males tend to become abusers. The ability to make proper, adaptive life decisions and to sustain careers, good personal relationships, and stability in the community can all be severely damaged by child abuse.

The human condition gives rise to fundamental fears in us, such as helplessness, loss, physical-mental deterioration, and extinction. Although individuals may vary widely in their perceptions of and reactions to these existential fears, and although the hurly-burly of our lives may distract our attention from them for a while, these fears are inevitable. In children who have been psychologically, sexually, or physically traumatized at a time in their lives when they are most vulnerable, these primal fears become greatly heightened. For many abused people, whether in childhood or after they become adults, their life contains little pleasure and even less joy. In attempts to master their terror, some of these traumatized children grow into adults who, in turn, victimize other children. Often, they sexualize the abuse in efforts to deny or to rationalize the painful origins of their behavior. W.H. Auden wrote in his poem "September 1, 1939,"

> I and the public know
> What all schoolchildren learn,
> Those to whom evil is done
> Do evil in return.

One of the highly psychologically damaging varieties of childhood abuse comes as a consequence of parents or caregivers who alternate between loving and abusing the child. Not all child abusers reject their children. Some child abusers love their children but, because of intense ambivalence, simultaneously hate them. Parents with poor parenting skills who were abused themselves or who become intoxicated with alcohol or drugs may harm children that they otherwise love. Children become totally bewildered by these utterly conflicting behaviors, further fostering the tendency to split off or dissociate the memories of their abuse.

Child abusers deal with the child as though he or she has no individual identity, and exploit the child exclusively for their own gratification. This kind of abuse is referred to as *soul murder*. Soul murder deprives the child of a personal identity and of the ability to experience joy in life. It is characterized by sometimes brutal, sometimes subtle acts of abuse against children that makes them act like whipped dogs—bonding them emotionally to their abuser because they can turn to no one else. The end product of the abuse is a tragic psychic and spiritual annihilation of the child's core self.

Soul murder is the defining kind of child abuse that we find in the background of most people who have MPD. As suggested earlier, 97% of people with MPD were abused during childhood. Of the remaining 3% of MPD patients, some appear to have the innate ability to dissociate, and others present with MPD symptoms after encountering life-threatening experiences such as a near drowning.

In the vast majority of cases, then, MPD develops as a way for people to cope with severe child abuse. When the child cannot assimilate the contradictory images of a loving parent or caretaker and the fact of being sexually or physically abused, the child feels helpless and unable to escape. A bewildering mind warp occurs. A young child tends to view self and others in all-or-nothing, good-and-bad terms. The idea that fair and foul can be mixed together is totally foreign to the mind of a child of 7 or 8. The abused child, overwhelmed with the terror, horror, and pain of the abuse, as well as with the inability to comprehend it, often copes psychologically by leaving the scene of the assault. Children do this by various means. Some MPD patients, for instance, describe autohypnotically focusing on an object or on a stream of light to mentally transport themselves to a favorite peaceful place such as the seashore or a pleasant wooded spot. When they are so transported, another part of the personality is left behind to personally experience the physical and emotional pain of abuse—and, not incidentally, to be the receptacle of the bad memory. Other patients dissociate from the abuse experience by mentally floating to the ceiling or to a corner of the room and watching the abuse from there, as if it were happening to someone else. By such mental mechanisms, the immense physical and psychological pain of abuse is temporarily escaped.

Memories of abuse couple with the intense feeling states of extreme fear, terror, and helplessness. These feelings are split off from consciousness by the psychological mechanism of dissociation. Dissociation can be thought of as a "horizontal" separation, in which the memory and the intense emotional trauma are split from one another. Thus disconnected and defused, like dynamite sticks from their fuses, the traumatic memories and feelings can be stored safely out of awareness, unless an external or internal trigger reconnects and ignites them. Severe psychological trauma may predispose persons to dissociate. By contrast, repression is a "vertical" separation mechanism that banishes unacceptable ideas, fantasies, feelings, impulses, or memories from consciousness, or that keeps in the unconscious dangerous thoughts and feelings that have never been consciously recognized or felt. Psychological conflict is often a precursor of repression. Repressed material is not subject to voluntary recall, although repressed memories may sometimes emerge in disguised form. Suppression, the conscious, temporary setting aside of a painful memory, may be a way-station to permanent, unconscious removal of the memory through repression. All of these *psychological defense mechanisms*, as they are called by therapists, work together to keep painful memories, feelings, and conflicts out of a person's awareness. These active mental defenses must be distinguished from ordinary forgetting. Our minds simply do not retain the day-to-day massive influx of data and information flooding into our brains every second. The vast volume of this influx is dumped. It is simply a myth that our brains record everything that has ever happened to us.

As with a piece of flotsam that is carried down a river, snags on the river bank, and gradually sinks into the mud, childhood memories and associated feelings of abuse become separated—dissociate—and are carried downstream and become buried in the back channels of the mind. It is not until some abuse survivors are in their 30s and 40s, and in therapy for depression, anxiety, or other personality disorders, that they are able to unearth or recall their abuse. For some, like Saul on the road to Damascus, revelation will come in a single blinding moment. In abuse sufferers, a stunning flashback is often triggered by a seemingly innocuous event, as in the following case:

> One lazy summer afternoon, a patient was lying on her living room couch and looking quietly at a picture on the wall. In one corner of the picture, she noticed some shrubbery at the edge of a lake. In a horrifying instant, she recalled having been sexually abused by her father on the farm where they lived. It had happened when she had accompanied her father on a walk through the farm's wooded area. Stunned, she recalled that her father had attempted sexual intercourse with her behind some bushes near the farm's lake. Paralyzed by the flood of terror that accompanied her newly found memory of the abuse, she lay motionless on the couch for hours.

More than the memories themselves, patients are very frightened and are loathe to reexperience the death-gripping terror and paralytic feelings that accompany memories of sexual abuse. If the right combination of thoughts, feelings, or situations is struck, terrifying memories of abuse long forgotten can be unlocked.

Sarah, whose story introduced this chapter, was a victim of extensive child abuse, a fact brought out at the time of the trial of Mark Peterson. Born and orphaned in Seoul, Korea, she was adopted at the age of 8 months by American parents, who raised her in Iowa City, Iowa. At the trial, Sarah testified that she had difficulty remembering her childhood, but that she did recall physical abuse from her father and mental abuse from her mother. Since age 4, she had heard "babbling" voices in her head, and as an adolescent she experienced severe mood swings and amnesia. Often, she felt compelled to place a blanket over her head and to hide in dark places. Her already compromised mental condition worsened at age 21, when she found her adoptive father crushed under a van.

The medications she received for severe anxiety and depression did not seem to help. With her mother, she moved to Oshkosh, Wisconsin, but was unable to keep her jobs as a dishwasher and a bakery sales clerk. Because of her illness, it was determined that she was unable to work, and she began to receive income from Social Security. She moved into her own apartment with her poodle, P.J., and her cat, Monster, though she maintained a friendly relationship with her mother. Sarah's illness was finally identified as MPD. Her rape occurred shortly thereafter.

At her trial, a psychiatric expert on MPD testified to the authenticity of Sarah's mental illness. In many ways, her disorder was typical, the expert noted, with the six main personalities exhibiting a full range of consistent behavior and memories, from the self-destructiveness of Ginger, Shadow, Patty, and Justin, to the protectiveness of Franny.

If her disorder was typical, however, her involvement with the law was atypical. Most often, when MPD cases reach the courts, it is because the destructive personalities of an individual with MPD have caused harm to others by committing assault, rape, or murder. The actual incidence of criminal acts perpetrated by persons with MPD appears to be quite small. Most of the time, the victims harm themselves in various ways.

Multiple Personality Disorder: A Controversial Diagnosis

Although the history of MPD runs parallel to the history of modern psychiatry, the diagnosis of MPD was first officially recognized by the American Psychiatric Association in 1980, as one of a group of stress-induced disorders that also now includes posttraumatic stress disorder, dissociative disorders, and somatization disorders. In the latest version of the official American Psychiatric Association diagnostic manual, the MPD diagnosis has been renamed *dissociative identity disorder*. Except when making a formal diagnosis, most clinicians use MPD as the preferred diagnostic term.

The clinical syndrome of dissociation into multiple personalities has been known about since the nineteenth century, and was noted in the work of Jean-Martin Charcot and Pierre Janet in Europe. In the United States, since the time of Benjamin Rush, the father of American psychiatry, eminent clinicians have had to deal with the complex issues now associated with the diagnosis of MPD. One source estimates that 1% of the U.S. population has some form of MPD. In psychiatric hospitals, the percentage of inpatients with MPD is thought to be about 20%, although MPD is often misdiagnosed as anxiety, depression, or schizophrenia. There are, however, well-qualified, experienced psychiatrists who doubt its existence. In Sarah's case, Dr. Harold Treffert, director of the Fond du Lac County Health Care Center in Wisconsin, testifying as an expert for the prosecution, said that "Multiple personality disorder is a very, very rare condition. Because of TV talk shows, it has become the disease of the month and plea of the year. It's a condition that's fairly easily induced in a very suggestible patient."

Such doubts are also expressed by juries and judges in court cases in which the victim or, more often, the accused claims to have MPD. Disbelievers in the MPD diagnosis maintain that the disorder is a fiction that has been created by zealous, trauma-seeking therapists who play upon the naïveté of suggestible, hysterical patients. On the other hand, proponents of the MPD diagnosis point out that it is a psychiatric entity noted by doctors for hundreds of years, which cannot be suggested to individuals because it is too complex and multifaceted to be induced by mere suggestion. They assert that mental health professionals who doubt the existence of MPD are resistant to recognizing the presence of severe childhood abuse in the backgrounds of MPD patients and the specific kinds of psychological damage that abuse can cause in adulthood.

The key to the controversy may lie in the fact, noted previously in this chapter, that severe childhood abuse or trauma is invariably found in the backgrounds of MPD patients. To some people in psychiatry, the epidemic of child abuse is also a fiction. Dr. Paul R. McHugh, emeritus chairman of the Department of Psychiatry at Johns Hopkins University, is a persistent critic of the plethora of child abuse allegations and the overuse of the MPD diagnosis. His critiques are worth exploring. Dr. McHugh claims that the flood of MPD cases reflects a prevailing social trend based on political hot buttons of the 1980s and 1990s, "particularly those connected with sexual oppression and victimization. Just as an epidemic of bewitchment served to prove the arrival of Satan in Salem, so in our day an epidemic of MPD is used to confirm that a vast number of adults were sexually abused...during their childhood."

Dr. McHugh has used polygraphs and extensive interviews with self-reported victims of child abuse and other informants to disprove allegations of child abuse. Both the symptoms that surfaced in the women of Salem 300 years ago and those today associated with MPD patients, Dr. McHugh argues, are really manifestations of hysteria, but not of a distinct psychiatric disorder. He believes that the symptoms of MPD can be explained by reference to hypnosis because "they are generated in a therapeutic, suggestive way, and they are eliminated in a way that shows their hysterical nature." Dr. McHugh is concerned because so often when a diagnosis of MPD is made, child abuse is then asserted, and soon afterward family members "are being accused of the worst kinds of sexual perversions with little children." To buttress his allegation, he points out that statistics show true abusers to be more commonly stepfathers than biological fathers, which is just the opposite of the patterns of abuse reported by MPD patients.

A second critic of the MPD diagnosis was Dr. Martin Orne. Until his death in 2000, he was a professor of psychiatry at the Institute of the Pennsylvania Hospital and an internationally recognized expert on hypnosis. Dr. Orne believed that the eliciting of childhood memories of sexual abuse in the treatment of MPD patients ruined the lives of people accused of having molested these patients. This ruination took place without any separate validation or evidence to support the allegation of abuse.

On the other hand, proponents of the MPD diagnosis point out that the diagnosis is based on established criteria developed over time by the American Psychiatric Association. Its existence has been discussed by many prominent and highly credible psychiatrists, among them Drs. Richard J. Lowenstein and Richard P. Kluft.

Dr. Lowenstein is medical director of trauma disorders services at Sheppard and Enoch Pratt Hospital in Towson, Maryland. He charges that the original nineteenth-century concept of hysteria was sexist and reflective of a male view of female personalities, and that to call all symptoms hysteria is to fall into an old trap. Furthermore, Lowenstein writes, "there isn't any evidence that the full syndrome of MPD can be created by suggestion." If there is some question about the ways in which childhood abuse is remembered and dissociated, he points out that this, not the existence of MPD, is still the area of ongoing research. He believes that those who oppose the MPD diagnosis and seek to discredit it are doing so to minimize the extent and damage done by child abuse in our society.

Dr. Kluft, clinical professor of psychiatry at Temple University School of Medicine, argues that "a therapist who dismisses the [alternate] personalities as unworthy of attention is avoiding serious scrutiny of much of the patient's mental life. It is a mistake to be preoccupied with alters as entities in themselves...but it is an equally serious error to suppose that engaging the alters reinforces the patient's psychopathology."

My own sense of the truth is that MPD is underdiagnosed, not overdiagnosed. As a psychiatrist, I have treated a number of patients with MPD and have spoken with many colleagues who have themselves seen many MPD cases. But I have also spoken with many colleagues who have never seen a case of MPD and who remain skeptical of its existence. In fact, MPD is hard, not easy, to diagnose accurately, and its existence may only be recognized in a patient years after that patient's treatment has begun. Several reasons can lead to the delay. According to Dr. Kluft, only about 20% of MPD patients spend the main part of their lives in an open MPD state. Another 40% may present signs that suggest MPD to the alert clinician but that may be missed by many therapists. The remaining 40% of patients diagnosed with MPD are so designated only after exploration done in the absence of signs that would strongly suggest it.

Reluctance to diagnose MPD is understandable. After all, the idea that numerous personalities can exist in one individual smacks of demonology and witchcraft. It also challenges the therapist's own sense of wholeness. Although most people are aware that there are many of us inside our heads, as mentally stable people we are able to maintain the unity of personality and memory. The notion that we may have dark, destructive personalities lurking in our minds (but beyond our awareness), and that these personalities could take control of us, is tremendously threatening. In a therapeutic situation, it can even threaten the therapist's equilibrium to listen as a patient's voice changes to that of a little girl and to see the patient then want to sit on the floor and play. It is as if a sudden time warp has occurred when an adult patient is psychologically transformed, before the therapist's very eyes, into a 3-year-old child. A profound sense of the uncanny may grip the therapist. At this point, even a good therapist may wonder if he or she is being conned. A more frightening facial transformation is a change from a normal visage to that typical of a psychopathic murderous personality; visions of Dr. Jekyll and Mr. Hyde dance in one's head. This is unnerving to the clinician. He or she must also realize that the transformation is extraordinarily frightening to the patient as well. In some instances, it can even lead to the patient fleeing the treatment or to an inexperienced clinician abandoning the patient. The clinician must always be aware that the patient is one person; alternate personalities do not exist separately from the patient.

The treatment of MPD is a complex, difficult, often daunting task. However, the results of achieving a reasonably integrated personality in the patient are extremely gratifying, both to patient and therapist alike. Because of the split-off personalities in MPD, the sum of the parts add up to one personality. It is a camp divided. The goal of treatment is to integrate the disparate personality elements. The patient's internal integration of personalities may take the form of a board meeting (with the host personality as chairman), a town meeting, a dictatorship, or some other form of processing internal communications, like a therapy group. Some patients achieve near total integration and oneness with the alternate personalities, a desirable result for both patient and therapist. In fact, a good deal of what happens to MPD patients has that quality of astonishing both the therapist and the patient. To observe the mind's adaptive ability to create various personalities in the effort to cope with overwhelming trauma is an amazing experience. The final creation appears as a brilliant piece of baroque art work, one that leaves both doctor and patient with a profound sense of awe and humility.

Multiple Personality Disorder and the Courts

Controversy among mental health professionals about the very existence of MPD, the fascinating and often dramatic nature of the disorder, the ease with which the disorder can be faked, and the natural disbelief of jurors make MPD a difficult legal defense to pursue in the courts. Nevertheless, in a number of cases, ranging from forgery and drunk driving all the way up to the more heinous crimes of robbery, rape, and murder, MPD has been raised as a legal defense and, on rare occasions, has been used successfully in an insanity defense.

Courts have generally taken the position that the mere presence of MPD does not relieve the patient of responsibility for his or her acts. In each case, a judge or jury must decide whether a person's disease affects his or her ability to stand trial and to assume responsibility for the crime in the eyes of the law.

Lewis and Bard (1991) described four major defenses presented at trial for crimes committed by alternate personalities:

1. The person had no control over the alternate personality committing the crime.
2. The person cannot remember the acts of the alternate personalities, and therefore cannot assist in his or her own defense and is incompetent to stand trial.
3. Because of the MPD, the person could not conform his or her behaviors to the law or tell right from wrong.
4. Like a sleepwalker, the accused person was unconscious of the alternate personality's behavior and thus cannot be held accountable for it.

The most often cited case on judicial theory having to do with MPD is *State v. Grimsley*. In this case, one of Ms. Grimsley's secondary personalities, named Jennifer, was arrested for drunk driving. Ms. Grimsley contended that her primary personality, Robin, "was not conscious of what was happening and lacked voluntary control over Jennifer's actions." The court rejected Jennifer's insanity defense on the grounds that "the evidence fails to establish by a preponderance that Ms. Grimsley's mental disorder so impaired her reason that she, as Robin or as Jennifer or as both, either did not know that her drunken driving was wrong or did not have the ability to refrain from driving while drunk." This argument upheld the long legal tradition in which the law judges a person's criminal liability according to his or her mental state at the time of the act. That is, in *Grimsley*, the court determined that both Robin and Jennifer knew better than to drive while drunk.

Three other cases are also noteworthy because of their judicial reasoning. In *Kirkland v. State*, in which a woman with MPD robbed a bank, the court agreed with the findings in *Grimsley*, echoing that "we will not begin to parcel criminal accountability out among the various inhabitants of the mind."

In *State v. Milligan*, the issue was more complicated. The 26-year-old man was arrested for a series of campus rapes. During pretrial incarceration, his behavior was inconsistent, and his attorneys decided that a psychiatric evaluation was needed. A variety of clinicians agreed that William Milligan had MPD. He was initially found incompetent to stand trial, but later he was deemed restored to competence and the trial proceeded. Further examination revealed that Milligan had committed the rapes while under the control of one of his alternate personalities, who was a lesbian, and that Milligan had not been aware of this alternate personality or of "her" actions. In fact, he was not generally aware of these other personalities, and on the rare occasions when he did become aware of them, he attempted suicide. Milligan was found not guilty by reason of insanity and was transferred to a psychiatric facility. It was determined that the alternate personalities had formed during his childhood to protect Milligan from severe abuse at the hands of his stepfather.

In the last case, *Rodrigues v. Hawaii*, a 23-year-old Marine was charged with three counts of sodomy and one of rape. Rodrigues, who pleaded not guilty by reason of insanity, was examined by five psychiatric experts. Four of them agreed on a diagnosis of MPD. The treating psychiatrist testified that Rodrigues manifested three personalities. "Rod" was his main or host personality. "David" emerged when Rodrigues was 16 and acted as a referee between Rod and the third personality, "Lucifer," who had come into existence when Rodrigues was 3. The treating psychiatrist testified that it was Lucifer who was in charge at the time of the offenses. The psychiatrist further asserted that although Rod and David knew that the sexual acts were wrong, Lucifer did not care if they were right or wrong. Similarly, Rod and David had the capacity to conform their conduct to the law's requirements, but Lucifer did not care about his conduct or about the consequences.

The trial judge granted Rodrigues' motion for acquittal by reason of insanity, but the verdict was reversed by the appellate court, which declared that MPD, by itself, does not automatically equate with insanity. Sanity was an issue for the jury to decide. The Supreme Court of Hawaii then ruled that MPD cannot be regarded in the same fashion as any other insanity defense and that "each personality may or may not be criminally responsible for its acts, [so that] each one must be examined under the...competency test." The court's analysis is reminiscent of Benjamin Franklin's admonition, "We must hang together or assuredly we shall all hang separately."

The Hawaii decision in the Rodrigues case reflects a growing tendency for the courts to view the person with MPD as if he or she were several people, each responsible for his or her own behavior. That is what happened in the case with Sarah (described at the beginning of this chapter): each personality was sworn in separately to testify. Unfortunately, this position, which is increasingly being taken by the courts, has an important drawback: it intrinsically accepts a central symptom of MPD, the disavowal of one's actions—and this can have the result of legally exculpating someone from responsibility for a heinous act.

In a bizarre twist, MPD was used as a defense in a rape case in which the criminal defendant testified that an alternate personality did it. He was charged with breaking into the apartment of a woman he met in group therapy and forcing her to have oral sex and then raping her. The defendant denied the charges, claiming that the sex was consensual between "Spirit," one of 30 personalities that inhabit his body, and "Laura," one of the woman's many personalities. Quoted in court papers, the defendant told investigators that "Spirit loved Laura." As noted earlier, a diagnosis of MPD does not preclude the main personality or any of the alters from being found criminally responsible if, in fact, the individual or any of his or her personalities committed the offense. The legal outcome of this case is unknown.

There is always a powerful incentive to decline responsibility in the litigation context, in which life, death, large sums of money, and personal reputations are at stake. In a treatment situation, a psychiatrist usually accepts an MPD patient's reality: that he or she experiences multiple personalities. Both therapist and patient strive toward integrating these personalities and toward having the patient assume responsibility for the behaviors of all of the personalities. In a litigation situation, however, the patient usually seeks a psychiatrist's assistance not for the purpose of treatment, but rather for help in mitigating punishment or possibly exonerating the patient of unlawful behavior.

The legal situation presents all sorts of difficulties for forensic examiners of an alleged MPD sufferer. For instance, there is the problem of conclusively demonstrating whether the alternate personalities—if they exist—are aware or unaware of one another, have or do not have control over one another, or are able or unable to distinguish right from wrong. Courts ordinarily do not accept amnesia as a defense in criminal cases, and, of course, amnesia is a vital aspect of what happens to a person with MPD. People who suggest for the first time at a trial that they are afflicted with MPD generally have a hard time convincing the court. A person who has been previously diagnosed with MPD can more effectively cite the illness as a defense in court, especially if the person can show that an experienced clinician treated him or her for the disorder before the criminal act occurred, or that a clear connection has existed between the host personality and a long-standing antisocial personality alternate that took control of the host and committed the criminal act. If a psychopathic alternate personality is truly present in a person with MPD, it most likely has appeared in the past and has committed antisocial acts that have been documented.

Multiple Personality Disorder, Hypnosis, and Malingering

Studies show that MPD symptoms can be fabricated. Even the experienced forensic examiner can have difficulty distinguishing faked from true MPD. Particularly in criminal cases, the possibility that MPD is being faked must always be considered. Also, an examiner must keep in mind the possibility that a person may have MPD and also malinger.

Ross Michael Carlson

The issue of possibly malingered MPD was the center of the case of 19-year-old Ross Michael Carlson, who forced his parents out of their car, ordered them to lie face down by the roadside, and then shot them in the head with a .38 Special. In one of the longest and most controversial criminal cases in the history of Colorado, Carlson pleaded insanity on the basis of MPD. His lawyers argued that because of the disorder, Carlson was not really present at the scene of the crime. Carlson alleged that he had no memory of the crime at all; that it was "Black," the protector, one of seven alternate personalities inhabiting

Carlson's body, who pulled the trigger in the execution-style murder of his parents. Carlson never came to trial. Following the murders and his arrest, Carlson spent 6 years of psychiatric hospitalization in a criminal facility before he was found competent to stand trial. However, Carlson died of acute leukemia before the legal proceedings could begin.

Psychiatrist Michael Weissberg served as an expert witness in the case. He examined both Carlson and the evidence. He noted that Carlson had never displayed any prehomicidal alternate personalities. Moreover, there was no evidence to corroborate Carlson's contention that he switched from one personality to another. For instance, his eyes did not roll upward in the movement known as *Spiegel's sign*, which is frequently seen in MPD patients when a personality switch is taking place. But seamless switches of personality do also take place, so the absence of the sign was not incontrovertible proof against MPD. Carlson also did not manifest loss of time, amnesia, or other symptoms associated with MPD. But MPD is hard to prove or disprove: there are no blood tests, X-rays, or other objective ways of discerning it. You cannot see, smell, or touch MPD. These factors are what give rise to the seasoned attorney's contention that MPD is a perfect "boutique" disease for the defense when no other exculpatory possibility is available.

Dr. Weissberg resisted pressure to use hypnosis in examining Carlson. Memories retrieved under hypnosis are more vulnerable to distortion and elaboration than are memories elicited through ordinary conversation. Contrary to the belief of laypersons, hypnosis can distort true memories and create false ones. Dr. Weissberg knew that descriptions of crimes developed under hypnosis are highly questionable. Many courts will not admit hypnotically enhanced memories as evidence. So Dr. Weissberg looked for other clues in Carlson's environment, and found some. He learned that shortly before the murders, Carlson had checked out library books that dealt with MPD. He also learned that Carlson had been born out of wedlock to religious parents. Dr. Weissberg theorized that his parents came to hate Ross as a reminder and projection of their own wickedness. In his book *The First Sin of Ross Michael Carlson*, Dr. Weissberg concluded that Carlson had been faking MPD. He speculates that instead, Carlson was really an emotionless psychopath who acted out the parents' death wish, absolving "his parents of nineteen years of guilt as he meted out their ultimate punishment."

Kenneth Bianchi

One of the most controversial and infamous cases in which MPD was alleged as a defense was that of Kenneth Bianchi, the so-called Hillside Strangler of Los Angeles. Bianchi and his cousin Angelo Buono were accused of raping and murdering at least 10 young women whose nude bodies had been left strewn along hillsides during a 4-month killing spree in 1977–78. Seven psychologists and psychiatrists examined Bianchi. Some offered opinions for a diagnosis of MPD and some against.

Some examiners used suggestive leading questions during the course of their interviews with Bianchi, both with and without hypnosis. Other examiners did not distinguish between their roles as therapists and as forensic experts. In treating a patient, a clinician usually accepts and works with the patient's perceptions of reality rather than attempting to independently verify the patient's story. In evaluating the patient for legal purposes, the clinician considers many information sources in conducting a diagnostic evaluation that can clarify and illuminate such strictly legal issues as competency to stand trial or criminal responsibility for actions.

Testifying for the prosecution, Dr. Martin Orne spoke of observing the lack of a prior history of dissociation, the overly dramatic presentation of Bianchi's alternate personalities, and their inconsistent presentation. Dr. Orne concluded for the court that Bianchi did not have MPD. He argued that Bianchi had been clever enough to defeat hypnosis and had also been able to con other psychiatrists into believing that he was not mentally responsible for the murders. Dr. Orne reminded the court that "contrary to popular assumptions, it is possible for untrained, naïve subjects to simulate deep hypnosis and fool even very experienced hypnotists by behaving in ways they think the hypnotist wants." He recalled for the court having advised Bianchi that real MPD sufferers always have at least three personalities. Up to that point, Bianchi had only claimed one alternate personality, "Steve." Later, on the day that Dr. Orne gave this information to Bianchi, "Billy" emerged—a con artist, a bounder who squirmed out of tight spots by lying. Dr. Orne concluded that Bianchi was sick but he was not legally insane. He diagnosed Bianchi as having "an antisocial personality disorder with sexual sadism," and described him as a man with a "perverted sexual need which allows him to obtain gratification from killing women." Bianchi was convicted and sentenced to prison; he later admitted that he had lied about having MPD.

This case and the others expose a fundamental difference between the litigation and treatment situations that affects the diagnosis of MPD. In litigation, what is sought is an external result—money, guilt or innocence, life or death. In treatment, what is sought is assistance in achieving an internal result, in becoming well. In this latter situation, then, the person presenting with MPD-like symptoms has no reason to fake the disorder. Persons with real MPD usually deny and conceal their symptoms, whatever the context. In fact, many MPD patients dissimulate their symptoms, either consciously or unconsciously, because they fear humiliation, embarrassment, or being thought of as "crazy" by others. Moreover, it is too horrible to recover memories of abuse and face the fact that one could be treated so miserably by parents or caretakers. For a child, it is unbearable to be hated by persons who are supposed to love you.

MPD patients tend to avoid help and to act against their own best interests. So dissimulation or the hiding of MPD symptoms is more common than simulating them, even in the litigation context. For the purposes of the courtroom, the diagnosis of MPD is made significantly more difficult because certain personality alternates mimic others or camouflage themselves behind more palatable others. Sometimes they deviously act together in a conspiracy to hide their own multiple existences, which, of course, renders it more unlikely that the forensic expert will diagnose MPD. In still other cases, the alternate personalities cannot agree on how to dissimulate, and symptoms may erupt that are initially more typical of psychosis than of MPD, such as audible thoughts or voices, or the expressed feeling that the person's body is under the control of outside forces. Such symptoms can naturally lead to a wrong diagnosis.

In the treatment situation, MPD patients receive an average of 3.6 erroneous diagnoses before they obtain the correct diagnosis. It takes, again on average, 6.8 years between the time of their first mental health assessment of symptoms that might be attributable to MPD and the accurate diagnosis of the problem. In the courtroom, there is no luxury of time or leeway for wrong diagnoses. But because the process of correct diagnosis requires time and sufficient latitude for exploration, limitations imposed by litigation may lead to either an erroneous overdiagnosis or an underdiagnosis of MPD among litigants and

criminal defendants. It is known, however, that MPD has a dispropor-
tionately high representation in the forensic population. This situation
is further complicated by those persons available (or unavailable) to
submit corroborating or controverting evidence. Lack of corrobora-
tion of a patient's MPD symptoms, for instance by family members,
may be evidence that MPD does not exist in that patient. But it may
also result from the patient's family having been involved in the childhood abuse that provoked the MPD into existence. Ultimately, the forensic examiner must rely on an intimate knowledge of the clinical pre-
sentations of MPD to make an evaluation for the court.

Hypnosis, the Legal Process, and Multiple Personality Disorder

The medical uses of hypnosis are well established and no longer controversial. Hypnosis (hypnoanalysis) can be used in psychiatric treatment to uncover painful feelings or buried experiences. Dramatic results have also been obtained through hypnosis in the treatment of
allergies, warts, asthma, insomnia, burns, and pain. However, the use
of hypnosis in questioning witnesses to enhance their memories and
thereby solve crimes remains highly controversial. Advocates of the
use of hypnosis in criminal cases point out that the nation's largest
mass kidnapping case was solved in this way. In 1976, in Chowchilla,
California, 26 children were abducted from a school bus and were buried in a pit. Under hypnosis, the bus driver recalled the license number
of the van in which the children were whisked away, and this led to
the solution of the case.

Laypersons, including some policemen, have a common miscon-
ception about hypnosis: they believe that hypnotized people must tell
the truth. This belief is false. Even some people who are deeply hypnotized are capable of resisting suggestions to be truthful and can continue to lie. Others are able to fake being in a hypnotized state, and
their fakery is good enough that it is only detectable through special
tests. In general, memories obtained under hypnosis, even when vivid,
are less reliable than those elicited through normal recall. The reason
for this is complex, but in part has been traced to the fact that the hypnotized individual is highly responsive to suggestions and may therefore translate his or her own beliefs, or even those of the hypnotist,
into pseudo-memories. Studies show that hypnotized persons can

readily accept, with total conviction, suggestions of happenings that contradict their actual experiences.

For this reason, the Council on Scientific Affairs of the American Medical Association (AMA) questions the usefulness of hypnosis to enhance memories in criminal and civil cases. Many state supreme courts have declared that hypnotically induced testimony is inherently unreliable and should not be admitted as evidence in criminal trials. The AMA council affirms that although subjects generally reveal more information under hypnosis, the recollections may contain many inaccurate details. The council has recommended that the use of hypnosis in the judicial process be limited only to the investigative stage. Other groups have pointed out that if the practice is relied on in court to provide validity to the testimony of witnesses, the use of hypnosis can lead to miscarriages of justice. Some forensic experts feel that hypnotic examination may be necessary in criminal cases because of the limited time available to question witnesses. The gain in finding important details, such as the van license number in the Chowchilla incident, must be balanced against the potential loss of credibility that can result when evidence has been obtained through hypnosis.

The people who are more responsive to hypnosis are usually those who are more adept than others at becoming totally absorbed in a fantasy. Approximately 15% of the population are highly hypnotizable, whereas 25% are thought not to be hypnotizable at all. The hypnotic state is merely an altered state of consciousness in which the mind's attention is sharply focused. People are considered to be in a hypnotic state when daydreaming. One common experience in self-hypnosis that most of us have experienced is becoming lost in thought while driving. After many miles, we awaken from reverie and cannot remember the drive. None of us can be hypnotized against our will, nor will we perform acts under hypnosis that we really do not want to carry out.

In the treatment of MPD, hypnosis can summon personality alternates in a way that is controlled and is not frightening. In the context of litigation, however, hypnosis—especially when it involves dealing with suspected personality alternates—is highly problematic. Particularly when leading questions are asked, hypnosis can cue the defendant to produce a false alternative personality for the purpose of avoiding criminal responsibility. Because we distinctly experience various aspects of ourselves, defendants who are in the "highly suggestible" category and are undergoing hypnosis may be able to personify these various aspects as independent personalities. To the untrained eyes of juries, these hypnotically induced personified states seem like MPD alternate personalities, even when they are actually artifacts produced by hypnosis and would not exist if the subject was not under hypnosis.

I do not mean to suggest that the forensic examiner who elicits these personified states through hypnosis does so maliciously. Experts are often fooled when using hypnosis, not realizing the extent to which suggestive questions can stimulate fantasy, distortion, falsification, and sometimes outright fabrication of memories. Clinicians who use hypnosis and then make a false diagnosis of MPD in the litigation context do so because 1) they lack clinical experience with dissociative disorders like MPD, 2) they are unfamiliar with hypnosis and its sometimes false artifacts, 3) their examination has been too brief, 4) they ask leading questions to the hypnotized subject, 5) they have not obtained enough collateral data about the existence or nonexistence of MPD in the subject, or 6) they have confused their own roles of therapist and of forensic examiner.

If hypnotically induced memories are untrustworthy, what about the trustworthiness of those memories that are only recovered and brought to light many years after events have occurred? This is a problem in therapy, and an even more difficult conundrum in the litigation process, because previously buried memories of childhood sexual and physical abuse have been at the center of high-stakes, hotly contested court cases. In all of them, the more general concern is the accuracy of memory—a subject critical to the understanding of child abuse and its long-lasting effects on people, and to the line that separates what bad men do from what good men dream.

8

The Ultimate Betrayal

Sexual Misconduct in the Helping Professions

I swear by Apollo the physician...never do harm to anyone.

—Hippocratic oath

Singer and songwriter Barbara Noël wakened slowly from sleep induced by the sodium amobarbital administered by her psychiatrist, Dr. Jules Masserman, former president of the American Psychiatric Association. Many times before, during the course of her 18 years of office treatments with Dr. Masserman, she had returned from deep sleep, but this time the awakening was shockingly different. A man was over her, and he was breathing deeply. As her consciousness brightened, she could feel his breath on her shoulder. Still under the influence of the amobarbital, she stirred and moaned. The breathing stopped and the man lifted his body carefully away. Fearing that the man might turn violent if he were discovered, Noël pretended to be asleep. Moments later, she opened her eyes a bit and saw a man standing at the sink, with his back to her. He was bald and tanned except for his white buttocks. To her horror, she recognized that it was Dr. Masserman. She could even hear the coins jingling in his pockets as he put on his trousers. Then she heard him walk over to her, pull up her underpants, and then carefully tuck the sheets around her and leave the room, closing the door behind him. She fell back to sleep. Some time later, the lights in the room flipped on and off. This was the customary way that Dr. Masserman had always awakened her from her amobarbital-induced deep sleeps.

In her book *You Must Be Dreaming*, Noël describes this scene and alleges that Dr. Masserman behaved toward her in other ways that were questionable and inappropriate to the doctor-patient relationship. Upon return from his travels, he would bring her coins, trinkets, Bach records, and other gifts. He gave her copies of his articles, poems, and music. He invited her to go sailing on his yacht and to fly in his airplane. Noël says she was uncomfortable but flattered by his attention. She accepted only one of his invitations while she was his patient, and that was to accompany him to Paris. There, as president-elect of the World Congress of Social Psychiatry, he was the host of an evening reception. She acted as his hostess.

Noël had no idea that Dr. Masserman, as president of the American Psychiatric Association, had condemned sexual relationships between psychiatrists and their patients. When she finally understood what had been happening to her, Noël had to overcome the disbelief of detectives, lawyers, and therapists, who dismissed her story as the erotic dream of an unstable woman infatuated with her psychiatrist. She finally managed to find attorneys who would bring suit on her behalf, and when she did, there was a firestorm because of Dr. Masserman's standing and prominence. He had written 16 books and 410 articles, had been president of the American Psychiatric Association and had previously been president of the American Academy of Psychoanalysis, the American Society for Group Therapy, the Illinois Psychiatric Society, the Chicago Psychoanalytic Society, the American Association for Social Psychiatry, and was an Honorary Life President of the World Association for Social Psychiatry.

Dr. Masserman denied all charges of sexual misconduct brought against him by Noël and three other former patients, all of whom described a similar pattern of having been sexually abused while they were under the influence of sodium amobarbital. Noël's attorneys later stated that 10 other women had also come forward with similar allegations against Dr. Masserman but had not wanted to join the suits. They did not want to undergo the further traumas that would be associated with litigation. Barbara Noël thought that her own childhood sexual abuse at the hands of her parents had set her up as a perfect, compliant victim for a powerful authority figure like Dr. Masserman. The four cases were all settled out of court. Noël received a $200,000 settlement. Dr. Masserman voluntarily surrendered his medical license and signed an agreement never to practice therapy in the United States again. He was censured and given 5-year suspensions from such organizations as the Illinois Psychiatric Society and the American Psychiatric Association.

Lozano v. Bean-Bayog

The case of *Lozano v. Bean-Bayog* received sensational, nationwide media coverage. It was alleged by the late Paul Lozano's family, in a malpractice and wrongful death suit, that Harvard psychiatrist Margaret Bean-Bayog had used an unorthodox method of therapy that fostered severe regression. They alleged that Dr. Bean-Bayog's treatment reduced their son—a medical student at Harvard—to the emotional stage of a toddler. The plaintiffs further claimed that she systematically manipulated and sexually abused him to the point that, 10 months after termination of his treatment, Paul Lozano committed suicide.

Unfortunately, the case was tried in the media before it ever got near the courts. Media reports, for instance, described items that had been retrieved from Paul Lozano's Boston apartment. These included children's books such as *Goodnight, Moon*, inscribed in Dr. Bean-Bayog's handwriting to "the baby"; tapes of the therapist instructing Lozano to repeat 10 times, "I'm your Mom, and I love you, and you love me very, very much"; and flash cards made by Dr. Bean-Bayog, one of which referred to missing "the phenomenal sex." The media displayed photographs, taken by Lozano, which showed the therapist snuggling a stuffed bear. Also revealed were a series of letters and stories that the psychiatrist allegedly wrote to Lozano in which fantasies of maternal love and devotion are played out. Dozens of pages of records in Dr. Bean-Bayog's handwriting described her sadomasochistic sexual fantasies in response to Lozano's bombardment of her with hideous fantasies of sexually torturing women. These pages also revealed that Dr. Bean-Bayog had consulted other psychiatrists about her treatment of Lozano.

The psychiatrist had explanations for all of these seemingly damaging items. For instance, she said that the flash cards had been dictated by the patient. She also said that the fantasies in her handwriting were transcriptions of her dreams and had never been intended for the patient to see. She alleged that without her knowledge, he had broken into her office and had stolen them.

Lozano's sister claimed that her brother had said that he and the psychiatrist had had an affair. Dr. Bean-Bayog categorically denied it. She claimed that treatment had been ended after Lozano allegedly refused to follow her recommendations that he be supervised by the Massachusetts Medical Society, which monitors impaired physicians. These services were also available to medical students. Her explanation for his death was that he had felt so rejected and angry after his therapy ended that he had taken revenge on her. She thought he had not committed suicide, but had died of an accidental overdose of cocaine. Dr. Bean-Bayog said that her treatment approach with Lozano had been unconventional but had also been necessary to treat a very disturbed patient with a history of severe childhood abuse. He had required at least 10 hospitalizations for suicide attempts, some before his treatment began with Dr. Bean-Bayog. Without such treatment, she said, the patient could not have functioned at all in the 4 years prior to his death.

From an outsider's point of view, what was most interesting about the pending court case was that the plaintiff and the defendant both cited the same documents in support of their opposing allegations. This was an extraordinary cache of 3,000 pages of documents filed by a lawyer for the Lozano family with the court. The key issue raised by the case was whether the psychiatrist had used an unconventional approach that was justified, given the nature of the patient, or whether she had gone beyond the pale of acceptable forms of care. Investigating the matter, the Massachusetts Board of Registration in Medicine found that there was not sufficient evidence to prove sexual misconduct. However, the board decided that Dr. Bean-Bayog's treatment "did not conform to accepted standards of medical practice," and that her failure "to terminate or otherwise address" her sexual fantasies that had been evoked in the treatment of Lozano was not acceptable.

Dr. Bean-Bayog had a choice. If she insisted on having a trial, and lost the case, she would be responsible for the enormous costs. Her insurance carrier advised her to settle. To avoid what she termed a "media circus," Dr. Bean-Bayog surrendered her medical license and settled the case out of court for $1 million. Decrying the storm of publicity, Dr. Bean-Bayog declared, "No male therapist has ever been the subject of such an assault." She will be able to continue to practice as a psychotherapist, a profession that does not require the therapist to have a license to practice medicine.

Critics who were close to the events of this case feel that Dr. Bean-Bayog's career was ruined by a combination of inaccurate, biased reporting by the news media, inept proceedings held by the Massachusetts Board of Registration in Medicine, and the threat of ruinous legal fees, which deprived her of having a fair day in court. A number of her colleagues stood by her. They cited the great difficulty in treating this very disturbed patient, Dr. Bean-Bayog's consultation with other psychiatrists, the need for an innovative treatment approach to her patient's unique problems, and the fact that the suicide took place 10 months after treatment ended, while Lozano was under the care of another psychiatrist, showing that he was unable to survive without the treatment provided by Dr. Bean-Bayog.

Sexual Misconduct by "Helping" Professionals

Crossing of sexual boundaries by those in the helping professions is probably the clearest example of how fine the line is between "good men" and "bad men." Abuses of professional power and authority occur across all of the helping professions. None are immune. Lawyers, clergy, teachers, physicians, psychotherapists, and other helpers have been censured, defrocked, and sued for committing a particular form of power abuse—sexual misconduct. Certain sensational cases that are reported in the media, particularly those that involve the abuse of children by such professionals, have fueled national scandals. Public trust has been undermined and the helping professions damaged by persons in prominent positions, usually men, who have betrayed the trust placed in them. The greatest harm has been felt by the victims of professional sexual misconduct. Their suffering is incalculable.

The vast majority of men and women in the helping professions are competent and trustworthy. And if they have sexual thoughts and feelings toward their patients and clients, it must be recognized that, as I demonstrate later in this chapter, such feelings and thoughts are quite common, and most of the time they are not acted out. In fact, the competent therapist is able to turn personal feelings to account for the benefit of the patient's therapy. It would compound the tragedy caused by abuse of power and authority to damn all professions and professionals because of the transgressions of the few. This said, the nature of sexual abuse and sexual harassment needs to be understood by both professionals and consumers to lower the incidence of sexual misconduct.

The law and legislation concerning sexual misconduct are continually evolving. Sexual abuse and sexual harassment are distinct from each other. Sexual harassment generally happens in the workplace. In sexual harassment, no special relationships or reasons for trust necessarily exist between the harasser and the person who is harassed. Some of the time, it is a matter of an employer taking advantage of an employee, as when the employer provides or withholds job-related benefits based on whether the employee complies or does not comply with sexual requests. Most of the time, sexual harassment occurs between coworkers, creating a hostile work environment.

Sexual misconduct by professionals, however, differs from coworker abuse because it is an exploitation of professional power and authority that arises from a special relationship that is inherently imbued with trust. Workplace relationships are not built on this implicit sort of trust: an employee does not seek "help" from the employer, only properly remunerated work. Lawyer-client, doctor-patient, priest-penitent, and teacher-student are all power-and-trust relationships. At the core of these relationships is the understanding that the professional will use the power and prestige of his or her position, along with the benefit of years of knowledge, training, and expertise, for the benefit of the person seeking help.

Abusing the Power and the Glory

In the past 20 years, more than 500 Catholic priests in North America were reported for molesting children. The Catholic Church in the United States has paid out over $1 billion in settlements to about 2,000 victims, and still more money in legal fees and bills for medical care of the errant priests. Many cases have attracted large-scale public attention.

Former Roman Catholic priest James Porter was accused of sexually abusing 32 boys and girls in the 1960s while serving as a priest in three Massachusetts parishes. He left the priesthood in 1974, married, and had four children before the charges were brought against him. In 1992 he pleaded guilty to molesting 28 of the Massachusetts children and was sentenced to 18 to 20 years in prison. Civil suits against him, alleging child abuse, were also filed in other states. In a separate court action, Porter was convicted of molesting a 15-year-old babysitter in 1992. In a similar case involving another former priest, 17 men who had accused him of sexually abusing them when they were children agreed to a $13 million settlement offered by several insurance companies.

There have also been abuses at higher levels of church authority. An archbishop in the Southwest expressed "profound sadness" after female parishioners said that they had had sexual relations with him. The much-beloved Archbishop Robert Sanchez, the first Hispanic Archbishop in the country, resigned in disgrace in 1993 after admitting that he had sex with at least five young women. Another American archbishop resigned in 1990 as head of a southern archdiocese after he was romantically linked to a 27-year-old singer. The highest ranking American Catholic official to be accused of sexual misconduct was Chicago Cardinal Joseph Bernardin, who was the target of a lawsuit that sought $10 million in damages. The Cardinal categorically denied the charges. They were later withdrawn and the suit was dropped.

Sexual misconduct among clergy exists in other denominations, of course. The sensational sex scandals of superstar televangelists Jim Bakker and Jimmy Swaggart drew national attention. More recently, the prominent minister of a large and venerable Protestant congregation in Washington, D.C., a man whose television program was also viewed worldwide, admitted to having had sexual contact involving "hugging and affectionate kissing," but not sexual intercourse, with several women in his congregation. After two women filed grievances, the minister was confronted and agreed to undergo counseling and retire. Clergy sexual abuse has occurred also among Jewish, Muslim, and Buddhist congregations—in short, it has occurred wherever it is possible for clergymen, vested in their power and glory, to go over the line that separates pastoral nurturing from sexual intimacy.

It is by virtue of their knowledge and training that professionals such as clergy hold their power positions. Clergymen are frequently viewed by their parishioners as the charismatic representatives of divine authority, knowledge, and sanctity. Some of the faithful view clergy as interceding on their behalf for reconciliation with God. Frequently, parishioners who feel guilt-ridden, deficient, or needy seek the help of pastoral counselors whom they hold in awe and veneration. These parishioners are vulnerable. Exploitative clergymen who have easy access to such parishioners will take advantage of them. As one sexually exploited victim put it, "They don't put a gun to your head, they put God to your head."

Advocacy Versus Intimacy

Persons involved in litigation have often experienced significant psychological trauma before consulting an attorney. Some of them may also be experiencing severe mental distress or may have a psychiatric disorder. The client's feelings of vulnerability can create considerable dependency on the attorney. The inevitable stress of litigation adds even more traumatic pressure, which also serves to enhance the client's vulnerability and the lawyer's power and authority. In these combustible circumstances, this power asymmetry is sometimes exploited by attorneys into sexual involvement with their clients.

The problem is even more acute when the litigation involves divorce, for matrimonial attorneys have to deal with clients who are often quite distraught over the breakup of a marriage. The stakes in such litigation are high. It may mean the potential loss of one's children and source of income for a spouse who has stayed at home to raise the children. Such a woman might well view her lawyer as the good, all-powerful parent who can rescue the client from calamity. Whether male or female, the client in such cases is highly dependent on the attorney and often is emotionally needy.

Even in cases that involve matters other than matrimony, lawyers can sometimes take advantage. In one instance, the attorney grievance commission of a state brought misconduct charges against a prominent attorney for allegedly kissing one client, spanking another, and repeatedly spanking his secretary, sometimes on her bare bottom. The case arose from a complaint by a client who had hired the attorney to bring a personal injury suit against a hunter who had accidentally shot her. When the attorney came to her house to view the scene of the shooting, the woman alleged, he told her she was a bad girl, placed her over his knee, and spanked her repeatedly.

In another instance, the power-and-authority abuser was a judge who was also the seven-term mayor of his town. He was convicted of violating the civil rights of five women by sexually assaulting them in his courthouse. Two of these felony convictions related to a woman who was trying to retain custody of her child. She testified that the judge had twice forced her to perform oral sex in his chambers. Five misdemeanor convictions involved instances in which four women testified that the judge had fondled them in his chambers.

In Loco Parentis

As with attorneys, teachers at all levels have power-authority roles. From earliest childhood, students often view teachers as role models and as parental surrogates. Such personal matters as positive feelings about oneself, good relationships with others, career choices, partner selection, and spiritual aspirations can be profoundly influenced by teachers. A positive encounter with an especially admired teacher can change the course of a student's life.

The negative side of this equation more regularly surfaces in college, where professors are similarly esteemed and wield tremendous power, especially in regard to students' chances for success when they graduate. For many women, success in what is still a man's world depends on the recognition of their ability by men in power who become their mentors. A top recommendation, a good grade, a phone call from the professor to an important person in business may seem of the essence to a student. The need to obtain these references by the student may be exploited by a professor for sexual purposes. According to several surveys, between 20% and 30% of all female college and graduate students have been sexually approached by their professors. One study reports that 17% of female graduate students in psychology report sexual intimacy with a professor, whereas 30% turned away unwelcome advances, particularly from female teachers.

Intense attachment between student and teacher can sometimes become sexualized. There have been a number of instances of female high school teachers becoming involved in sexual relationships with their male students. The most sensational was that of Mary Kay Letourneau, a married 34-year-old mother of four who seduced a 12-year-old. Letourneau was pregnant with the 15-year-old's child when she was sent to prison. Released for a few days, she was again caught with him and returned to prison, where she birthed a second child. Upon her release from a 7-year jail term, she married the former student, then 22.

In other such cases, Debra Lafave, a 25-year-old middle-school reading teacher, pleaded guilty to having sex with a student and received a 3-year house arrest. Kimberly Merson, a substitute teacher and cheerleader, admitted in court to "sexual contact" with nine male students ages 15 to 17, and was sentenced to 18 months in jail. And San Bernardino, California teacher Tanya Hadden ran away to Las Vegas with a 15-year-old student from the high school where she taught; she was sentenced to 2 years in prison.

Helping Others or Helping Ourselves?

A national survey of fourth-year psychiatric residents found that 4.9% of the 548 respondents reported sexual involvement with their educators. The same survey also reported that 1.2% of the male students and 0.4% of the female students acknowledged sexual contact with their own patients. The abuse of patients by psychotherapists is of great concern to everyone. It is discussed in detail in the following section because it provides a model for understanding professional sexual misconduct in general.

The common thread that runs through the sexual misconduct in the helping professions is that professional relationships produce certain role expectations in the people being served. The therapist, professor, lawyer, or clergyman are all fiduciaries to the people they serve. A fiduciary is a person who acts for another in a capacity that involves confidence or trust. That fiduciary role does not include the establishment of an intimate sexual relationship, such as we understand those relationships to exist in a context of love. Love relationships differ from fiduciary ones in the following way: in love relationships, the presumptions exist that two relatively equal individuals are joining together, that they are doing so by freely given consent, and that they do so for the purpose of meeting their *mutual* needs.

A key factor in a fiduciary relationship gone awry is vulnerability. People who do not possess the power or resources to choose or to act for themselves are deemed vulnerable. Age, gender, education, cultural background, race, role, current life situation, and a number of other individual psychological factors all affect a person's vulnerability. The judge who allegedly forced the woman seeking to retain custody of her child to perform oral sex exploited many of these factors. The relationship between the judge and this woman cannot be considered a love relationship because, among other things, it lacked her freely given consent. When sexual activity is induced through fear, coercion, or manipulation that is imposed through a position of power or authority, the meaningful consent that is so necessary for an emotionally satisfying sexual relationship is absent.

Female vulnerability and sexual coercion are woven into the fabric of our society. Efforts to understand sexual exploitation solely by means of individual psychological analysis of the particular victim or perpetrator often may overlook important societal-cultural factors. Such an analysis fails to recognize that sexual coercion is embedded throughout the structure and processes of most human culture. It would be a naïve error to conclude, however, that female professionals do not sexually exploit persons who seek their help. Nevertheless, female exploiters among professionals are in a distinct minority. Why male professionals are the perpetrators in the majority of the sexual exploitation cases is an extremely complex question. The answer involves cultural factors; for instance, men are acculturated to test boundaries, whereas women have been taught to accept boundary testing. There are also biological factors, for instance, the role of testosterone in producing sexual aggression. The evolutionary fact that men were hunter-predators may make some contribution to the male psyche. But cultural factors alone do not provide a satisfactory answer—the fact is that most male professionals do *not* sexually exploit their clients. This means that individual psychological factors play key roles for male professionals who *do* cross the boundary between maintaining their fiduciary role and sexual intimacy.

Therapist-Patient Sex

No accurate figures are available concerning the actual percentages of mental health professionals who commit acts of sexual misconduct. Most of the surveys that have attempted to ascertain the incidence of therapist-patient sex fall short on two counts: 1) the acts committed may be too narrowly defined, and 2) the survey methods are notoriously unreliable. Only about 15% to 25% of the therapists surveyed bother to respond. Also, the truth of what they have said on the survey cannot be verified independently. It can safely be assumed that most of the offenders do not respond to the survey, so that the real incidence must be higher than the reported incidence. That said, it must be pointed out that the reported figures are high enough to be of concern. A nationwide survey of 1,442 psychiatrists revealed 7.1% of male and 3.1% of female respondents acknowledged sexual contact with their own patients. Eighty-eight percent of these sexual contacts occurred between male psychiatrists and female patients, 7.6% between male psychiatrists and male patients, 3.5% between female psychiatrists and male patients, and 1.4% between female psychiatrists and female patients.

There has also been therapist sexual contact with child patients. In one study of 958 patients who were sexually exploited, 5% were minors. In another study exclusively of minors, the average age of sexually exploited children was 12 for male patients and 14 for female patients. Generally, psychiatrists, psychologists, and social workers have equal rates of sexual involvement with their patients.

Let me say it plainly: sex between a therapist and a patient *always* is unprofessional, is unethical, and constitutes malpractice. Psychiatrists, as physicians, pledge to first do no harm to their patients when they take the Hippocratic oath. Sex with a patient is *never* an acceptable form of treatment. Patients who come for psychiatric or psychological treatment are experiencing mental and emotional suffering that is painful and can be debilitating. Their decision-making capacities and judgment are usually impaired to some degree. Although the patient may not be incompetent to make major life decisions, he or she may have vulnerabilities and psychological blind spots that can be exploited. Moreover, the patient seeks out the therapist as a critically important source of help and hope. Under such circumstances, the patient frequently comes to idealize the therapist as the all-good, all-powerful parent figure. The patient, who is experiencing mental pain, is highly influenced by early, powerful yearnings to be comforted or cared for by the loving parent. Barbara Noël described her feelings for Dr. Jules Masserman by characterizing him as "my 'healthy' father figure." Along with idealization of the therapist as a good parent comes the patient's fear of losing this newly important figure in his or her life—a fear that increases the patient's vulnerability to exploitation by the therapist.

Transference is narrowly defined as the primary unconscious tendency of *all* individuals to assign to others in the present those feelings and attitudes that were originally connected to important figures in the course of their early childhood development. A more expansive, totalistic definition of transference includes the entire conscious and unconscious responses of the patient to the therapist. Transference occurs to some degree in all relationships but is particularly strong in fiduciary-type relationships. Mismanagement by the therapist of the patient's powerful feelings from the past and the present is a key factor in the treatment boundary violations that lead down the slippery slope to sexual intimacy with the patient.

Therapists' and Patients' Thoughts of Each Other

The differential of power and authority that exists in professional-patient relationships intensifies transference. In psychotherapy, the patient usually identifies the therapist with his or her parents or other important early figures. Carolyn Bates, in the book *Sex in the Therapy Hour*, which she cowrote with psychologist Annette M. Brodsky, described the growth of her feelings toward her therapist:

> Over the months, in my weekly 45 to 50 minute sessions, I have no doubt that much of the trust and love I had for my father was directed toward Dr. X, for I perceived him as having both wisdom and an unconditional concern for my well-being.

Unfortunately, Ms. Bates later found that her intense feelings toward Dr. X were exploited by him. That is not the usual case. Transference feelings can be an important part of the patient's treatment. On one end of the spectrum, some patients may resist or deny transference feelings; on the other end, some patients may wish to live out transference feelings with the therapist.

Therapists sometimes egregiously mismanage transference feelings when they accept at face value the patient's expressions of love, adoration, and dependency. The well-trained therapist knows that, as with dreams, transference expressions are a surface presentation that hides a patient's darker passions and attitudes. Feelings of love for the therapist may mask deeper feelings of hostility and anger that the patient must work out in the therapy. The psychodynamic, "insight" psychotherapist is trained to know how to manage the transference therapeutically and knows better than to exploit it for his or her own benefit. But insight psychotherapy is only one form of therapy. Although important, its use by itself has been declining in recent years. Today, the number of psychotherapeutic approaches, or "schools," is above 450 and climbing. In all therapies, however, transference plays a role, either directly or indirectly, which means that all therapists, no matter what method of treatment they use, must be aware of the importance of transference in their work with patients.

Therapists must also be sensitive to their primarily unconscious emotional responses to the patient—*countertransference*—which can also present a danger to patients. In a strict sense, this is the therapist's transference to the patient; that is, the therapist reexperiences feelings, thoughts, and behaviors toward the patient that have their origin in the therapist's past relationships. More generally, the term countertransference refers to the totality of the therapist's conscious and unconscious thoughts, feelings, and behaviors toward the patient. For example, the therapist's countertransference to the patient may contain compelling erotic, incestuous feelings from early childhood that may be currently fueling a sexual interest toward a prohibited person—the patient. As with transference, countertransference exists in all relationships but is a particular problem in professional interactions. It can fuel the therapist's temptation to exploit a position of power and commit sexual misconduct. As former secretary of state Henry Kissinger once observed, "Power is the great aphrodisiac."

The inevitable countertransference feelings induced in the therapist regarding the patient can become a therapeutic window into the conflicts of the patient and into his or her characteristic ways of interacting with others. Insights gained through examining countertransference can assist the patient's recovery. But countertransference feelings, particularly of the erotic variety, can also be occasion for the therapist mismanaging the patient's treatment. Therapists get into trouble with patients when they are unable to hold, contain, and analyze their own feelings toward the patient. This is what the medical board in Massachusetts alleged had happened with Dr. Bean-Bayog, as they pinpointed her failure "to terminate or otherwise address" her sexual fantasies evoked in the treatment of Paul Lozano. The board found that her inability to deal with these issues was unacceptable.

Sexual exploitation of patients does not necessarily arise from transference or countertransference. Some therapists are—plain and simple—predators who pounce on vulnerable individuals. These therapists usually have severe malformations in their character and personality. In general, therapists who undertake long-term psychotherapy with patients should undergo their own psychotherapy or analysis, although this is not an absolute prerequisite. But the therapist must have or develop the ability to turn his or her mind on itself for the purpose of understanding personal problems, particularly in relation to the treatment of other people. For example, the lure for the therapist of having illicit sex with patients often has its roots in the therapist's early incestuous desires. Understood and controlled, these feelings can prove useful in alerting the therapist to the nature of the material coming from the patient that may be stimulating incestuous feelings in the therapist. Misunderstood and uncontrolled, the feelings may lead to therapist-patient sexual misconduct.

With psychotherapists especially, the notion that bad men do what good men dream is of the essence. This notion is confirmed by a study showing that whereas 95% of the male psychotherapists and 76% of the female psychotherapists among 575 surveyed felt sexually attracted to their clients, only 9.4% of the men and 2.5% of the women acted on such feelings. Other studies show that nearly 75% of therapists have had sexual fantasies about a patient and 58% have become sexually aroused during therapy. Slightly more than 25% have had fantasies about a patient during sex with someone else.

When the Therapist Is a Woman

A significantly lower incidence of sexual misconduct by female therapists is a consistent finding of many surveys. Among those female therapists who do become sexually involved with their patients, the most common form of involvement is heterosexual relationships. Some female therapists, however, do develop what have been described as "tea and sympathy" relationships with female patients. These therapists are usually heterosexual and become overinvolved with the patient and overidentify with the patient's problems. Their offers of tenderness and closeness may turn into hand-holding, kissing, fondling or even suckling the patient.

Numerous reasons (though not necessarily accurate ones) have been proffered to explain the lower incidence of sexual misconduct by female therapists:

- A strong mother-son incest taboo is unconsciously operating in the therapy, for both parties.
- Female therapists tend to have practices in which a higher proportion of their patients are women and children.
- The effects of maternal-child feelings generated by the treatment are sexually inhibiting for both parties.

- Women have been acculturated into nonpredatory roles; there is no female equivalent of the "macho" man's role.
- Gender differences in the biological bases of aggression (e.g., the presence of more testosterone in males) affect incidence of sexual misconduct.
- The female therapist's response to desperate, needy patients of the opposite sex is less likely to be erotically tinged than is the male therapist's response because of acculturation and gender differences.
- Female therapists who are older are less likely to view themselves, and to be viewed, as sexual beings within the treatment context.
- Females, as a group, are more compassionate, nurturing, sensitive, and empowering of others.

Treatment Boundaries and the Slippery Slope

All professions establish professional and ethical guidelines for the conduct of their practitioners. For example, the Hippocratic oath taken by all physicians states *primum non nocere*—first, do no harm. The purpose of such guidelines is not only to protect the consumer from exploitation but also to provide good care. That is certainly true in the mental health field. All psychiatric therapies, regardless of their philosophical or theoretical orientation, are based on the fundamental premise that the therapist's positive interaction with the patient is aimed toward alleviating psychic distress, positively changing the patient's behavior and, in a meaningful way, altering the patient's perspective on the world. In short, the therapeutic equation is a unique opportunity for a patient to obtain much-needed help. Exploitation of patients by therapists destroys this potential.

There are basic guidelines for the maintenance of treatment boundaries that are commonly accepted by most therapists. The concept of treatment boundaries, in fact, began in the twentieth century, largely as an outgrowth of psychoanalysis and psychodynamic psychotherapy. As early as 1909, the founder of psychoanalysis, Sigmund Freud, strongly disapproved of his disciple Sandor Ferenczi's sexual involvement with his patient "Frau G" and her daughter "Elma." Treatment boundaries were further defined by the ethical principles developed by the mental health professions and by the legal duties imposed on therapists by courts, by statutes, and by regulatory agencies. As a case in point, the therapist's duty to maintain the patient's confidentiality derives from three distinct sources: good professional care, ethical codes, and legislative mandates. Treatment boundaries are set by the therapist and not by the patient. It is the therapist's professional duty to establish and maintain boundaries that define and secure the therapist's professional relationship with the patient. Sound boundaries promote a trusting working relationship between therapist and patient.

Psychiatry continues to be highly receptive to innovative treatments that offer the hope of helping the mentally ill. But what is an inviolable treatment boundary to one "school" of psychotherapy may seem like nonsense to another. Some people fear that restricting treatment boundaries can pose impediments to therapeutic innovation. The new hope for helping the mentally ill, they argue, depends on innovative and possibly boundary-defying techniques. I am not persuaded by that argument, nor do I believe that maintaining basic treatment boundaries is any impediment to responsible innovation.

Rules, however, cannot always be hard and fast. Exceptions exist for mental health professionals practicing in small communities and rural areas, who encounter unique situations and customs that may require appropriate adjustments of treatment boundaries—for example, where "everybody knows everybody else." There is a general boundary guideline that physical contact between therapist and patient should be minimized. In the case of alcohol and drug-treatment programs, an exception to this rule must be made because part of the therapeutic process is the hugging of patients. Also, therapists who work with children, the elderly, and the physically ill frequently have need to touch their patients. As long as this is done in a nonerotic, clinically supportive manner, it is appropriate to the treatment process. In every instance, when trying to fashion a boundary for treatment, what needs to be taken into account is the nature of the patient, the therapist, the type of treatment, and the status of the relationship between therapist and patient. Despite the wide variety of psychological treatments, a general consensus does exist among practitioners concerning the necessity of appropriate treatment boundaries. There is never a circumstance in which "anything goes."

As a forensic psychiatrist, I have had the opportunity to review a number of sexual misconduct cases sent to me by lawyers. Almost without exception, I have found that treatment boundaries are not violated suddenly, except in the reported instances of forcible rape.

Rather, the violations are gradual and progressive—especially those that lead eventually to sexual intimacy. Sometimes the erosion of the boundary is barely noticeable. Even if sexual relations are not the eventual end product of the boundary violations, other sorts of exploitation may be produced. The patient may be used to provide services or to perform chores for the therapist. The therapist may involve the patient in business dealings, exploiting the patient monetarily. It is my experience that patients are more frequently exploited over money than sex. Sometimes it is both. All such boundary violations invariably impede or destroy the patient's treatment.

Therapists who are boundary sensitive may breach a barrier in a minor way, then awaken to the fact that it is being violated and take actions to properly restore the treatment boundaries. But there are therapists who are not boundary sensitive. With them, what is the patient to do? In many instances, the patient may feel that a boundary is being violated but may not be able to escape from a therapy that is heading toward sexual exploitation. Consider the following case:

> A 56-year-old male therapist began individual psychotherapy of a 32-year-old woman who was attractive, divorced, and depressed. Just prior to starting this therapy, the therapist had recently concluded a bitter divorce that ended his 25-year marriage. During the initial 6 months, the therapy progressed and treatment boundaries remained intact. Thereafter, an easy familiarity blossomed between the therapist and patient, who had started to address each other by their first names. A handshake at the end of a session replaced the simple good-bye that had been the standard at parting. The tenor of the therapeutic sessions became more social, with mutual sharing of experience. On one occasion, the psychiatrist talked about his divorce and loneliness. On another, he shared his sexual fantasies and dreams with the patient. She responded by describing the various social functions available to divorcées. The handshake at session's end progressed to a hug. Then, in their embraces at the end of each session, the therapist and patient began to linger. Because the patient felt she was receiving special attention from the therapist, her depression appeared to improve dramatically. She stopped questioning some of the therapist's behaviors toward her that were initially troubling. In due course, the patient's sessions were scheduled for the end of the therapist's day when they could spend uninterrupted time together. Before long, therapist and patient occasionally dined together. Movie dates followed, with hand-holding and kissing. Eventually, a sexual relationship "just happened."

It did not "just happen," of course: the sexual relationship was but one more, albeit critical, boundary violation in a series that had begun almost imperceptibly. In the case example, the sex was the culmination of many earlier, progressive boundary violations. Boundary violations frequently begin insidiously "between the chair and the door." During this segment of the therapy session, patients and therapists are more vulnerable to committing boundary crossings and violations. Therapists must be aware of the potential for boundary violations to begin during this interval when both patient and therapist can slip into a social relationship. Studies also show that therapist self-disclosure of personal information to the patient, particularly of sexual fantasies and dreams, is highly correlated with eventual sexual misconduct. Therapist-patient sex is never the only deviation in the patient's care. There are invariably other transgressions, many of which are not explicitly sexual: for example, medication mismanagement, failure to correctly diagnose, breach of confidentiality, poor record keeping, improper billing. Consider the following instance:

A 38-year-old single woman with symptoms of generalized anxiety entered therapy with a 41-year-old male therapist. Unbeknownst to her, this therapist had sexually exploited several of his other female patients. This patient suffered from very low self-esteem and had a great need to please others. The therapist diagnosed the patient as having dependent personality disorder. He prescribed for the patient a combination of psychiatric drugs that had the effect of keeping the patient oversedated much of the time. Within a few months of having started once-weekly psychotherapy, the patient was returning the therapist's library books for him "as a favor." Gradually, the therapist convinced the patient to do other menial chores. When the patient began having trouble paying her treatment bill, she agreed with the therapist's suggestion that as partial payment she clean the therapist's office twice a week. Because her therapy sessions were scheduled at noon, the patient agreed to fetch the therapist's lunch before each session from a nearby delicatessen. If the lunch was unsatisfactory, the therapist would scold the patient. He also frequently expressed displeasure with the way she cleaned the office. Fearing rejection, the patient gradually slipped under the therapist's total control. The last vestiges of supportive psychotherapy vanished. When the patient appeared crushed by the therapist's criticisms, she would be directed to sit on the therapist's lap, where he would stroke and rock her. By then totally dependent on her therapist, the patient was emotionally incapable of resisting his subsequent sexual advances.

Patients with low self-esteem and intense rejection sensitivity are easy marks for unscrupulous therapists. In this case, the sexual activity that occurred relatively late in the patient's "treatment" can be seen to be within the context of increasingly serious deviations from the norm in care of the patient. Treatment boundaries were gradually but inexorably breached as the therapist gratified his own needs through exploitation of the patient. Oversedation was done primarily to attain control over her. Abuse of medications occurs in a number of malpractice cases that also allege sexual misconduct. In this particular case, the patient's mind was repeatedly raped before her sexual abuse ever began.

Another case presents a different type of breach:

> A 61-year-old male therapist had been treating a 48-year-old woman for marital problems for approximately 1 year. During this year, he saw the patient twice weekly for supportive and insight psychotherapy sessions. The year before treatment began, the therapist had lost his wife to a lingering illness. As the woman's treatment progressed, the therapist gradually began to share more of his own thoughts, feelings, and experiences with the patient. Just as gradually, she took on a supportive, confidante role with him. Occasionally, when speaking of his dead wife, the therapist would break down and cry. When this occurred, the patient would place her arm around the therapist and reassure him in a soothing voice. Most of the sessions became devoted to the therapist's problems. Eventually, the therapist and patient began to see one another outside of the therapy sessions. The therapist's depression improved. As for the woman, feeling neglected in her own marriage, she now found renewed meaning in her relationship with the therapist. She assumed the position of a doting maternal figure for the therapist. When sexual relations occurred between them, these were secondary to the caretaking role of the patient. The complete switching of positions of therapist and patient had been achieved.

Basic Boundary Guidelines

Psychotherapy is an impossible task. It cannot be done perfectly. In psychotherapy, boundary *issues* inevitably arise from the patient and form an essential ingredient in the treatment. Boundary *violations*, however, are another matter, for these arise not because of the therapeutic situation but because of the therapist. They are damaging to the treatment process, particularly if they go unchecked and if they become progressively more serious. Unrestrained, progressive boundary violations usually reflect the acted-out conflicts of the therapist. Incidents of boundary violation, often called boundary *crossings*, that are both brief and quickly recognized and rectified by the therapist can provide important insights into conflictual issues for both the therapist and the patient. An example: the therapist begins to self-disclose, then checks himself. The patient asks why the therapist stopped. The therapist turns the question around and asks the patient about why he wants to know more about the therapist. This leads to a helpful discussion about the patient's resistance to self-scrutiny.

Several basic, interlocking principles provide the underpinning for the establishment of boundary guidelines. One is the rule of abstinence. The therapist must refrain from obtaining personal gratification at the expense of the patient. It is understood, in consequence of this rule, that the therapist's main source of personal gratification comes in the form of the professional pleasure derived from the psychotherapeutic process and the satisfactions gained from helping the patient. The only material gain obtained directly from the patient is the fee for the therapist's professional services. Other principles underpinning the guidelines include the therapist's duty to maintain therapeutic neutrality, to support patient autonomy and self-determination, to uphold the fiduciary relationship between therapist and patient, and to respect human dignity. Out of these principles, the following general guidelines have been elucidated as a necessary treatment frame for the conduct of most psychotherapies:

- The therapist maintains relative therapeutic neutrality, withholding his or her own personal views.
- The therapist fosters the independence of the patient by maintaining the patient's psychological separateness from the therapist.
- The therapist preserves the patient's confidentiality, an essential element of trust in psychotherapy.
- The therapist works collaboratively with the patient and obtains informed consent for treatment and procedures.
- The therapist interacts with the patient primarily through talking.
- The therapist takes pains to ensure that there are no previous, current, or promised future personal relationships with the patient.
- The therapist makes sure to minimize physical contact with (and possible erotic stimulation of) the patient.
- The therapist avoids burdening the patient with personal disclosures and preserves relative anonymity.

- A stable fee policy is established, and the therapist accepts only money as payment for treatment.
- A consistent, private, and professional setting is provided for the therapy—usually, a therapist's office.
- Length and time of sessions are clearly defined. Stability and consistency are therapeutically important. Also, clear time definition of sessions eliminates the possibility of extended sessions that may be a part of progressive boundary violations.

Many of these principles and guidelines apply equally for all physician-patient, lawyer-client, pastor-parishioner, and other professional relationships.

The Therapy Predators

Based on my experience assessing what has happened in many cases of alleged sexual misconduct, I can divide the exploitative therapists into five main types: 1) personality disordered, 2) sexually disordered, 3) incompetent, 4) impaired, and 5) situationally stressed. These categories often overlap. I cannot speak authoritatively for all professions, but it is likely that groups such as lawyers, professors, and clergymen contain similar clusters of exploitative individuals.

Predator therapists are the repeaters, those who sexually exploit numerous patients. These therapists usually display manipulative and exploitative characteristics of a borderline, narcissistic, or antisocial personality disorder. Approximately 40% of the therapists who abuse a patient have abused more than one patient under their care. *Sexually disordered* therapists are often likely to be repeaters as well. They are subdivided into three categories: frotteurs (compulsive sexual touchers), pedophiles (who use children as sex objects), and sexual sadists. *Incompetent* therapists may be poorly trained or have persistent boundary blind spots. Sexual misconduct, however, occurs at all levels of training and of professional experience. *Impaired* therapists' mishandlings of patients can be traced to abuse of alcohol, drugs, or their own mental or physical illness. *Situationally stressed* therapists are those who because of painful personal circumstances—such as the loss of a loved one, the experience of marital discord, or a professional crisis—may turn to the patient for repair of their psychological wounds.

Warning: Patient Vulnerable!

It is *never* the patient's fault when therapist-patient sex takes place. It is *always* the therapist's responsibility to maintain the integrity of the treatment and to protect the patient from therapist-induced harm. Approaching the problem of therapist-patient sex as though it might be the patient's fault is tantamount to "blaming the victim." Yet it is essential to study all elements of the interaction between therapists and patients that culminate in sexual intimacy to understand how to prevent such sexual abuse from occurring.

In a study that reviewed more than 2,000 cases of therapist sexual misconduct, no factors were found that predicted patient involvement with therapists. Predictive characteristics were found only for therapists. Nevertheless, the experience of a number of forensic psychiatrists identifies certain patients who appear to be more vulnerable than others to sexual exploitation:

- Patients with current depression and a recent loss of a love relationship
- Patients with dependent personalities
- Patients who have been sexually and physically abused as children
- Patients with serious psychiatric illnesses or with alcohol and drug abuse problems
- Patients with impaired mental and personality functions; these patients have low self-esteem, are dependent, have difficulty separating reality from fantasy, are self-destructive, or have impulsive or other maladaptive traits
- Physically attractive patients with low self-esteem
- Mentally retarded patients
- Patients who have had chronic illnesses as children

Most of these categories are self-explanatory. The terrible combination of impaired mental functioning, low self-esteem, and loneliness often places a patient at risk for sexual exploitation. Any history of childhood sexual and physical abuse, even of severe childhood illness, creates special vulnerabilities. Seductive behavior toward the therapist, for instance, is frequently a consequence of childhood sexual abuse. According to the College of Physicians and Surgeons of the Ontario Task Force Study, 23% of incest victims who seek psychotherapy are sexually abused by the therapist. An additional 23% are victims of other forms of abuse by the therapist. These are shockingly high figures. Only 30% of these patients receive any help from their first therapist. Indeed, the average incest victim sees 3.5 therapists in the course of treatment.

Childhood sexual abuse tends to create the need to master the original trauma through repetition. It sexualizes subsequent relations, distorts boundary maintenance in the patient's personal relationships, and induces low self-worth and feelings of guilt. Frequently, patients who were sexually abused in childhood will test treatment boundary limits through seductive behavior in their attempts to determine whether the therapist can be trusted. Also, patients who have suffered child abuse have learned to mentally dissociate themselves while being abused. When such vulnerable patients are sexually approached directly by a therapist, they may psychologically and physically freeze. These patients may mentally dissociate to a corner of the room or feel like they are floating to the ceiling to watch what is occurring, as if it were happening to someone else. In this psychological state, they are easy prey for the predator therapist.

Patients who have had extensive medical and surgical procedures as children may also be vulnerable as adults to sexual exploitation. They have had their bodies frequently exposed to numerous medical personnel as well as to family members. Also, they have endured intrusive medical procedures that distort body privacy boundaries. These intrusions set the stage for later sexual intimacies with exploitative therapists who do not maintain appropriate boundaries.

Patients with certain dysfunctional personality characteristics sometimes attempt to manipulate the therapist and draw him or her out of the treatment role. With these patients, therapists are tempted to make frequent exceptions to the rules of treatment. Such patients tend to induce in the therapist the desire to do better than the patient's parents or other caretakers or to undo the damage to the patient done by them. If the therapist takes this bait, he or she commits a major error. Attempting to "re-parent" the patient is almost always disastrous. Aside from the realization that it is an impossible task, the endless demands that come from the patient when the therapist attempts to reparent interfere with the patient's more important need to mourn the losses of childhood and move on with life.

Therapists are trained and expected to appropriately manage difficult patients so that patient exploitation does not occur. If a therapist cannot manage the patient appropriately, and harm threatens the patient, the therapist should refer the patient to a competent therapist.

After the Bubble Bursts

The harm caused by therapist-patient sex can be enormous. The psychic pain and damage become particularly apparent after the patient discovers that he or she has been sexually exploited by the therapist. Psychological harm includes worsening and exacerbation of the patient's preexisting psychiatric conditions; creation of new conditions such as anxiety, depressive disorders, or even psychosis; damage to personal relationships; possible destruction of future treatment possibilities; and suicide. Almost invariably, the patient who has been sexually exploited only becomes fully aware that he or she has been abused after a real or perceived rejection by the therapist. Such feelings of rejection may come as a consequence of the therapy being terminated, the therapist going on vacation, learning that other patients are having sex with the therapist, the refusal of the therapist to leave a spouse or to marry the patient, or any number of other real or perceived acts of rejection. The realization may be sudden or gradual, but it is always devastating. New psychological symptoms may appear, or old ones may be magnified when the sex between patient and therapist stops, termed by some the "cessation phenomenon." Some patients regress dramatically and become profoundly depressed and suicidal. As for the therapist, there is no golden parachute, no easy disengagement from the situation. Invariably, both patient and therapist are harmed. The patient in a sexual relationship with a therapist is harmed in many ways by the boundary violations that almost always precede actual therapist-patient sex. In such situations, the patient's original problems, for which he or she sought treatment, are worsened, and an important opportunity to treat those problems is lost. Moreover, when the patient becomes aware of having been exploited, the patient's sense of being special to the therapist evaporates, leaving instead feelings of profound betrayal, rage, and loneliness.

The cornerstone of any therapy is trust. Patients who have been sexually exploited by their therapists may have great difficulty undertaking meaningful therapy again because their trust has been shattered. The exploitation strikes at the heart of the patient's psyche: the critical ability to trust oneself and others. The foundations for basic

trust are established in the first few years of life. For example, fundamental beliefs such as that the world is a predictable and rational place,
that bad things do not happen to good people, that we have control
over life events, and that persons in positions of trust and authority are
beneficent and trustworthy develop early in the child raised by good-
enough parents. Most people make gradual adjustments in these assumptions as they encounter life's vicissitudes. It is when fundamental
beliefs are dashed suddenly and traumatically that psychic harm results and trust is shattered. Some level of basic trust is necessary in the
conduct of almost every aspect of life. For example, we could neither
leave the house nor cross the street without trust. The paranoid psychotic individual usually is debilitated by the inability to trust.

Many exploited individuals do not seek therapy again, losing once
and for all the opportunity to regain their mental health. Even if they
do try therapy again, the exploited patient's sense of appropriate treatment boundaries has been gravely distorted. As part of any new therapy, there will have to be hard work both by the patient and the new
therapist to reestablish treatment boundaries. If that work is not done,
such patients remain quite vulnerable to being exploited yet another
time. To break the cycle, it is sometimes useful to refer a sexually exploited patient to a same-sex therapist to allay some of the patient's
anxiety concerning his or her continued vulnerability to exploitation.

As for the therapist, a clear-headed look at the matter would show
any therapist that sexual involvement with a patient is tantamount to
committing professional suicide. Such therapists' professional reputations are usually damaged, if not outright destroyed, when the exploitation of the patient comes to light. The therapist risks having his or
her professional license suspended or revoked. Professional organizations may bring up the therapist on ethical charges and even expel the
therapist. The therapist risks great collateral damage to his or her family and colleagues. Studies have shown that the knowledge that a close
and trusted colleague has had sex with a patient is as great a stress on
the clinician as having a patient commit suicide. For the therapist
whose sexual exploitation becomes known, he or she is likely to be hit
with a civil suit and with attendant sensational media coverage. In certain states, criminal charges may be brought. Financial damages levied
against the therapist by the court may not be covered by the therapist's
malpractice insurance. In the end, the abusive therapist may lose everything because he or she had sex with a patient.

The exploited patient, in addition to being able to seek legal redress through the courts, has recourse through professional organizations and state licensure bodies. However, the patient will need to explore his or her psychological readiness to pursue any of these avenues with a therapist because they are fraught with considerable emotional pain and stress. The patient must resist the temptation to act impulsively and must summon the psychological resources necessary to stay a very difficult course. In many instances, an accused therapist will use all legal means available to fight the patient's charges. The abused patient's journey through the legal system is usually another abusive experience. The law is a blunt instrument.

Here are the legal and professional actions that can be brought against an exploitative therapist at the instigation of a harmed patient:

- Civil suit
- Breach of contract action
- Criminal sanctions
- Civil action for intentional tort (e.g., battery, fraud)
- License revocation
- Ethical sanctions from professional societies
- Dismissal from professional organizations

At issue in some of these matters is the statute of limitations. In most cases, the time frame within which a party is permitted to bring a suit is 1 to 2 years after the discovery of an injury. In some cases of sexual exploitation, the law recognizes that the therapist's negligence may have impaired the ability of the patient to become aware of the psychological injuries that have been produced. The issue of the patient's competency in this regard may toll—that is, stop—the statute of limitations from running out. Fraudulent concealment by the therapist may also toll the statute of limitations. Patients have been sexually exploited for years without realizing the terrible emotional consequences to themselves, because the power differential between therapist and patient has strengthened the patient's denial mechanisms. Fraudulent concealment may occur when the therapist misinforms the patient that sex is therapy, or when the therapist fails to inform the patient that what the patient feels for the therapist is not love but transference at work.

And Ye Shall Know the Truth

Effective psychotherapy is a joint enterprise based on mutual trust between therapist and patient. But the public is not yet completely aware that therapist-patient sex is malpractice. Prospective patients need to be educated about the establishment of appropriate treatment boundaries. The patient who is well informed can enhance his or her chances of successful treatment by being knowledgeable about what is expected between a therapist and a patient. Radio and television programs, books, and special educational materials can educate people on these matters. The Internet is a useful tool for checking the credentials of a prospective therapist, as well as any adverse actions brought against the therapist. Licensure board websites should be consulted.

Many patients who enter therapy, particularly for the first time, do not know what constitutes appropriate treatment, nor do they have clear ideas about treatment boundaries. There is also a need for education about what a patient can or should do if he or she has been sexually exploited or feels that the therapist's behavior has been inappropriate and harmful. Studies show that sexually exploited female patients lack knowledge of complaint procedures rather than lacking motivation to take action on their own behalf.

It is a matter of "uh-oh" versus "ah-ha." Patients who sense that they are being exploited often have an "uh-oh" reaction about what is happening to them. However, patients who are receiving proper benefit from their therapy will often have an "ah-ha" reaction to insight and psychological growth.

For patients who want to evaluate their own therapy experience, the Wisconsin Task Force on Sexual Misconduct has published guidelines, recommending protective options for patients who feel they are threatened with exploitation or who have already been exploited.

The following questions can alert patients, or therapists themselves, to the possibility that therapeutic boundaries are being crossed:

1. Is the therapist requesting or pressuring the patient to perform any personal task, or to join in any activity that appears to be for the primary benefit of the therapist?
2. Is the therapist-patient relationship becoming less professional and more social over time?
3. Is the therapist revealing highly personal information about himself or herself?

Prevention requires diligent efforts in several directions, in addition to public education. Among the other directions are the selection of appropriate candidates as future therapists, the professional education and supervision of practicing therapists, and the toughening of ethical, professional, and legal sanctions against offending therapists. Prevention will never be total or perfect. All therapists are human and therefore imperfect. Sexual involvement of therapists with patients, though reprehensible, is likely to remain an occupational hazard for therapists and a danger for patients. Humankind's darker side ensures that this danger can never be completely eliminated.

9

You Only Die Once—
But Did You Intend It?

The Forensic Psychiatrist As Sleuth

> Doubt is not a very pleasant condition, but certainty
> is absurd.
>
> — *Voltaire*

Was It Really Suicide?

Vincent W. Foster, Jr.

On Tuesday, July 20, 1993, as White House Counsel Vincent W. Foster, Jr., walked out of his office in the west wing of the White House, he told his secretary to help herself to some M&M's candy left on his lunch tray. He then drove his car to Virginia, taking the George Washington Parkway to a scenic and secluded spot in Fort Marcy Park, and shot and killed himself.

In many ways, Foster was a modern version of "Richard Cory" in the poem by E.A. Robinson. As a corporate lawyer in Little Rock, Arkansas, Foster had earned professional acclaim and was earning $300,000 per year. But in Washington, D.C., at the side of the Clintons, life was different for him, and difficult. In the week before his death, he was worried about a possible congressional investigation into the White House travel office. His connection to that discredited office had been condemned by such newspapers as *The Wall Street Journal*. Foster sought the names of psychiatrists but feared that his sessions with them might be taped. He talked to his wife about resigning and returning to Little Rock, to their former, comfortable life. On Friday, July 16, Foster confided to his sister that he was fighting depression. She gave him some names of psychiatrists to call in Washington. He attempted to reach one of the psychiatrists twice but failed to make contact.

Foster took a getaway weekend, which seemed to refresh him, because back in his White House office he appeared rejuvenated. On the day before his death, he called his family physician and obtained antidepressant medication, but to the very end, Foster exhibited few outward signs of mental distress.

Foster's death roiled Washington. He left no suicide note and had not spoken to anyone about suicide. People who knew him were gripped with utter disbelief. How could a man of such stature and apparent stability, a man whom President Clinton called "the rock of Gibraltar," have killed himself? Foster's judgment and intellect had been so respected by his White House peers that he was considered a potential Supreme Court nominee. The park officer who found Foster's body commented that his slacks were creased, his white shirt was starched, and every hair on his head was in place.

Foster's injured professionalism has been advanced as the single cause of his death, but as a forensic psychiatrist I reject that explanation as too simple. Stock ideas about suicide have no place in a true understanding of this complex subject. At best, the broadest statement that can be made about suicide is that its goal is to escape intolerable and excruciating mental pain and problems of living, considered to be solvable only by self-destruction.

The specific circumstances of every apparent suicide are unique and must be thoroughly investigated. In Foster's case, the more plausible explanation is an unrecognized and untreated psychiatric disorder. On June 30, 1994, Whitewater Special Counsel Robert Fiske, citing conclusive forensic evidence, officially determined that Foster's death was a suicide. The report describes his severe depression and symptoms of panic. Consumed by depression, he could not eat or sleep. Panic caused his heart to pound and his stomach to boil. He could not concentrate.

I have seen patients who have tolerated depression for years but who could not tolerate both depression and panic. It is one thing to feel depressed and hopeless, but life can become intolerable when one is also constantly terrified. The combination of severe depression and debilitating panic attacks likely proved fatal for Vincent Foster. Both disorders are associated with an increased risk of suicide. It is particularly tragic because both conditions usually can be effectively and simultaneously treated with antidepressants. But it is likely that conspiracy theories will proliferate because definite answers are themselves improbable in apparent suicides.

Vincent Foster's death was quickly judged a suicide. So, too, for a time, were the deaths of two other notables, Marilyn Monroe and Robert Maxwell. On August 5, 1962, at 4:30 A.M., the Los Angeles police found Marilyn Monroe dead in her home. The cause of her death was unknown, but some considered it a suicide. On November 4, 1991, publishing tycoon Robert Maxwell's naked body was found floating in the calm waters off Grand Canary Island. Similarly, some considered Maxwell's death a suicide. But were these really suicides? Let us first examine the facts of these two deaths.

Marilyn Monroe

On that morning in 1962, Marilyn Monroe was found lying nude, face down, with a sheet pulled over her body. Her habit was to sleep naked. No suicide note was found. The night before her death, no disturbance had been heard by her neighbors, who knew her and considered her a good neighbor. On the morning after her death, an autopsy was conducted by Deputy Coroner Thomas Noguchi, M.D. Five days later, the Los Angeles coroner rendered a preliminary judgment that Monroe had died of a possible barbiturate overdose. On August 17, that judgment was amended to probable suicide. Ten days later, the coroner issued his final judgment, saying that Monroe died of acute barbiturate poisoning that followed an overdose.

The coroner's decision was based on toxicologic analysis, for no external signs of violence to the body were found. Blood analysis revealed 8 mg of chloral hydrate, a non-narcotic sedative, and 4.5 mg of pentobarbital, a sedative barbiturate. A much higher concentration (13 mg) of pentobarbital was found in the liver. It was theorized that the chloral hydrate may have interfered with the metabolizing of the pentobarbital and increased the pentobarbital's lethal potential.

Many drug bottles were found at Monroe's bedside table, some full, others half-empty. One bottle contained antihistamines for a sinus condition. An empty canister, dated August 3—only 2 days before her death—had previously contained twenty-five 100-mg pentobarbital capsules. There were also ten 500-mg capsules of chloral hydrate, and the remainder of a 50-capsule bottle dated July 25 and refilled on July 31st, which had been prescribed by Monroe's longtime psychiatrist, Dr. Ralph Greenson.

Dr. Greenson spoke with a suicide prevention team that the coroner had assembled to compile a psychological profile of Monroe at the time of her death. This was done so the coroner could more judiciously consider whether there had truly been a suicide. Neither Dr. Greenson nor Monroe's caretaker, Eunice Murray, believed she had deliberately taken her life. Other evidence assembled by the team showed that Monroe had not been mentally unbalanced or physically dependent on drugs. Her drug intake was considered to be light to medium. Pressed to make a decision—as one member later admitted—the team concluded that Monroe had either committed suicide or had made a suicide gesture that had turned lethal. The coroner's office was reportedly anxious to have the investigation completed, to issue a death certificate, and to put the Monroe matter behind them.

Because the controversy over her death has continued to this day, that last aim was never achieved. The haste with which the suicide investigation was conducted almost ensured that the case would, at least in the mind of the public, remain open. It has been reported that Dr. Noguchi and other forensic experts familiar with the facts at the time did not believe that Marilyn Monroe committed suicide. For example, they had learned that Monroe had made positive plans for the future. Also, the difference in drug levels in the blood and liver suggested that she had lived many hours after ingesting the pentobarbital. Further, the forensic experts cited the fact that no trace of the drugs had been found in her stomach or duodenum. To them, this meant that a lethal dose of pentobarbital could not have been taken by mouth or by injection. (An examination of the body with a magnifying glass concluded that there were no needle marks.)

In a biography of Monroe, author Donald Spoto examined carefully and rejected all the fanciful theories that contend Monroe's death was ordered because she "knew too much" about the Kennedy family. However, Spoto was convinced that her two caregivers, an attendant and Dr. Greenson, were accomplices in her death. He theorized that they could not tolerate Monroe's emerging independence and capacity to achieve happiness apart from them. Spoto believed that Dr. Greenson had become so enmeshed in Monroe's life that her plan for imminent departure to a new life was an intolerable rejection of him, one that impaired his professional treatment of her. Spoto contended that the chloral hydrate enema ordered by Dr. Greenson for Monroe capriciously imperiled her. There is no evidence, however, that Dr. Greenson consciously attempted to harm Marilyn Monroe.

Was Marilyn Monroe's death a suicide, murder, or an accident? We may never know, because there was no opportunity to do a complete forensic psychiatric autopsy or postmortem evaluation drawing on how she lived her life in the days and weeks prior to her death.

Robert Maxwell

A few days before Robert Maxwell's death, he had suddenly ordered the captain of his yacht to sail for Madeira and Tenerife Island, off the northwestern coast of Africa. The captain reached Grand Canary Island and sailed around it, since Maxwell had decreed no particular course. At approximately 5 A.M. on that morning in 1991, Maxwell called the bridge to complain that his room was too cold. Then, unseen by anyone, he made his way up to the deck and either fell, jumped, or was pushed to his death. Was it suicide? An accident? Murder? Or natural causes? The answer was not an academic matter, for if it could be determined that Maxwell's death was accidental, his family could collect $36 million from his life insurance.

Maxwell had been a billionaire, the exuberant wielder of enormous power through his newspapers and other businesses, and through statesmen whom he had befriended. Given Maxwell's previously demonstrated ability to rebound from personal scandals and business disasters, suicide seemed out of character for him, although he—much more than Marilyn Monroe—seemed to have had reasons for committing suicide. Adversity had always inspired him. He seemed to crave challenges. Many who knew him, however, came to the conclusion that his death was not an accident, or by natural causes, such as cardiac arrest either before his fall into the ocean, or by the shock of the water. They believed he had committed suicide to avoid complete personal disgrace and jail that might await him upon his return to England. Outraged bankers and members of his own corporate board were scheduled to confront him about the disappearance of corporate assets and monies from pension funds. These intimates believed that for Maxwell, who desperately sought the respect of people in high places, the humiliation that would have followed revelations about the disappearing assets would have been unbearable—and, therefore, pushed him to a shame suicide.

Some believed that Maxwell had not died at all and that the body identified by family members was that of someone else. The Spanish authorities who recovered the body refused to do a dental plate comparison. They could not use fingerprints on file because the files were too old. The autopsy that they performed was suspect because it described the corpse as having chestnut-colored hair, when Maxwell's was gray and dyed jet black. Other people—members of Maxwell's family—advanced the theory that Maxwell had been murdered by a treasonous crew member or by a frogman assassin.

What was known about Maxwell's personality gave rise to these and other theories because he was an enormously complex man of myriad contradictions, capricious behaviors, mood swings, and dark corners of mind. Some intimates thought he possessed multiple personalities; one, a former editor, believed him to have had as many as 20, each struggling with the others for control.

Evidence that Maxwell lived in a fantasy world of some sort was not hard to find. He had invented his background, his name, and parts of himself. Born Jan Ludwik Hock, he changed his name at various times to Leslie DuMaurier, James Maxwell, Ian Maxwell, and finally Robert Maxwell. He told people that he had been with the Czech underground in World War II, fighting the Nazis. But his tales were unsubstantiated and also at odds with the facts of the underground activity in the area of Czechoslovakia where he had lived at that time. Maxwell once refused to be interviewed by a Jewish magazine, asserting that he had joined the Church of England, but later claimed that the conversion was only a prank played on a journalist.

The most likely theory of Maxwell's death is that he killed himself because he was at a point in his life where the final identity that he had created for himself was about to be destroyed. The idea of Maxwell having multiple personality disorder also provides a theory if, in fact, Maxwell suffered from this disorder. It was not beyond possibility that because of the extreme stress of events, a murderous alter personality could have emerged and killed Maxwell. The explanation of his death could also be a lot simpler: a Spanish pathologist took note of the fact that Maxwell's stomach contained a barely digested banana and surmised that he could have slipped on a banana peel and fallen to his death.

Suicide, Accident, Murder, or Natural Death? Enter the Forensic Psychiatrist

What happened in the deaths of Vincent Foster, Marilyn Monroe, and Robert Maxwell—that despite the availability of sophisticated scientific analyses, the intent to suicide has not been definitively established but also cannot be definitively dismissed—is often true of suicides. Although most suicides are intentional, some are not, as I explain later in this chapter. What appears to be a suicide, even if unintended, may be murder. For example, preliminary results of a recent forensic examination on the exhumed body of germ warfare researcher Frank R. Olson appear to contradict government conclusions that he jumped to his death in 1953 from a Manhattan hotel after unwittingly taking LSD in a CIA experiment. This recent finding at last verified the suspicion, long held by Olson's family, that he was murdered.

Murder Masquerading as Suicide

Murder masquerading as suicide is not rare. It is less likely to occur with a public figure or celebrity, however, because close scrutiny may uncover the deception. Murder masquerading as suicide is more likely to remain unsolved when the individual murdered has a history of mental illness.

> Angela, a 36-year-old married but separated woman, was found hanging naked in her bedroom closet by her landlord. Her knees were approximately 4 inches off the floor. The police found no signs of a struggle in the apartment, and no suicide note. Angela had told friends and coworkers that she was taking a few days off to put the finishing touches on a novel she was writing. A manuscript was found on her desk. She did not have significant financial problems.
>
> The body was cut down so as to preserve the knot made for the noose. Fingerprints were obtained but were inconclusive. The forensic pathologist retained by the prosecution opined in her report that the death was suspicious. She noted that suicide by hanging is not a preferred method for women. The slipknot that was used contained clumps of the deceased's hair tangled within the knot. The forensic pathologist stated that persons who hang themselves usually do so with a simple slipknot that is not intertwined with their hair. The slip-

knot is tied first and then the noose is placed over the head without entangling the hair in the knot. The rope around Angela's neck was on a horizontal plane, as if it were tightened first before any strain was applied. The forensic pathologist explained that a diagonal misplacement is more pronounced in suicides. The rope's impression on Angela's neck was not as pronounced as seen in hanging deaths. Moreover, the forensic pathologist observed that women who kill themselves do not ordinarily do so in a naked state. Furthermore, it could not be determined whether Angela sustained any trauma to her body because of advanced bodily decay. There was no evidence of a sexual assault. Blood analysis did not indicate evidence of drugs or alcohol. The pathologist concluded that Angela was murdered.

The defense's forensic pathologist's report states that it is not uncommon for hair to become entangled in a noose, that no conclusions should be drawn from the knots used, and that his experience was that women hang themselves in various states of undress. Also, the angle of the ligature was an equivocal piece of evidence. This pathologist concluded that Angela's death was a "garden-variety" suicide.

After further investigation, the police learned that Angela's husband, age 49, a retired military officer, had a police record for spousal abuse. After 10 years of marriage, Angela was planning a divorce. A year prior to her death she had obtained a protective order against her husband for stalking. Witnesses testified that Angela was afraid of being stalked again by her husband, who had once threatened to kill her. She had begun a new romantic relationship at work. Angela had told friends that her husband said that he would kill her rather than "give her up" to another man. Neighbors provided sworn statements that they had heard loud, angry voices and the sound of furniture falling over at about the time of Angela's death. One witness saw the husband's car in the parking lot and observed him entering the apartment building where Angela lived at around the time of her death. Hair samples found in Angela's apartment matched those of her husband.

The husband was questioned but denied any knowledge of Angela's death. He claimed that he had not spoken to his wife in more than a year. He stated that she had an extensive psychiatric history, and had attempted suicide on several previous occasions. His alibi was that he was out of town attending a regatta during the time his wife had died, but the alibi could not be substantiated.

Because of the suspicious circumstances, the district attorney requested a postmortem psychiatric assessment to determine the presence or absence of suicide risk factors at the time of Angela's death. Witness statements and medical and psychiatric records were obtained and reviewed. The records indicated that she had developed bulimia nervosa at age 17. The breakup of a romantic relationship had resulted in depression, superficial wrist cutting, and a brief hospitalization at age 19. A maternal grandmother had attempted suicide during a postpartum depression. The inpatient psychiatrist had made a diagnosis of Angela as having an adjustment disorder with depression.

Angela had married at age 26 after graduating from college with a master's in business administration. Because of psychological and physical abuse by her husband—a particularly violent beating—she then sought outpatient treatment. Her physical injuries included six fractured ribs and a facial fracture. Her husband was arrested, briefly jailed, and ordered to attend a treatment program for wife abusers. Angela's new psychiatrist diagnosed dysthymic disorder (chronic depression). He noted that Angela had experienced brief flurries of unbidden suicidal thoughts after being assaulted, but had no suicidal intent or plan. As a way of medicating her marital stress symptoms, she occasionally drank wine excessively. She received 3 years of psychiatric treatment, which ended 1 year before she obtained the protective order.

Further information of note came from Angela's parents, who revealed that she was about to receive a $500,000 inheritance from an aunt who had recently died. Angela and her husband knew of this bequest. Angela's husband was a secondary beneficiary of the inheritance as long as the couple remained officially married.

The estranged husband was indicted for second-degree murder, convicted, and sentenced to life in prison.

Did You Intend It?

An individual may have no intention of dying when he or she makes a suicide gesture—the sole purpose of the gesture may be as a cry for help or to bring about a desired result, in a relationship or in the external world.

Friedrich Nietzsche, in *Beyond Good and Evil*, said, "The thought of suicide is a great consolation: by means of it one gets successfully through many a bad night." For some very disturbed patients, the freedom to terminate one's own life is a fundamental solace. It is conservatively estimated that 30,000 people kill themselves each year. In fact, the actual figure is likely much higher. The World Health Organization estimates that nearly a million people around the globe take their lives each year, The same organization also estimates that 10 to 20 million people attempt suicide each year. Almost everyone has thought of suicide at one time or another, usually when seriously depressed or during a difficult personal crisis. Although there is quite a spectrum of intent among those who have contemplated suicide, often only a fine line exists between those who think about suicide and those who actually commit it.

In my clinical experience, patients may be suicidal for just seconds, minutes, or hours. Other patients have been seriously suicidal for days, weeks, months, years, or much of their lives. Sometimes a quirk of fate makes the only difference in whether a person survives a suicide attempt. One of my patients, prior to coming to me for treatment, survived a massive overdose of pills that she took as she lay in a bathtub full of water. It was in the middle of winter. The water rapidly cooled as she lost consciousness, lowering her metabolism enough so that she survived until the next day, when she was discovered by her housekeeper. Having attempted suicide once and failed, she never again had the urge to harm herself. However, of those who do commit suicide, anywhere from 9% to 33% have made previous attempts. It is estimated that 8 to 25 suicide attempts occur for every completed suicide. Between 7% and 12% of patients who make suicide attempts commit suicide within 10 years, which means that attempted suicide is a significant risk factor for suicide.

In the United States, the statistics on suicide provide some hard facts. The rate of suicide in the general population in 2005 was 11 per 100,000 people per year. The rate has remained steady for many years. For persons with schizophrenia, mood disorders, or those who abuse alcohol or drugs, the rate soars to 180 per 100,000. In one study, the leading methods of suicide were

- Firearms, 60% (males 65%, females 40%)
- Hanging, 14% (males 15%, females 12%)
- Gaseous poisons, 10% (males 8%, females 11%)
- Solid/liquid poisons, 9% (males 6%, females 27%)
- All other methods, 7% (males 6%, females 10%)

The family and friends of suicide victims are at increased risk of suicide themselves. They are also more vulnerable to physical and psychological disorders. Suicide intent is frequently an issue in criminal cases in which it must be determined if the victim was murdered or committed suicide. In civil litigation, determination of intent is necessary to recover death benefits under insurance policies, in legal actions involving workers' compensation benefits, in malpractice claims, and when suicide is alleged to be the result of injurious actions by third parties. The most insidious tangle is in regard to insurance benefits.

Insurance companies that suspect suicide may invoke a policy's exclusionary clause to deny responsibility to pay benefits, whereas the deceased individual's estate may contend that the death was accidental and not suicide. Stakes regarding suicide intent can be as large as the $36 million riding on the cause of Robert Maxwell's death.

Why Naked Suicide?

Legend has it that when Cleopatra committed suicide by allowing the bite of an asp, she was naked. A famous painting of Cleopatra's death reveals an obvious erotic theme. Both Marilyn Monroe and Robert Maxwell were naked when discovered dead, she in her bed, he floating in the ocean. There is little mystery about Monroe's naked state, since she was known to sleep in the nude. Why Maxwell was naked when he died is a mystery, and the authorities seemed to take little note of it in their autopsy. They should have. As an expert witness in a number of suicide cases in litigation, I found that in approximately 5% of my cases, the individual committed suicide naked. Even so, attorneys and other experts in most of the cases showed little interest in the fact of the suicide's nakedness. Only in one case did it make a difference; the attorneys for the defense in a suicide malpractice case postulated that the patient was found hanging naked as the result of an autoerotic asphyxia gone wrong. The case was settled.

Most naked suicides are fraught with psychological meaning, if that meaning can be divined. The professional literature has little data on the topic. Most information is anecdotal, coming from individuals who have attempted suicide naked, but survived. The reasons given reflect highly individual psychodynamics in each instance. I have asked a number of experienced psychiatrists for their interpretation of naked suicide. Many spontaneously recited Job 1:21: "Naked came I out of my mother's womb, and naked shall I return." Other psychiatrists postulated that naked suicide symbolizes a new beginning, a rebirth and cleansing or a sloughing off of an intolerable world. Naked suicide challenges the forensic psychiatrist's sleuthing abilities.

Mysterious Deaths: The Psychological Autopsy

The psychological autopsy originated in 1958, from the Los Angeles Suicide Prevention Center, to assist the Los Angeles County Medical Examiner's Office in distinguishing drug overdoses from suicides. The basic principles for performing the psychological autopsy were established, as was its goal: the psychological autopsy is a procedure that assists in the classification of equivocal deaths, where the manner of death is unclear. A lack of standardization of the psychological autopsy procedures is a significant limitation on the practice, raising admissibility issues in criminal and civil cases.

Forensic psychiatrists are experts who understand the pertinent legal issues as they apply to psychiatric cases before the court. They translate psychiatric principles into the language of intent as it is defined by the legal system. Forensic psychiatry is a recognized subspecialty of psychiatry, and specialists can earn board certification. Years ago, forensic psychiatrists were known primarily for their work with criminals. Today, they also consult on a wide variety of administrative, legislative, and civil law matters, some of them involving suicide.

The forensic psychiatrist is frequently called upon in insurance litigation to evaluate suicide intent, sometimes by the plaintiff—the estate that is bringing the suit—and sometimes by the defendant—the insurance company. Although, as Oliver Wendell Holmes once observed, "Even a dog knows the difference between being tripped over and being kicked," the forensic psychiatrist's job in establishing suicide intent can be a complex, daunting task. The basic problem comes from the fact that psychiatry and law have views that differ in trying to understand the conundrum of suicide intent. Psychiatric theories of behavior tend to be deterministic; that is, they say that the individual contends with psychological forces that are often beyond his or her control. On the other hand, legal theories are based on the belief that humans have free will—that they are not deterministic. In evaluating suicide intent, therefore, the forensic psychiatrist must keep both understandings in mind, adapt psychiatric principles to the legal framework, and perform what is, in essence, a psychological autopsy.

The *intentional injury exclusion* of insurance policies is designed to prevent enrichment for immoral or illegal acts that have been performed by a *competent* individual. Competency itself is vague and complicated. When is someone competent, and when not? It is necessary in individual suicide cases to determine whether the victim intended to end his or her life. Approximately 90% to 95% of all those who commit suicide are suffering from a mental disorder. In a given case, did the individual understand that the self-destructive act would end his or her physical existence or was he or she not able to understand that?

One factor affecting the legal definition of *intent* is the presumption against suicide that is maintained in many jurisdictions. This presumption is a legal restatement of the common belief that the instinct for self-preservation in a rational person renders suicide improbable. This, of course, is not always true. So-called rational suicides occur, for example, among individuals who have terminal illnesses.

In elderly persons or persons suffering from chronic or terminal illnesses, deciding when a contemplated suicide is rational can be a very tricky business. I have been asked to assess elderly persons who were refusing food, water, and essential medications. In a number of instances, the elderly person's caretaker assumed that the patient had decided that he or she has lived long enough and has made a rational decision to die. Yet a majority of these persons were depressed and, in reality, were committing silent suicide. Their response to antidepressant medications was often rapid and gratifying.

Evidence of intent is generally derived from two basic sources. The first is from the persons who knew the individual's behavior and desires for some time prior to the moment of death—such as family members, friends, neighbors, coworkers, and treating physicians. The second source is forensic, and is provided by experts and based on the development of all relevant information about the individual at or around the time of death. In an insurance claim contest, this latter information will be given by forensic psychiatrists, who attempt to determine the *most likely* psychological reason or cause for the insured person's death.

In doing our forensic psychiatric work in an equivocal suicide case, we attempt to reach a detailed understanding of the deceased person's life because the way a person lived has a bearing on how and why he or she died. The key to the establishment of intent, then, depends on the establishment of motive. What could have been the reasons for wanting to die, that is, to have an intent to commit suicide? A terminally ill patient who refuses further medical treatment may seem to be, but is not necessarily, committing suicide. He or she may not intend to die, but rather, to live free of useless, burdensome, or painful medical treatments. Especially in regard to the elderly and chronically ill, the forensic psychiatrist must distinguish between suicide and the desire not to prolong the process of dying. Suicide notes may establish a motive, but such notes are found in only about one-third of all cases.

To reconstruct the psychological life of an individual who is suspected of having committed suicide is to perform a psychological autopsy. In systemic risk assessment, forensic psychiatrists thoroughly examine the person's lifestyle, circumstances, and the feelings, thoughts, and behaviors that existed during the days and weeks prior to death. This permits a better understanding of the psychological events of those last weeks and the circumstances that might have contributed to the death, considering both suicide risk and protective factors. Table 9–1 is a conceptual model of suicide risk assessment used in assessing suicidal patients and in determining whether a person committed suicide or died of other causes. Other models of suicide risk assessment are available, but none have been tested for reliability and validity.

In a psychological autopsy, what we look for are ways to evaluate the ability of the deceased to *conceive*, *plan*, and *execute* suicide, and to evaluate that within the legal concept of *intent*. A failure in any one of these three basic phases of mental functioning may indicate that the deceased lacked the mental capacity to intend suicide. However, the presence of ability to conceive, plan, and execute suicide does not necessarily ensure that the deceased had sufficient mental capacity to intend suicide. For example, one could conceive and plan violent acts with the greatest diligence and execute them with remarkable elegance, and still be mentally deranged by delusions and thereby be considered as lacking the mental capacity to fully intend a violent act. In some jurisdictions, the presence in the deceased of serious mental illness may negate any finding of intent. In other jurisdictions, even if the person has been totally psychotic, he or she can still be determined to have had suicide intent. If the psychotic individual did not understand what he or she was doing, would that mean intent was absent? For example, was there intent to die if a person on LSD was convinced that he or she could fly off a building and not be harmed? In that instance, I would conclude that the intent was not to commit suicide.

Complex and nuanced medical-psychiatric issues are often present in determining intent to commit suicide. The psychiatrist who only treats patients, or who seldom thinks along the lines necessary for forensic evaluation, has a tendency to overidentify with the family of the bereaved and give a judgment that favors the family over the insurer. Forensic psychiatrists, trained in clearly separating the treatment component from the role of evaluator, are more able to minimize or to avoid emotionally biased conclusions in litigation.

It is important to evaluate the person's state of mind in relation to the legal question at hand, for example, to evaluate intent to commit

TABLE 9–1.	Systematic suicide risk assessment: a conceptual model		
Assessment factors[a]		**Risk**	**Protective**
Individual			
Distinctive clinical features (prodrome)			
Religious beliefs			
Reasons for living			
Clinical			
Current attempt (lethality)			
Therapeutic alliance			
Treatment adherence			
Treatment benefit			
Suicidal ideation			
Suicidal intent			
Suicide plan			
Hopelessness			
Prior attempts (lethality)			
Panic attacks			
Psychic anxiety			
Loss of pleasure and interest			
Alcohol/drug abuse			
Depressive turmoil (mixed states)			
Diminished concentration			
Global insomnia			
Psychiatric diagnoses (Axis I and Axis II)			
Symptom severity			
Comorbidity			
Recent discharge from psychiatric hospital			
Impulsivity			
Agitation (akathisia)			
Physical illness			
Family history of mental illness (suicide)			
Childhood sexual/physical abuse			
Mental competency			

(continued)

TABLE 9–1. **Systematic suicide risk assessment:**
a conceptual model *(continued)*

Assessment factors[a]	Risk	Protective
Interpersonal relations		
Work or school		
Family		
Spouse or partner		
Children		
Situational		
Living circumstances		
Employment or school status		
Financial status		
Availability of guns		
Managed care setting		
Demographic		
Age		
Gender		
Marital status		
Race		
Overall risk ratings[b]		

[a]Rate risk and protective factors present as low (L), moderate (M), high (H), nonfactor (0), or range (e.g., L–M, M–H).
[b]Judge overall suicide risk as low, moderate, high, or a range of risk.

Source.   Adapted from Simon and Hales 2006. Used with permission.

suicide as defined in the insurance policy signed by the deceased and by the laws of the jurisdiction. The legal context evaluates *motive, intent,* and *act* in regard to a particular happening. In clinical psychiatric contexts, it is *conception, planning,* and *execution* that must be assessed, and the two sets of notions are only roughly similar. Here, as in other clinical-legal contexts, an imperfect fit exists between psychiatry and the law.

Conception (Motive)

How, when, and why the idea of attempting or completing suicide arises in a person must be critically analyzed, especially in a court case.

Was it a sudden and impulsive act, or was it planned in considerable detail? Was the suicide committed in a fit of rage or during a bout of drunkenness? Was the suicide the outgrowth of depression or schizophrenia? Can one find evidence of a plan to commit suicide, say, in the fact that an individual was mired in financial problems and might hope by death to provide for his or her family through insurance death benefits? Consider the following case:

> A 57-year-old chairman of the board of a once successful manufacturing company, which he had built up through years of hard work, is facing difficult choices. Business reverses and intense competition have brought on a crisis. Banks are demanding payments on loans that are overdue and are refusing to refinance those loans. The chairman sinks his personal fortune into the company in the fight to keep it afloat. He takes a substantial cut in his own salary. His wife of 28 years is worried, because in all that time, she has never seen him so upset. He seems "panicked" about their personal finances.
>
> The couple's three children are in college, and he wants to keep them there. He himself never had the benefit of a college education. He cannot bear the thought that if the financial situation continues to worsen, he might not be able to pay the balance of their tuitions. He hints to his wife and friends that he has a plan to improve his financial situation. At work, he seems to function without difficulty. He does not seek out a mental health professional, nor does he seem to co-workers to be depressed.
>
> One morning, the chairman works until 11 A.M. and then departs in his car for a meeting in another part of town. The weather is clear. En route to that meeting, and traveling at 80 miles per hour, his car strikes a bridge abutment. He dies instantly in the crash.
>
> Police examination of the scene reveals no skid marks from his car. No other vehicles were involved in the crash. It could not be established that there were any pre-crash mechanical problems with his car. An autopsy finds equivocal evidence that he had had an acute heart attack. No suicide note is found. The death certificate states that the cause of death is natural. The workers' compensation insurance carrier, however, conducts its own investigation and concludes that the death was a suicide. It refuses to pay out on his policy.
>
> The forensic psychiatrist retained by the family of the deceased, and charged with the task of performing a psychological autopsy, does not automatically accept the death certificate finding, nor does she reject it. Death certificates frequently do not address the matter of suicidal intent or lack of it. The death certificate is a document whose purpose is to provide vital statistical data. It is not based on the totality of evidence that may later become available. The forensic psychiatrist

cannot simply accept the postmortem finding of a possible heart attack either, because it is not in keeping with the weight of the other evidence. For instance, it was discovered that shortly before his death, the deceased had put all of his affairs in order.

The forensic psychiatrist's examination of the chairman's life reveals a man who was very disciplined and who rarely acted impulsively. He led a quiet life, had conservative habits and tastes. No history of alcohol abuse, drug abuse, or gambling was present. Family, financial stability, and occupational success and gratification are no longer protective factors against suicide.

The workers' compensation law in the deceased's state reads that the insurer could refuse to pay compensation "if the injury or death resulted from the person's intent to injure or kill himself." The forensic psychiatrist concludes that despite the absence of evidence of a mental disorder such as depression or psychosis, the preponderance of the available evidence (more likely than not) showed that the chairman had intended to kill himself, in a suicide staged as an accident, to provide financially for his family. The chairman's *conception* or *motive* for killing himself was likely the result of his declining financial status and the perception that further decline would produce dire consequences for his family. His *plan* was to cause his death through a staged accident and thereby enable his family to cash in on his large insurance policy. *Execution* of the plan of suicide was carried out by crashing the car into the bridge. The three conditions required to find intent to suicide were thus met. The forensic psychiatrist presented her findings to the family. They discharged her and decided to seek another expert opinion.

In the matter of conception or motive, there are suicides that are not motivated or not intended. Some people who suffer from brain disorders may be considered unable to conceive or to have a motive for suicide, but they occasionally randomly or impulsively kill themselves—or others. Trauma to the head or drug and alcohol intoxication can cause acute brain dysfunction accompanied by the unleashing of violence. The resulting acts, even when directed against the impaired person, may not meet the legal criteria for intent to commit suicide, in part because it is so obvious that the other two conditions, planning and execution, have not been met.

Certain "suicides" are also just as clearly not intended, although they involve no physical brain disorder. For example, a person may plan a suicide gesture. The motivation may show the intent is only a cry for help or the desire to manipulate a situation or another person, but, through miscalculation, the suicide gesture may result in death.

Miscalculations also occur in other kinds of death that initially may appear to be suicides, such as in autoerotic asphyxia. This is an attempt by young men to enhance sexual pleasure by decreasing the flow of oxygen to the brain. If miscalculated, it can result in death by hanging, even though the real motive was only to produce a heightened sexual experience while masturbating.

Planning (Intent)

One can conceive the idea of suicide but fail in the intent or planning of it. Persons driven by impulse, by psychosis that produces a break with reality, or by intoxicants may have lost the ability to plan a violent act, even though they have thought about it for some time. The event may still happen, however, even if it is not actually planned. Intoxicants may destabilize the person and prematurely precipitate a violent act. For example, consider this case:

> A 33-year-old minor league baseball player harbors a grudge against a former major league coach. The player has often been heard by other players to threaten physical harm to that coach, who he feels has thwarted the player's major league career. One evening, while intoxicated with alcohol and cocaine, he takes a baseball bat and bludgeons to death a different person, the coach of an opposing minor league team, and then fatally shoots himself.
>
> Citing the intentional-injury clause of the player's team liability insurance, the carrier disallows payment to the deceased coach's family. Litigation follows. The forensic psychiatrist conducts interviews with players from both teams, which reveal that the murdered coach was liked and admired by the player who killed him. Postmortem blood analysis of the player reveals the presence of cocaine and a blood alcohol level of 0.23 (intoxicated).
>
> In this case, forensic psychiatric analysis reached the conclusion that the player's toxic mental state, brought on by cocaine and alcohol, had caused the release of a violent act against an unintended victim. This indicated the inability to plan. The murder-suicide, then, was unintended; it was, instead, an impulsive act.

Another case illustrates a different cause for failure of intent:

> A 28-year-old depressed, devoutly religious woman, a week after the birth of her first child, awakes to intense command auditory hallucinations. She writes a note to her husband: "God commanded me this morning to bring myself and the baby to Him immediately. God said

we will not die but live forever. I must obey God. I know you will understand." Leaving the note for her husband, she gathers their child in her arms and jumps from the 18th-story apartment.

Forensic psychiatric examination reveals that the woman had a stable personality prior to the birth of the child, but that a severe psychotic depression emerged after childbirth. The suicide note clearly indicates an acute postpartum psychosis. Having a newborn child was not a protective factor against suicide in this instance, as it is in many others. The psychiatrist reports to the court that in this instance, the planning phase of suicide was nonexistent because the woman heard the auditory hallucinations that compelled her to act immediately. Such command hallucinations can be extremely powerful psychotic symptoms that can force action in the here and now. Another factor that affects the psychiatrist's understanding of the case is that women who intend suicide often do not use a method of suicide that will leave them disfigured. They choose a method that does not involve smashing themselves on the ground. This testimony is challenged by the opposing expert as not having any scientific merit. The court rules that the deceased did not intend suicide because when she jumped, she did not want or expect to die.

Execution (Act)

An individual may be able to conceive and to plan a violent act, but the way in which the violence is manifested may indicate impairment of the individual's capacity to execute. Unintentional death, bizarre actions, and the inability to delay or to control behavior are strong indicators of the presence of severe psychiatric disorder. Consider the following case:

> A divorced rancher squanders his inheritance, runs into financial difficulties, and is in danger of losing his ranch. His older brother, by contrast, has invested his portion of the inheritance wisely and has accumulated considerable wealth. The two have had a falling out. The wealthy brother refuses to lend money to the rancher brother. The rancher conceives the idea of killing the brother's beloved wife and then shooting himself. This is no idle fantasy, for the rancher has been in frequent fights throughout his life and has a reputation for violence.
>
> The rancher waits until the brother is out of town on business and sets out to do the deed. He drinks three martinis before he goes. He

also leaves a note detailing his intentions. The note contains rambling comments about past grievances against the brother but also mentions "the good times" with him. The rancher hopes that he will change his mind about killing the sister-in-law before he arrives at her home. On his way to kill his sister-in-law, the rancher is involved in a minor automobile accident. An altercation develops. The rancher shoots and kills the other driver, and then kills himself.

The estate of the slain driver brings a claim against the rancher's excess liability insurance policy. This policy contains an exclusionary provision, which denies coverage for bodily injury or property damage "intentionally" caused by, or at the direction of, the insured.

The forensic psychiatrist interviews friends, acquaintances, and employees of the deceased rancher. He also culls the available records. The rancher's history of intense envy and ambivalent feelings toward his brother are revealed, as are his spendthrift and impulsive-spending ways. School, military, and police records demonstrate years of alcohol intoxication and fights. His blood-alcohol content at the time of death was 0.15 (intoxicated). Few, if any, protective factors against suicide existed, especially abstinence from alcohol.

The psychiatrist concludes that the rancher had the mental capacity to conceive and plan a violent act but lacked the capacity to execute the plan in the way that he had intended. As the rancher drove to his sister-in-law's house, the psychiatrist testified, his envy and rage were so great that the minor accident and altercation in which he was involved, combined with the alcohol that he had ingested, ignited the violence prematurely toward an unintended victim and himself.

The court decides to apply a narrow view of intent and makes a determination that the murder-suicide was the result of the altercation that came out of the accident. The court ruled that the rancher had known that he was firing a gun at the other driver and had wished to bring about a fatal result. The ambivalent feelings expressed in the note, the court opined, meant that the deceased might have changed his mind about his original target. The court's decision, therefore, was to uphold the injury exclusion clause of the policy and to deny payment to the family of the deceased driver of the second car.

Is Every Suicide a Murder?

As the various cases in this chapter make clear, the forensic psychiatrist's role in the retrospective assessment of lethal acts is a difficult and arduous task. It is also one in which the psychiatrist's judgment is not the final word. The law is pragmatic. It only requires testimony of "reasonable medical certainty," but reaching any sort of certainty is often hard to do. The evidence is often conflicting, and it is up to the court to decide what weight to give to each part of it. Moreover, the legal determination of whether a suicide occurred may depend heavily on criteria of intent applied by the courts. Ultimately, psychological interpretation of the web of facts and fantasy surrounding a mysterious death is an art based on a science, and art is a subjective undertaking. It is left to the courts to make the legal determination of suicide, accident, or murder.

In the world of the psychiatrist, distinctions are not and cannot be clear-cut. Violent rage reactions can change direction in a second. A person's murderous rage that erupts against someone else may, at the very last moment, be turned upon himself. Conversely, at the last second, a person who intends suicide may turn murderous rage outward and kill someone else. Or both things may happen: after committing a murder, and as part of the same violent act, the murderer may turn the same murderous impulse against himself or herself.

Many years ago, Karl Menninger, the famous American psychoanalyst, observed that almost every suicide is a murder. The recognition that murderous rage can go either way—directed outward or inward—is critically important in assessing the last mental stage in suicide and in murder. Suicide is often attempted or completed among a welter of unclear, confusing, and ambivalent feelings. In fact, only one thing about suicide is clear: the intent to kill oneself is hardly ever absolute.

10

Messianic Madness

Killer Cults to Holy Warriors

From fanaticism to barbarism is only one step.

—Diderot

On the morning of September 11, 2001, 19 members of an al-Qaeda suicide group board four passenger planes in three American cities. They have been told by their leader, Mohammed Atta, "The sky smiles, my young son," an expression of joy in death. Shortly, the cult members will hijack the airliners and fly them into the World Trade Center towers in New York, into the Pentagon in northern Virginia, and into a field in western Pennsylvania, killing themselves, hundreds of other passengers on the planes, and more than 3,000 people in the targeted buildings.

At Ranch Apocalypse, near Waco, Texas, the self-proclaimed messiah David Koresh gathers cult members from Israel, Jamaica, Great Britain, New Zealand, and Australia, as well as from the United States. He tells them no one will survive the coming battle, that it will be Armageddon. In Jonestown, Guyana, the Reverend Jim Jones calls his flock together over the loudspeaker for their last communion and tells them, "We're going to meet in another place," which they all understand to be heaven. At Rancho Santa Fe, California, the leader of the Heaven's Gate cult Marshall Herff Applewhite claims to be "King Do," the same celestial spirit that once occupied Christ. He convinces 39 members to commit suicide by drinking a cocktail of vodka and tranquilizers; they believe their deaths will bring them passage to a UFO trailing the Hale-Bopp comet. And in three separate incidents spanning several years, as many as 69 burned bodies of members of the mysterious Order of the Solar Temple are found, some having been murdered and others having committed suicide, in three locations in Quebec and Switzerland. Members of the international doomsday cult, thought to still be in existence, with fewer than 1,000 members, believe that ritualized suicide leads to rebirth on a planet called Sirius.

Armageddon in Texas

The Branch Davidians began with the visionary prophecies of a defrocked Seventh-Day Adventist minister, Bulgarian-born Victor Houteff. He declared that he had been appointed by God to "cleanse" the denominations of false believers. There were an estimated 2,000 to 3,000 Branch Davidians in the United States, some of whom followed David Koresh when the group split off. Those in the Waco sect included a Harvard-schooled lawyer, a nurse, a carpenter, and a computer expert.

Koresh had the ability to captivate his audience with a soft voice and a soothing Texas drawl. His marathon sermons frequently went on for 15 hours at a time. He had long preached the prophecy of Apocalypse Now: most of his sermons were drawn from the Book of Revelations, which contains the terrifying Four Horsemen of the Apocalypse, the forerunners of the Last Judgment. Koresh claimed that he could open the "seven seals" on the scroll in God's hand, a scroll that prophecies the calamities that will precede the apocalypse.

On February 28, 1993, officers of the federal bureau of Alcohol, Tobacco, and Firearms (ATF) first tried to enter the Davidian Mount Carmel compound near Waco, Texas, or Ranch Apocalypse, as it had been named by Koresh. They planned to arrest Koresh for illegal possession of automatic firearms and explosives. Their search warrant permitted the ATF agents to look for grenades, explosive devices, machine guns, and military assault rifles. The armed Davidians opened fire, killing four ATF agents and wounding sixteen others. Six cult members died in that confrontation, and many were wounded, including Koresh.

There followed weeks of frustrating negotiations between the Davidians and the federal authorities. During this time, families who had members within the cult compound, as well as former cult members, warned the authorities that the group was preparing for a final confrontation and were prepared to commit mass suicide. As the siege wore on toward the end of its second month, Koresh became increasingly erratic in his behavior, speaking constantly about the end of the world. In prolonged Bible study sessions, Koresh would make odd biblical interpretations and ramble in an incoherent manner. He was convinced that the ATF had infiltrated his group and was out to get him. He was ready, with enough arms to supply a small army, in a well-fortified compound with a fail-safe bunker.

On April 19, 1993, after a 51-day siege by the FBI and other federal authorities, agents using specially equipped tanks burst holes into the walls of the Mount Carmel compound, flooding it with a non-lethal, disabling gas. Within a short while, the compound burned to the ground, consuming an estimated 82 Branch Davidians, including Koresh and a number of children. Nineteen of the Davidians (including Koresh) were reported to have gunshot wounds, some self-inflicted. There was strong evidence that the fires had been deliberately set by the cult members. Later, criminal indictments would charge that in early April, several weeks before the government's assault, Koresh and his lieutenant, Steve Schneider, had decided to burn down the compound. At the trial of surviving Branch Davidians, one witness testified that Koresh had planned mass suicide.

Lethal Communion in Guyana

On November 18, 1978, the Reverend James Warren Jones summoned the more than 900 members of the Peoples Temple in Jonestown, Guyana, to their last communion in the central pavilion, where he told them that they all must die. "If you love me as much as I love you," Jones said, "we must all die or be destroyed from outside." Learning that Armageddon was at hand, mothers cuddled their children and asked, "What have they done?" On Jones's order, the medical team brought out the "holy wine," a battered tub containing a concoction of strawberry-flavored Kool-Aid and cyanide. As guards armed with guns and bows and arrows stood at the fringe of the crowd, ready to shoot anyone who tried to escape, Jones commanded that the babies be brought up first. Then the older children came together and followed his orders, lining up to accept their communion cups of poison. Parents and older folks followed. The "white night" mass suicide pact had been practiced many times before. As they stood in the gathering darkness, each person was given a small glass of red liquid. They were told by Jones that death would come in 45 minutes. The last communion was no rehearsal. Cult members were told that they would die today but be resurrected tomorrow. Some families came forward voluntarily. When some resisted, guards snatched babies from resisting mothers, holding them up so that "nurses" could spray cyanide down the babies' throats with hypodermic syringes. Sticking a gun into the ribs of a mother who would not stop clutching her 1-year-old son, a guard shouted, "You dumb bitch. You better do it or we're going to shoot your ass off." Tears running down her face, she injected the cyanide mix herself into the baby's mouth. Almost immediately, the child began to convulse and scream. An old man who resisted violently was knocked to the ground, his jaws pried open and cyanide poured down his throat. All the while, Jones was on the loudspeaker, exhorting his flock. "There is great dignity to dying," he called out. "It is a great demonstration for everyone to die."

Cult members who had drunk the Kool-Aid were taken away by guards and instructed to lie down in rows. Families and groups of friends grasped hands. Some embraced. Soon, they all began to gasp for air and retch. Blood poured out of their noses and mouths. Jones continually gave his benediction, repeating over and over, "I tried. I tried. I tried." Finally, he called out "mother," six times. A shot was fired, and Jones careened backward with a fatal bullet wound to his right temple. When the silence descended completely over the jungle commune, and the "service" was over, some 914 members of the cult were dead.

Definition of a Cult

What is a cult? It depends on who you ask and at what point in a group's lifespan the question is asked. Today the term *cult* is largely pejorative. To call a group a cult is a subjective judgment and not one that people inside the group might choose to make. Some Muslims consider the politically radical al-Qaeda group, which encourages suicide missions, a deviant cult. The early Christians were considered deviant cultists and persecuted accordingly. No one today would consider Christianity to be a cult. However, when the Protestants separated from the Catholic Church, they were treated as a heretical cult. Also considered cults at one time were the Church of Jesus Christ of Latter-Day Saints, the Christian Scientists, and the Jehovah's Witnesses. All these are now established, respected, denominational religious groups. Today, there are many nonreligious, charismatic treatment groups that emphasize the use of contemporary psychology. For example, Transcendental Meditation, the rage of the 70s and 80s, continues to gain adherents. Is it a cult? That, again, depends on who you ask.

Perhaps the most dispassionate understanding comes from social scientists, who divide religious groups into three categories: churches, sects, and cults. *Churches* tend to be large denominations with an open, welcoming approach to life and an identification with the prevailing culture. *Sects* follow their denominations in most aspects but are more strict on doctrinal matters and in the demands they make on an individual's behavior. Quaker and Mennonite sects, who have disavowed war, come to mind: many conscientious objectors have come from these sects. *Cults* follow an altogether different religious structure in that they are foreign and alien to the main stream of religious communities. Among the more widely known entities in this category are The Church Universal and Triumphant (Summit Lighthouse), Elan Vital (Divine Light Mission), The International Society for Krishna Consciousness ("Hare Krishnas"), the Unification Church (its members are called "Moonies," after their founder Sun Myung Moon), and the Church of Scientology. But it is important to remember that what may appear to be a cult for one person, may for another be a religion.

Psychiatrist Marc Galanter refers to cults as "charismatic groups." Such groups usually contain at least a dozen members and often many more. The members adhere to a strongly felt, mutually accepted belief system. They are highly enmeshed. Cult members are strongly influenced by the group's behavioral standards. They seek or undergo altered consciousness experiences, and they attribute charismatic (divinely inspired) power to the group or its leaders.

According to J. Gordon Melton, the author of the *Encyclopedic Handbook of Cults in America*, there are approximately 500 to 600 cults in the United States. Of these, about 100 are principally ethnic groups composed of first- and second-generation immigrants who only recruit within their own ethnic base. Other estimates put the total number of cults in the United States as much higher, in the range of 2,500. Cult Hotline and Clinic estimates the number of cults at 3,000 to 5,000 and says that 5 to 7 million Americans have been associated with cults or

cult-like groups at some point in their lives. Contrary to popular opinion, cults are just as prevalent today in the United States as they were
in decades past. Today's cults are more sophisticated, taking on new
names or mimicking established groups; they also splinter into other
groups, shut down, and morph into another configuration. The Hotline estimates that there are 180,000 new cult recruits every year.

Close observers have noted that cults perform both terrible and
positive deeds. Some cults have perpetrated horrible acts on their
neighbors, whereas some have provided people with productive and
uplifting experiences. Most cults fall in between the two extremes of
negative and positive, and their practices and aspirations are quite
common and ordinary. Killer cults are at the deviant extreme of the
cult spectrum. But many of the things that killer cults do—for example, how they attract members and how they are led—are represented
all along the spectrum. In many instances, what is common to the
most benign is also present in the most lethal of cults.

Most cults have reasonably stable structures and functions. They
generally have a written body of ideas and beliefs that govern relationships with others, the leader, the world, the cosmos, and God. *The Divine Principle*, the so-called *Moonie bible*, was written by the Unification
Church's Reverend Sun Myung Moon. As with similar tracts by other
cult leaders, this is considered to be divinely inspired. In the cult, "all
for one and none for the self" is the motto. The individual's self-worth
and survival are seen as intimately interwoven with the group's survival. Although most cults have leaders who are charismatic, it is not
required that a leader have charisma. Some groups themselves are
charismatic, evangelical, and very demanding of their members. Leaders can be old or young, male or female. The Divine Light Mission's
Maharaj Ji was 15 years old at the height of his popularity. The Reverend Moon is in his late 80s. Although male leaders are more common, female leaders are also found, principal among them Elizabeth
Clare, Prophet of the Church Universal and Triumphant.

Cults emerge whenever the structure of society is seriously threatened. During the upheavals of the Industrial Revolution in England,
the French Revolution, and the westward migration of large populations in the United States, for example, many such cults formed.
Closer to the present, when American society was disrupted by the
Vietnam War in the mid-1960s, many young people were attracted to
charismatic politicians and religious leaders. This was also a time

when there was fragmentation of the fundamental structures of society—the family, schools, and established churches. Many people were left susceptible to the seductive appeals of cults that provided total answers for life here and in the hereafter. The need to belong somewhere is irresistible to most humans. For many people in that era, the need was met by joining a "new" group.

Who Joins a Cult, and Why?

From this psychiatrist's perspective, the dangers in joining a cult are the stunting of one's personal growth and the surrendering of responsibility in exchange for what at best is spiritual security and what at worst is passive dependency. As Erich Fromm suggested in his book *Escape From Freedom*, to leave one's thinking to another is unlikely to be an enriching life experience.

Most cults look for specific kinds of recruits. Charles Dederich, the Synanon guru, specialized in rehabilitating drug addicts who were willing to make a life commitment to the cult. Jim Jones recruited the oppressed, particularly poor blacks, prostitutes, and other disaffected individuals interested in communal living and the pursuit of a socialist utopia. The Hare Krishnas, the Moonies, and the Children of God prefer idealistic, intelligent, college-educated recruits who will bring honor to the cult.

Most people who joined cults in the 60s and 70s reported that they came predominantly from upper middle-class socioeconomic backgrounds. They were young (median age 22), white, reasonably well-educated, and from intact families. The majority of members of such diverse cults as Elan Vital and the Unification Church attended college. They reported that at least one of their parents had also done so.

Psychiatrists have done studies to determine the mental health or illness of persons who join cults. Some outsiders may argue that anyone who joins a cult is deranged, but the studies do not confirm this proposition. A liberal estimate of significantly mentally troubled or disordered individuals among those who join cults is no more than one-third of the members. Some psychiatrists and psychologists argue that there is no evidence at all to suggest that members of cults are any more disturbed than are comparable peers who are not members.

Nonetheless, a significant number of sect members have reported themselves as being psychologically troubled. In fact, psychological distress has been found to be an important precursor to joining a cult. Psychological distress does not necessarily indicate the presence of mental disorder. Interviews conducted by clinicians among cult members, former members, and relatives of members paint a picture of young adults who are experiencing depression and serious personality disorders. New members have described experiencing feelings of inadequacy, sadness, loneliness, and rejection just before joining; many had limited social connections at the time. For people in the midst of a personal crisis, joining a cult has led some to experience a significant diminishing of their personal psychological suffering—at least, for a time. Yet many people seek and join mainstream religions for these very same reasons.

Cults can be powerfully seductive to individuals who have strong conscious and unconscious yearnings to be loved and nurtured. For such psychologically needy persons, cults may provide the guidance, purpose, love, nurturance, sense of belonging, relief from conflict, and self-control that they desperately seek. Much of this is done as the recruit establishes a personal relationship with the cult's charismatic leader. Religious cults offer direct contact with God through their own charismatic leaders. This appeals to recruits who seek a transcendent or enlightened spiritual experience.

The cult as a whole is an extension of the leader's personality and teachings. The leader's grandeur, as well as his or her association with divinity, provides an essential feeling of specialness and importance to cult members. For people who do not fit in anywhere or see themselves as misfits or outcasts, this connection to the leader is very compelling. Their relationship with the leader can "cure," or at least alleviate, some of the personal losses and deprivations that they may have experienced with their own families. Symbolic of this connection, the cult leader is often addressed as father or some version of the word, such as "baba." The leader's teachings offer all-encompassing prescriptions for having a world and cosmic view, as well as strict codes for day-to-day living. In these ways, the powerful parent figure provides a supplementary conscience for members who need support against their own aggressive, sexual, and drug-seeking behaviors that in the past have threatened to go out of control. Thus, the structure and direction provided by the cult restrains the dark side of some of its members.

It then becomes understandable why many members find it very difficult to extricate themselves from a cult or reject a leader who has been defrocked and exposed as a sham. To do so is to risk losing an idealized and idolized figure who has provided self-cohesion, life-meaning, and psychological support to the cult member. The highly troubled, vulnerable persons in Charles Manson's "family" found him to be a vitalizing force in their aimless, desolate lives. After their imprisonment, "family" members continued to espouse Manson's beliefs. Without the connection to Manson, they likely believed that their lives would shatter.

According to Melton's *Encyclopedic Handbook of Cults in America*, approximately 90% of those who join a cult leave within 1 year. More than 1 million people took the Transcendental Meditation course, yet the number of members in the United States remained steady in the 1980s at 10,000 to 20,000. Several hundred thousand people took the Unification Church's basic weekend introduction course; 30,000 to 40,000 joined up, but by 1990, fewer than 6,000 remained as members. Many members leave cults voluntarily, without having been deprogrammed—and also, it seems, without significant psychological consequences. For the fortunate who come out unharmed, it becomes just a phase they were passing through. When considering the spiritual and psychological experiences of cult members, one is reminded of William James's classic *The Varieties of Religious Experience*. James wrote that the religious experience can be normal or pathological, and that the spiritual experience can be sublime or painfully distorted by mental dysfunction. Similarly, according to the psychological needs of the cult member, a cult can be used for the purposes of illness or of health.

Cult Practices

Recruitment

One of the chief duties of cult members is recruitment. It is absolutely essential to the cult's survival and is practiced by most cults as both an art and a science. When seeking converts, timing is a key factor. Recruiters for cults come to college campuses, for example, when the students are most vulnerable, usually around exam time, or in the first months that students start to attend a college. Recruiters sit in libraries, waiting to make eye contact with students who exhibit some difficulty, hoping to find in such students the detritus of a broken romance, poor grades, or uncertainty about future goals. In cities and resorts, recruiters scope the scene, looking for backpacking students who have declared a moratorium on schoolwork or who are struggling with identity problems. Experts on cults recognize that everyone is susceptible to some form of organizational recruitment during their lives. UCLA law professor Richard Delgado, an expert on cults, says that "everyone is vulnerable. You and I could be Hare Krishnas if they approached us at the right time."

Cults speak to the universal dreams of mankind for nurturance, security, and certainty. The Grand Inquisitor of Dostoyevsky's *Brothers Karamazov,* when Christ returned to earth and spoke of giving mankind unlimited freedom, told the "stranger" to go away and never come back again. The Grand Inquisitor argued that people cannot bear the burden of freedom and responsibility for their own actions throughout life. They would prefer to cede direction for their lives over to some other authority. In the story, Christ appears to agree that that "burden" was best borne by the church of which the Grand Inquisitor was a high-ranking representative.

The Unification Church has perhaps the most sophisticated methods for acquiring potential cult members. The first phase is called "love bombing." A lonely student is spotted, drawn into friendly conversation, and invited to dinner. The student is soon surrounded by smiling faces and warm hands, and inundated with compliments. An invitation to a weekend retreat is extended. At the retreat, guests are urged to take part in endless exercise, singing, games, and oblique religious discussion. Little time is left for the potential recruit to sleep. Any probing questions by the potential recruit are discouraged. Monitors accompany them everywhere, including the bathroom. When Sunday arrives, potential converts are urged to stay for one last party. If the potential recruit calls family members or an employer to say that they will not be present on Monday, the Moonie recruiters know that the individual will stay for the full 7-day program.

That recruits stay for the entire program is essential, from the recruiters' point of view, because a basic tenet of most cults' conversion process is to isolate the recruit from the outside world, especially from family and friends. During the intense phase of conversion, recruits are made to feel guilty about their lives and past deeds. They are exhorted to become reborn and join their already cleansed and omniscient "brothers and sisters" in the cult family.

Many cults give converts new names. The Heaven's Gate cult added "ody" to its members' names to distinguish them from ordinary people. Some cults emphasize the new reality for recruits by defining time differently. For example, the day is divided by prescribed tasks and duties but is otherwise timeless. Other cults try to produce a new personality in the recruit through sensory deprivation, special diets, sleep deprivation, and by forcing the recruit to take part in endless, exhausting chants, prayers, and indoctrination sessions that focus on the cult leader's vision.

Although many cults recruit vulnerable people, the popular sense has been that they are the downtrodden of society—as indeed, they were in Jim Jones' Peoples Temple, in the cult led by ex-convict Charles Manson, and in many others. But the Branch Davidians came from a higher stratum of society. The Heaven's Gate cultists were so well educated that they had a business designing websites. One might hope that a cult made up of reasonably well-educated, well-off recruits from the middle and upper classes, from intact families, would not fall under the suicidal thrall of a deranged cult leader. Unfortunately, this has happened as a result of the power of cult psychology and of the deviant leader's dominance.

Location Is Everything

All cults try to maintain established meeting places for their activities. Even when a cult has a number of groups that are distributed far and wide, their meeting places display a remarkably uniform appearance. This phenomenon can also be observed in the uniform appearances of the churches of any more-established denominational religion, even though they are in different cities, and, sometimes, in different countries. Similarly, the Hare Krishna temples and the Divine Light Mission ashrams maintain a comforting uniformity that bespeaks continuity and certainty, and that exists regardless of location. When a cult maintains many branches in a country or throughout the world, it is less likely to deteriorate into a killer cult. What keeps it alive and functioning is contact with other cultures and dispersion of authority, both of which serve to counter the regressive forces within a cult.

However, when a cult goes into physical isolation, watch out. Such isolation allows deviant leaders and their teachings to fester. The Jim Jones group was relatively harmless when it was meeting regularly in a converted auditorium on Geary Street in San Francisco. But it became far more than that when its members retreated to a vastly different compound in the Guyana jungle. Similarly, when the Branch Davidians took up residence near Waco, Texas, where 77 acres had been purchased years earlier, more was changed than just their venue. The Heaven's Gate group was not dangerous when they first met in a hotel on the Oregon coast, but when they moved to an isolated location in southern California, they were ready for death and transfiguration.

Earthly Treasures

In their locations, whether isolated or not, the cults promulgate rules and regulations that are rigidly applied and observed by cult members. Many of these are calculated to foster fund-raising activities. Money, seemingly so unimportant in the spiritual life of the cult, is really of the essence because it is needed for running day-to-day operations. Members may be exploited for their labor or may have their personal incomes expropriated for the benefit of the cult and of the leader. In several instances, cult leaders—who are generally excused from following the rules to which members must adhere—live in opulence, whereas members learn to do without basic comforts. Followers of the Bhagwan Rajneesh, of the Osho Foundational International, gave him a fleet of more than a hundred Rolls Royce automobiles so he could enjoy daily rides. David Koresh had his own private suite with electronic equipment, television, and air conditioning, whereas the other Davidians lived communally in a compound where toilets and running water were substandard. The cult leader, because of his divine connection, is exempted from the worldly restrictions and travails that are the lot of ordinary cult members. The indulged leader's excesses are but a worldly metaphor for the spiritual rewards that await aspirants.

In return for giving up the material and comfort rewards of this world, the cult members are promised salvation and healing. Many members even like the altruistic rewards of a stripped-down existence. Promised rewards in the hereafter, many say that they feel happy, content, and spiritually fulfilled. Focused on the group and its ideals, committed cult members come to believe that their own personal difficulties are insignificant and must be ignored.

The Road to the Apocalypse

Killer cults are not born, they are shaped over time. The leaders of killer cults are generally either psychopathic, psychotic, or both. As they sink into madness, they pull their followers down with them. Deviant leaders take a generally benign group of adherents and gradually transform them into followers of a self-fulfilling fatal vision in which, at least for them, the ultimate apocalypse occurs within the cult members' lifetimes.

How does a group or cult transform itself into a killing machine? Can cults, like individuals, become sick and die? Is there a way of identifying a cult that is beginning to show the early signs of becoming a killer cult?

For the purposes of discussion, cults can be divided into two categories: nondeviant ("healthy") and deviant ("sick"). This division is already arbitrary because, by definition, cults deviate from the mainstream of society. Moreover, the idea of anything being divided into baskets of healthy or sick is a fiction. For individuals, psychiatrists are fond of saying that normality does not exist. How, then, could it exist for a group? Nevertheless, using the healthy–sick distinction may help us understand some fundamental differences among cults and possibly identify those that are heading for trouble.

The theoretical healthy cult is less authoritarian and more benevolent in style of leadership than the sick one. In it, humane and charitable practices flourish in harmony with the cult's espoused ideals. In healthy cults, members feel a stronger allegiance to the ideals of the cult than to the personage of the leader. Such a cult maintains open communication with mainstream society. Honesty, candor, and benevolence mark the relationship of members with one another and with the outside world. The cult is not at war with the outside community or country, and a siege mentality does not exist within it. This cult's spiritual message is universal, not idiosyncratic. Members seek, and possibly find, spiritual peace and fulfillment. Genuinely happy with their lives, they do not require coercion to remain within the cult. Members are free to leave at any time. Such a cult serves to empower its members personally and to facilitate their own journeys toward spiritual enlightenment. The healthy cult channels the dreams of good men and the acts of bad men into constructive outlets.

Cults become sick when their leaders become deviant or mentally ill. The worst problems often surface because a deviant or mentally troubled cult leader may attract equally dysfunctional cult members. Jim Jones of the Peoples Temple recruited many who were disadvantaged psychologically, socially, and economically. These members' personal needs were so great that it was relatively easy for them to hand over their lives—and eventually, their deaths—to the deviant whims of a mentally disturbed leader.

It is possible for a cult to be chronically ill without the illness becoming terminal. Some cults remain in this sick condition. The leadership of a sick cult is authoritarian and harsh. The real value system of such a cult, hidden behind an idealistic cover, is guided by the leader's pursuit of power, money, and sex. Rather than seeking spiritual enrichment of its members through humane, charitable practices, the cult demonstrates to the astute observer that such practices are only superficially espoused and that the leader seeks only self-aggrandizement. In such a cult, the spiritual message is frighteningly apocalyptic and promises unique benefits only to people who are and remain members of the cult. Members are exploited rather than enlightened. They are subject to mind control. Information coming into the cult and going out of it is censored. Sharply drawn boundaries hide the cult's secrets from the outside world. A siege mentality is induced by the leader's "sick" mind, and the cult may arm itself for the final battle. In the sick cult, the dreams of good men and the acts of bad men are inflamed, and both are harnessed to the nefarious purposes of the deviant cult leader.

MOVE was a cult in Philadelphia that preached a poorly defined mix of primitivism and anarchy. Armed and dangerous, MOVE had bad relations with its inner-city neighbors and city authorities for years in the early 1980s. In a final, tragic confrontation in 1985, the city decided to try and dislodge cult members from their barricaded row houses. The police used several hundred thousand gallons of water, shot through high pressure hoses, and 7,000 rounds of ammunition in the attempt, which failed. It was then decided that the police ought to "neutralize" the bunker on top of the building. A helicopter dropped a bomb containing an incendiary blasting substance. The fire that erupted destroyed 61 adjoining homes and left 250 families homeless. In the conflagration, 11 MOVE members, including 4 children, died.

A Tale of Two Killer Cults

For a cult to become a killer of its own members, as with the Peoples Temple and the Branch Davidians, the leader must become deviant and deranged in the extreme. Jim Jones constantly preached an apocalyptic end for his followers at the hands of the FBI, CIA, Ku Klux Klan, and through nuclear war. Toward that end, he had the members practice the "white night" ritual of mass suicide by poisoning. Nearing the time when that end actually came about, Jones could not separate reality from fantasy. He believed that he was the reincarnation of Christ, Lenin, and other historical figures. David Koresh also spoke repeatedly of an apocalyptic finale to his ministry. He referred specifically to the seven seals of God's prophecy for the unfolding of the Apocalypse. There was eyewitness testimony at the trial of the Branch Davidians that this cult, too, had rehearsed and prepared for mass suicide.

A misunderstanding of several important factors about the mentality of killer cults contributed to the terrible ends of both the followers of Jim Jones and of David Koresh. The power of apocalyptic prophecy was not properly weighed. Nor was the fact that the more a group perceives itself to be under the threat of persecution, the stronger the group bonds become. Cult cohesion under conflict ought to be expected, as well as the paranoia that accompanies and is part of a siege mentality. Then, too, the suspiciousness, isolation, and "us-versus-them" perception of reality further create a self-fulfilling prophecy of inevitable destruction. It waits only for the trigger event.

Reports filtered out of Guyana about secretive activities of the Peoples Temple—extensive firearms acquisitions, abuse of members, keeping members in virtual captivity. Such reports brought U.S. House of Representatives member Leo Ryan and a group of reporters to Guyana to investigate. Jim Jones viewed the appearance of Representative Ryan and his group as a confirmation of his own belief that the Peoples Temple was about to be attacked by U.S. government forces. Cult members killed Ryan and two reporters and wounded 16 others at the Jonestown airstrip. When news of this reached Jones, he activated the mass suicide procedure.

The accumulation of sophisticated weaponry began at Ranch Apocalypse long before ATF agents approached its gate. Driven by paranoid expectations of an apocalyptic ending, Koresh decreed military-type drills and construction of bunkers. When the ATF agents tried to force their way into Ranch Apocalypse to confiscate the weapons, the event triggered Koresh's self-fulfilling prophecy of apocalyptic destruction.

Both Koresh and Jones had declared that they were God. When a cult leader makes such a statement, it is evidence of a serious mental disorder. Gods do not have to abide by the rules of mere mortals. Thus, Koresh and Jones had numerous sexual partners among the cult members. Koresh was alleged to have had sex with many girls in his sect, some as young as 12 years old. He is also alleged to have sired most of the young children in the compound—12 of the 17 who died, by one account. Jones reportedly had sex with both males and females in his cult. Both men had sex with the wives of cult members. They broke up existing families so there would be no other groups competing within the cult. Jones ordered some marriages ended and arranged new ones. All the while, Jones ordered cult members to abstain from sex, which was considered evil except when he engaged in it. It was reported about Ranch Apocalypse that Koresh freely took whichever woman caught his fancy, whereas the other men of the cult lived in "anguished celibacy." In other words, in both cults, sex was used along with many other matters as a way of controlling cult members.

Sexual activities were an integral part of a gradual, general regression of the cult and its members toward primitive functioning and thinking. In each instance, the signs of this regression were clearly present. In 1987, Koresh was charged with the attempted murder of a competing cult leader but was acquitted. Jim Jones had been involved in a paternity suit brought by a cult member. He had also been arrested for making lewd advances to an undercover officer in an adult movie theater.

As the leader becomes more and more tyrannical, demanding allegiance to himself rather than to cult ideals, serious encounters with the law occur. Suspiciousness and paranoia grow. The wagons are drawn into a circle. In Guyana, armed guards patrolled the Peoples Temple commune. Access to Ranch Apocalypse in Waco was also carefully controlled. The paranoia spills over into observation of cult members, too, for any sign of possible betrayal. Spying was rife inside the Waco and Guyana compounds. Jim Jones had his members sign undated suicide notes, which would be used as part of cover stories should he later need to eliminate those members.

Inside the compounds, violence escalates. Child beatings become more brutal and frequent. In Jim Jones's last days, he had little children dunked into deep wells on the end of a rope for even minor infractions of his rules. Children present serious problems for cult leaders. Although they are seen as those who will carry on the life of the cult, they are also perceived as burdens by "sick" leaders. They require considerable time and effort, they bring in no money, and they detract attention from the leaders. Rebellious children may challenge the leader's authority when adults have long since stopped doing so. Moreover, during times of crisis, children react to stress with disruptive, acting-out behavior. One reason to break up families is to render children vulnerable and then to raise them communally, so that their only allegiance is to the group.

In the last phases, Jones and Koresh gave endless sermons and harangues. Members were exhausted by their leaders' incoherent, emotional exhortations to prepare for the Apocalypse. Jones spent an average of 6 hours per day on the loudspeaker, calling attention to the "fascists" who were coming. Koresh drew attention to the ATF agents, who were sure to attack again and prove his prophesied cosmic conclusion.

As the leader's mental state deteriorates, paranoia and a siege mentality escalate. Cult members are worked to exhaustion, made to make do with a subsistence diet. They are once again deprived of sleep, this time by the endless harangues. The whole idea of escape is made to seem impossible. No one could escape the sound of Jones's loudspeaker-amplified voice in Guyana, telling the cult members that although everyone must die, they would all soon be resurrected and given the means to remain together, rather than being hounded, persecuted, and dispersed here on earth. In Waco, Koresh decided who could leave and who must stay. During the first 4 weeks of the siege, 34 cult members, including 21 children, came out voluntarily. But in the last 2 weeks, no one was allowed to leave. Later, after it was all over, the FBI believed it had evidence that 20 Davidians who had wanted to leave had been shot as a warning to others.

Members who might want to leave are at war with themselves. The anxiety and fear that has arisen in the cult member is denied, displaced onto other cult members who are suspiciously perceived as possible defectors. The image of the all-powerful, all-knowing leader is preserved through increased acts of devotion and submission. Cult members often project their anger and disappointment at the leader onto the outside world, increasing their own paranoia. Such psychological defenses paradoxically lead cult members to rely even more on the cult leader. Though the emperor has no clothes, none of his subjects is psychologically able to admit it.

In the final weeks, the prospect of death may be welcomed by cult members, for whom life has become so wretched. Deprived of food and sleep, working grueling schedules with no time for relaxation or even spiritual refreshment, cult members may believe that a permanent rest is desirable. They fear the wrath of their now-deranged leader and his certain punishment should they deviate from his instructions. Cut off from the rest of the world and from former family ties, they are hardly able to resist the prospect of mass suicide. Deborah Leighton, a confidant of Jim Jones in Guyana, managed to escape the Peoples Temple but explained that in the last days there, "The concept of mass suicide for socialisms arose. Because our lives were so wretched anyway, and because we were so afraid to contradict Reverend Jones, the concept was not challenged."

Near the end, the minds of cult members have fallen totally under the tyrannical control of the leader. Members have become wholly dependent and have long ago stopped thinking for themselves. When the call to die is given, most of the members go unflinchingly to their deaths by poison, fire, or gunshot, self-inflicted or given by others. The Apocalypse has arrived.

The Lethal Leader: Inside the Deviant Psyche

Throughout the history of mankind, lethal leaders have led their groups to destruction. In our century, Adolf Hitler charismatically enthralled an entire nation in the cultist pursuit of Aryan supremacy. In the process, he plunged the world into war and ordered the murders of millions of innocent people. Joseph Stalin, whose reign was later labeled by his successor, Nikita Khrushchev, as "the cult of personality," murdered more than 20 million of his country's people. Jim Jones and David Koresh led their followers to murder and suicide. Charles Manson's domination of his "family" led to the grisly bludgeoning, stabbing, and shooting of seven people. The nation was appalled that Manson's young men and women would murder repeatedly at his command. Cult leaders who cause death have variously been considered psychopaths, psychotics, or, at best, borderline personalities. It is likely that the above-named lethal leaders have manifested all of these conditions at various times (see Table 10–1), or all at one time, especially as the end neared.

Diagnostic certainty is hard to achieve because most cult leaders were never examined psychiatrically. Adding to the difficulties of making a proper diagnosis are the special circumstances under which their

TABLE 10–1.	Typical psychological characteristics of killer cult leaders

- Mentally disordered
- Deity complex (Christ)
- Sexually deviant/exploitative
- Persecutory beliefs
- Primitive psychological defenses (splitting, projection, denial, regression under stress)
- Charismatic
- Apocalyptic vision (suicide)
- Attracts dysfunctional cult members
- Seeks isolation and control
- Childhood abuse history
- Materialistic

mental aberrations occurred. Even people on the outside can appreciate the mind-warping effects of having to function under extreme stress.

When cult leaders are isolated from the normalizing influences of other communities, they are subject to mutual validation between themselves and their members. The leader's grandiose conception of self, and the fears, paranoia, and sense of an apocalyptic vision waiting to be fulfilled, are all mirrored back to him and further distort the mental processes. When the cult is actually under siege, as the Branch Davidians were in Waco, fact and fantasy begin to merge. All the deviant mental processes are heightened. As the end approached, Koresh's behavior became more erratic. He slept until mid-afternoon while cult members worked. At night, when cult members were exhausted and ready for sleep, he raced through the dormitories, ringing a loud bell as a signal for beginning marathon Bible study sessions. During these sessions, Koresh frequently made no sense. It is always possible that the leader, when dealing with elements outside of this cataclysmic pressure cooker, may appear quite normal and may seem to behave rationally.

Psychotic cult leaders blur the boundaries between reality and fantasy. They exhibit grandiose ideas about themselves, persecutory beliefs, and a conviction that the end of the world is nigh. The man originally named Vernon Howell combined the names of two Biblical kings and, like David Koresh, declared himself to be the "sinful" incarnation of Jesus Christ. Vernon Howell had been an abused child, an itinerant carpenter, and a would-be rock star. David Koresh was different. He was convinced that he could open the seventh seal of the book held in God's right hand, as described in the Book of Revelation, which prophesied all the calamities that would take place before the Apocalypse. Charles Manson, when arrested, insisted that he be booked as "Charles Manson, aka, Jesus Christ, God."

The problem created for the person identifying with Jesus Christ is that he or she has to die before resurrection can take place. When authorities are in confrontation with a psychotic leader who claims that sort of divinity, they would do well to remember this potential problem and to defuse paranoid and grandiose delusions by backing away. De-escalating intimidation and removing the crisis from the limelight are often useful when dealing with a person who has identified so openly with a deity.

Psychopathic cult leaders who are not psychotic never reach such delusional heights (or depths). Throughout their tenure, they maintain a basic sense of reality. Their leadership is based on self-aggrandizement, the exploitation of cult members, and the accumulation of money, power, and sexual indulgence. If cornered by the authorities and unable to see any way out, psychopathic leaders may impulsively choose suicide, taking others with them, if the leaders can no longer stay alive.

Cult leaders may display some of the following characteristics of a borderline personality, particularly during a crisis:

- The tendency to split the world, people, and themselves into good and bad
- Unstable yet intense personal relationships that alternate between extremes of idealization and devaluation
- Impulsiveness in sex, spending, and substance use
- Rapid mood swings
- Intense but poorly controlled anger
- Recurrent suicidal threats or behavior
- Frantic efforts to avoid real or imagined abandonment
- Uncertainty about personal self-image or sexual identity
- Under stress, temporary breaks with reality or manifests transient paranoid thinking

All of these personality traits become exacerbated as cataclysmic psychological stress takes hold and the cult's end draws nearer. These reactions are also intensified by the psychology of the cult as a whole. The good-bad splitting occurs on a wider basis. The world is divided into us and them. The outside is seen as threatening and evil, whereas the cult inside is seen as threatened and good. Mutual reinforcement of this view by the cult leader and followers can fire up hostility and aggression against the outside world. Hitler saw the Jews as evil and required their elimination. His followers did not disagree with the task he set out for them. Jim Jones saw the enemies as the CIA, the FBI, and the Ku Klux Klan.

Charles Manson looked upon blacks as the source of evil and destruction. He hoped that his murders would provoke blacks into starting a race war and bringing about Armageddon or, as he called it, Helter Skelter. Manson and his white followers would be transformed into deities and rule the Earth when the blacks discovered that they were incapable of managing it themselves. For Charles Dederich, the leader of Synanon, the government and the news media constituted the evil empire. For other militant religious cults, the enemies are their members' natural parents.

Three prominent psychological defense mechanisms are frequently used by deviant cult leaders: 1) good-bad splitting, 2) projection, and 3) projective identification. These mechanisms are particularly evident in persons with borderline personality disorder.

In *good-bad splitting*, the cult leader devalues and rejects the "bad" parts of the world (and oneself), and idealizes and embraces the "good" parts. Jim Jones saw his cult as a socialist utopia. He hated the outside evil forces that would, in his belief, destroy that utopia. For those who so split the world, awareness of the hated part of the self is submerged and *projected* onto the world outside. In a cult, this mechanism impels the cult leader to further distance his or her group from society. Such projection of the bad and hated self onto the outside world also contributes to the group's suspiciousness and to its siege mentality. Once it became apparent to Jim Jones that his cult's boundary could no longer be secured, he made the deranged but clear choice to preserve the cult's identity in spirit, even if he could no longer preserve it in reality—and chose mass suicide.

An understanding of *projective identification* also is crucial to deciphering the sorts of massacres that occurred at Jonestown and Waco.

Projective identification is a primitive mental mechanism that goes through three steps:

1. The person projects (attributes to others) intolerable inner feelings while still maintaining a certain awareness of what is projected.
2. The person who projects tries to control the individual on whom the unacceptable feelings have been projected.
3. Unconsciously, when interacting with that individual, the projector leads that individual to experience what has been projected onto him or her.

This process is made clearer by the following example:

> John, a person who fears loss of control over his aggressive impulses, is persuaded to accompany friends on a hunting trip. While walking with the hunters, John is seized by the fear that they could turn their guns on him. Even though he recognizes his own past fears that he might shoot someone, if he had a gun and momentarily lost control, John nevertheless continues to be anxious that he could be killed. He attempts to control the hunters by dissuading them from doing any more hunting, suggesting that they go home earlier than planned. The hunters, noting John's anxiety, sense his fear of guns and also become briefly concerned about their own safety.

Projective identification produces a self-fulfilling prophecy. In denying one's feelings and attributing them to someone else, the individual behaves in a way that causes others to respond in kind. Thus, when the borderline person's hostility is returned, he or she finds confirmation of his or her original paranoid thinking.

Negotiating with the Devil

The negotiator handling a cult crisis must have an understanding of the defense mechanism of projective identification. Lack of awareness of this defense may well play into the self-fulfilling apocalyptic prophecies of a mentally disturbed cult leader. Given their knowledge of projection, mental health professionals may help negotiators in crisis situations. What is needed is a critical window into the cult leader's mental state. Usually there is one negotiator who is in regular contact with the cult leader. If the feelings engendered in that negotiator by the cult leader can be psychologically held, examined, and properly interpreted—without immediate action being taken—it is possible to obtain important data about the cult leader's state of mind, and to gather it on a continuing basis.

For example, a cult leader stressed by a confrontation crisis may experience an increase in feelings of helplessness, fear, and rage. The leader, although conscious of these threatening feelings, may misperceive their origins and project them onto an adversary. The leader's efforts to control the adversary may create similar feelings of helplessness, fear, and rage in the negotiator. What needs to happen is for these feelings to be deciphered and taken into account before any action is taken. What sometimes occurs, though, is that these feelings are reflexively acted upon by the authorities, themselves triggering an attack that fulfills the leader's projections as well as the apocalyptic fantasies.

No one can know with any certainty the extent to which such mechanisms as good-bad splitting, projection, and projective identification played parts in the mass murders and suicides of the 82 Branch Davidians. But it is likely that they played a prominent role. For example, it had been alleged that Koresh had been abused as a child. It was the reports of his increasing physical and sexual abuse of the children at Ranch Apocalypse that produced a realistic sense of helplessness in the authorities. They perceived a need to act, ostensibly to protect the remaining children. Could it be that the escalating child abuse at the hands of Koresh was also a sign of increased good-bad splitting within himself and of his projecting the bad aspect onto certain cult children?

Adding to the authorities' mounting sense of frustration were Koresh's repeated promises to surrender peacefully, promises that he never kept. Koresh, rather than the authorities, seemed to be in control of the situation. Inside the compound, as a cult member later testified at the trial of surviving Branch Davidians, Koresh "told the ladies to do 50 pushups, 50 situps, 50 deep knee bends, every two hours…to make us strong, to stop the American Army, the Assyrians, from raping us, the ladies." Koresh likely saw the Branch Davidians as all good and the world outside as all bad. From Koresh's psychological perspective, evil did not lurk in his heart but resided in the minds and intentions of the government agents who were besieging him. Cult members shot the ATF agents because they "knew" the agents would kill them. The members did not fully comprehend that they were stockpiling arms intended to kill other people because Koresh had projected his (and their) fear, hate, and rage at the outside world. Koresh projected his terrible feelings onto the FBI and then attempted to control the FBI and the likelihood of FBI retaliation against him and his followers.

Finally, according to a spokesman for the FBI, "there was simply an accumulation of frustrations: the negotiations had gone nowhere, they were convinced that Koresh was stalling and feared he was spoiling for a confrontation." To what extent was this statement a true assessment of David Koresh's thinking? Is it possible that the decision to assault the compound was driven by feelings Koresh had communicated in his deranged mental state and that these feelings had not been properly psychologically assessed?

In both instances, with Jim Jones and with David Koresh, government officials grossly misunderstood the psychological forces operating inside the cults and in the minds of their leaders. The authorities did not comprehend the siege mentality or the suicidal intent of the cults. They did not seem to know how to evaluate or decipher such mechanisms as good-bad splitting, projection, and projective identification. As a result, 15 years after Representative Leo Ryan set foot on a Guyana airstrip and provided an unwitting trigger to Jim Jones's apocalyptic end for over 900 of his cult members, the government authorities replicated their mistake in that first assault in which four ATF agents were killed. Once government agents had been killed, the fiery apocalyptic fate of the Branch Davidians was all but signed and sealed. It was later delivered on national television.

During the 51-day siege, the FBI's Behavioral Science Unit composed a psychological profile of David Koresh. In a detailed memo, these behavioral experts concluded that a high probability existed that the cult leader would commit suicide if directly confronted by the FBI. Nonetheless, the FBI agents on the scene handling the negotiations reportedly grew impatient and disregarded the advice of their own behavioral science experts. When the government forces attacked, the apocalypse took place as Koresh might have wished—live for a national television audience. The futility and folly of using intimidation and then of mounting a frontal assault upon a would-be martyr with an apocalyptic vision ought to have been apparent to the authorities, but it was not.

After the fires cooled, a psychiatric expert on the panel who reviewed the government's handling of the siege disagreed with what had been done to "resolve" the crisis. He criticized the FBI for using pressure tactics and tear gas that may well have pushed Koresh into triggering his plan for mass suicide. In the future, it is hoped that negotiators in similar situations—and there will be others—will use the psychological knowledge that is available about cult leaders and their followers to avoid unwittingly becoming the executioners of a cult leader's self-fulfilling death wish.

Analysis of the psyches of cult leaders has its limitations, however. Cult leaders are not available for psychiatric examination at the time of crisis. Moreover, cult leaders' personalities vary greatly, particularly in their motivations and degree of mental aberration. Cultural and ethnic differences, if present, may also complicate psychological analysis. Moreover, psychiatrists cannot draw clear distinctions between mystical experiences of the sort that cult leaders say they have and deviant mental states. Nevertheless, when a cult leader becomes psychotic, it is reasonably certain that tragedy is likely to be a result.

Forensic Psychiatrists and Cults

There are many types of litigation involving cult members and cults in which forensic psychiatrists can and do become involved. For example, forensic psychiatrists may testify in suits alleging fraud, unlawful imprisonment, or the intentional infliction of emotional distress. We try to grapple with some of the following questions: Was the alleged emotional trauma caused by the cult experience, or can it be traced to some other cause? Did the emotional trauma exist before the person's joining the cult? Was the trauma exacerbated by joining a cult? What is the extent of the psychological damages that have been incurred?

All psychiatric interventions involving involuntary evaluation or treatment of a cult member are fraught with thorny ethical and legal dilemmas. Some psychiatrists who have given adverse testimony about a cult member's mental competency and against the cult itself have been hit with civil suits and even with threats of physical violence. No involuntary examinations of cult members should be attempted without prior consultation with psychiatrists and attorneys who have had experience dealing with cults.

Forensic psychiatrists can also lend a hand in incidents involving cults during a developing crisis or confrontation. Most forensic psychiatrists have acquired knowledge and experience concerning the always murky relationship between mental illness and the emergence of violence. Psychiatrists do not possess the ability to accurately predict violence but, in association with other mental health experts, forensic psychiatrists are sometimes called on to attempt to assess the risk of violence.

Mental health professionals can be of consultative assistance to negotiators, generally in hostage situations, whether domestic or terrorist. A critically important role for mental health professionals is the treatment and management of those who have been psychologically traumatized by terrorist events.

Al-Qaeda and the Mind of the Jihadist

Psychiatrists and other mental health professionals cannot perform the same consultative roles when dealing with terrorist groups like al-Qaeda. As noted above, psychological profiling of terrorists lacks reliability. Psychiatrists and psychologists have taken part in interrogations of captured terrorists. This is a highly controversial role. It is unnatural and unethical for a psychiatrist to participate in the torture of detainees for interrogation purposes. But psychiatrists and psychologists have acted as consultants to interrogators—and there is no bright line separating consultation from participation.

Is al-Qaeda, translated as "The Base," a killer cult? At first glance, it appears to share similarities with the killer cults discussed above. For example, Osama bin Laden is a charismatic leader. He is considered by many in the Islamic world to be the *Mahdi,* the missing and long-awaited Messianic deliverer, the mighty warrior of the apocalypse. Like killer cults, some of bin Laden's group and other al-Qaeda groups live in distant isolation, hiding from their enemies. As do killer cults, al-Qaeda espouses a death ethic, but for reasons of Islamic revolution. Suicide bombings are its trademark. The terrorist feels enraged, humiliated, and besieged by the "crusaders" who occupy Arab lands. A prominent Saudi imam has issued a *fatwa,* or religious ruling, granting bin Laden and other Islamic terrorists permission to use nuclear weapons to kill 10 million Americans. Bin Laden's vision is not a self-destructive apocalypse but a nuclear Armageddon visited on the United States. It includes a worldwide Islamic revolution at the tip of a sword, if conversion to Islam is not voluntary.

The Muslim–infidel dichotomy is a classic example of good-bad splitting. This is a psychological mechanism that allows demonization of "infidels," that is, persons of other religions. Good-bad splitting is endemic to the human condition, but is taken to extremes among killer cults and terrorist organizations. There is, however, little similarity between al-Qaeda and killer cults such as the Peoples Temple and the Branch Davidians. Al-Qaeda is governed by a leadership council, and major decisions made by the core group are approved by bin Laden. There is a known second-in-command, Ayman al-Zawahiri, an Egyptian surgeon. Unlike killer cults, which consist of members trapped within the delusion (and control) of a deranged leader, al-Qaeda has a distinct governance infrastructure based on cells organized for sharply defined purposes including logistics, fundraising, and sophisticated media management. To launch a single suicide bomber requires many levels of assistance, for example a quartermaster who obtains explosives and other materials (nails, ball bearings, nuts, bolts), a technician to make the bomb, a reconnaissance operative, and someone to identify the specific target. Before the operation, a handler sequesters the bomber in a safe house, away from family and friends, sees to it that a film crew helps the bomber make a martyrdom video for propaganda and recruitment purposes (and so the bomber will not back out), and then places the bomber as close as possible to the target.

The administrative infrastructure is very sophisticated; al-Qaeda is run much like a multinational corporation whose reach and scope extends to many countries. Instead of manufacturing a product, al-Qaeda aims to export Islamic revolution and death. It is innovative, resilient, and determined. Losses of personnel are replaced by a seemingly never-ending stream of loyalists and recruits. Al-Qaeda learns from its mistakes and constantly reinvents itself.

Another difference between al-Qaeda and killer cults can be seen in al-Qaeda's interaction with the wider world. Killer cults are often isolated microcommunities that have little contact with the outside world. The vision of the killer cult has to do with defense and survival. Recruitment of new members has long since ceased by the time the leader sinks into madness and the cult begins to disintegrate. No leadership structure remains to counter the leader's paranoia and enable the group to survive. Al-Qaeda's strong organization belies the wishful thinking of critics who believe it is only an offbeat killer cult that will sooner or later self-destruct. Moreover, its leadership differs. Although killer cult leaders are often disadvantaged, marginally functioning individuals, al-Qaeda's leaders are educated and come from the middle and upper classes, frequently from prosperous families. Some of the 9/11 hijackers also came from such backgrounds. Osama bin Laden himself is a multimillionaire. And despite the beliefs of many outsiders to the contrary, there is no evidence that bin Laden or others in leadership positions of al-Qaeda are manifestly mentally ill.

What is most difficult for Westerners and Christians to understand about Islamic terrorists is the desire, even the yearning, that they display for death. This desire, we think, goes against the primal human instinct for life. The suicide bomber believes otherwise. He (or in some cases, she) is overjoyed to join Allah's jihad against infidels, for the reward is great—eternal bliss in paradise's garden of sensual delights. As Ayatollah Ruhollah Khomeini of Iran put it, "The purest joy in Islam is to kill and be killed for Allah." Martyrdom is the only certain path to paradise. Honorable actions, good deeds, and devotion to God do not guarantee entrance to paradise.

People who survived a suicide bombing on a bus described the terrorist as going to his death with a smile. He acknowledged passengers, smiled, then activated the bomb. In the Shia Islamic tradition, this is known as the "smile of joy," anticipating one's imminent martyrdom and entrance into paradise. In his last will and testament, the 9/11 hijackers' ringleader Mohammed Atta used the phrase, "The sky smiles, my young son."

Radicalized by feelings of injustice, humiliation, and rage by the "crusader" occupation of Arab holy lands, the "holy warriors" accept martyrdom in the cause of Allah. They know that death is inescapable, the common lot of all mankind, and choose to sacrifice their lives because of love for Allah and in submission to Allah's cause, which is the highest expression of their Islamic faith. The Islamic fundamentalist terrorist willingly exchanges a few paltry years on earth for eternal bliss in paradise.

When the failed car bombings in England and Glasgow in the summer of 2007 were revealed to have been conducted by Islamic terrorists who were physicians and medical students, it seemed inconceivable to Westerners. How could physicians dedicated to saving lives undertake the mass murder of civilians? The Hippocratic oath, cornerstone of medical ethics, enjoins physicians to "First, do no harm." The contradiction between that oath and the attempted deeds of the car-bombing physicians boggles the Western mind.

However, a number of physicians have become lethal revolutionaries. Che Guevara, a physician, was a Marxist revolutionary. George

Habash, a pediatrician, led the Palestinian militant group the Popular Front for the Liberation of Palestine. Radovan Karadžic, a psychiatrist who wrote poetry and books for children, led the Bosnian Serbs and was held responsible for the "ethnic cleansing" of tens of thousands of Muslims. And, as noted above, the surgeon Ayman al-Zawahiri is the al-Qaeda second-in-command. There is no evidence of overt mental illness in any of these physician terrorists.

Although Islamic physicians are devoted to a humanitarian ethic, they are not immune to becoming radicalized and may be drawn to serving Allah above all else. Such a physician terrorist might explain that adherence to God's laws supersedes all allegiance to mere man-made ethics.

As the example of the physician suggests, there is no reliable psychological profile for identifying Islamic terrorists in general or suicide bombers. The job description for a terrorist would include that the work is demanding. The would-be terrorist must be able to conceive, plan, and execute often complex actions. The suicide bomber is the ultimate smart bomb, and the terrorist must handle the bomber well. The suicide bomber, however, must be capable only of commitment to killing and dying for the Islamic cause. Younger people, flush with zeal and idealism, are the most frequent perpetrators of suicide bombings. In the schools known as madrassas, even young children are groomed to be suicide bombers. Older men and women usually do not take such roles. Age tempers idealism. Family relations—spouse, children, extended family—become earthly ties. There are exceptions; a few suicide bombers are middle-aged, married, and even have children.

There is no doubt that individual psychodynamics play an important role in choosing to be an Islamic terrorist. Dr. Varnik D. Volkan, a psychiatrist and psychoanalyst who has studied the psychology of suicide bombers, states, "Reports show that those who select suicide bomber candidates have developed an expertise in sensing whose personal identity 'gaps' are most suitable for filling with elements of large-group identity." Furthermore, Dr. Volkan writes, using "borrowed elements sanctioned by God [to replace] one's internal world makes the person omnipotent and supports the individual's narcissism."

A word of caution. Psychiatrists do not examine or clear individuals for the role of suicide bomber. That would be an abomination to the Jihadist. Nor are suicide bombers who have lived because the detonators on their bombs malfunctioned examined by psychiatrists— that would be an even greater abomination. Thus, little can be known factually about the individual psychology of suicide bombers until mental health professionals have an opportunity to examine them.

I look to my psychiatric colleagues raised and educated in Muslim society to shed light on the mind of the Islamic terrorist, a subject that this Western psychiatrist finds opaque. The psychological workings of the Islamic terrorist's mind is of immense interest to mental health professionals. The history of humankind shows that no class of individuals, rich or poor, educated or uneducated, old or young, is immune from radicalization that can empower them to kill for God's cause. Throughout history, ordinary, good men and women of many faiths, have committed terrible crimes against humanity while acting in the name of God.

Anticult Organizations

The emergence of cults has been balanced to some degree by the creation of anticult organizations. An original, informal network made up of parents whose children have been cult members, the American Family Foundation has become a leading anticult organization that acts as a coordinating center for the anticult movement. It disseminates information, provides families with a support system, conducts educational programs, and publishes newspapers and reports. The Cult Hotline, the Jewish Board of Family and Children's Services, and the Watchman Fellowship (a Christian group) also provide up-to-date information on cults. Anticult organizations originally supported the deprogramming of cult members, but this practice has been in decline.

Sometimes, when a family member joins a cult, the family is seized with an anticult fanaticism. This can further alienate the cult member and be a hindrance to communication with him or her. Family members' understandably strong but disruptive feelings need to be productively tempered. This can be done with the assistance of knowledgeable mental health professionals and with the support of the groups and informational sources noted above. A major problem with regard to combating cult groups is that religious practices are protected by the First Amendment. No matter how unacceptable a cult's religious exercises may be to the family of a cult member, such practices are considered legal. The only legal way to contest a cult is to prove that it has used coercive mind control methods that have reduced a victim's mental capacity to the condition of being legally impaired.

Many mental health professionals hold an anticult bias. This is understandable because of their humanistic bent, which favors individual autonomy and freedom. Moreover, mental health professionals generally do not interview, and thus have no familiarity with, people from cults who had had positive experiences. Rather, they are usually charged with the treatment of current or past cult members who are mentally disturbed, and with the treatment of their families, who are often devastated and in psychological pain.

It is a fact that some people are psychologically damaged by their cult experience. No doubt there are some who also benefit in various ways from their time in a cult. The statistics on influx to and outflux from cults suggest that the majority of people who enter and then exit cults emerge basically unfazed, going on with their lives after a brief fling with social and personal experimentation.

Apocalypse Now: The Future of a Delusion

Apocalyptic killer cults exist today at various stages of incubation. Some time—sooner rather than later—a new killer cult will burst violently into our consciousness. Similar killer cults, with their apocalyptic messages, have been part of humankind for hundreds if not thousands of years. They will be with us forever because some people will always need to attribute their darkest impulses to others whom they must then kill or escape from through suicide. In Japan, an apocalyptic cult named Aum Shinrikyo, or Supreme Truth, conducted a fatal nerve gas attack on Tokyo's subway. The Sarin gas killed 12 commuters and sickened about 5,500 more. Shoko Asahara, the doomsday guru of Supreme Truth, said that he had been attacked by the CIA with poison gas. Asahara made repeated predictions that the world was about to end. He listed among his many enemies the Japanese and U.S. militaries. Asahara and a number of his top disciples were arrested and charged with murder and attempted murder. Several, including Asahara and the member who made the Sarin gas, were convicted and given death sentences.

Once a killer cult self-destructs, the violence does not necessarily end. On April 19, 1995, the second anniversary of the government raid that led to the death of 82 Branch Davidians at Waco, Texas, Oklahoma City's Alfred P. Murrah Federal Building was bombed. Investigators believed that revenge for Waco was the main reasons that

Timothy McVeigh and his co-conspirator targeted the federal build-ing, which housed offices of the Bureau of Alcohol, Tobacco and Fire-arms as well as a children's day care center. The Oklahoma City bombing focused attention on the emergence of civilian militias onto the American scene. They now exist in almost every state. Some of the more virulent militias have ominous, killer-cult-like traits such as apoc-alyptic vision and an angry, paranoid view of the government and the world. Unlike most cults, some militias espouse racist and anti-Semitic views.

The future of the "apocalypse now" delusion is a self-fulfilling ca-lamity as horrible and as terrifying as that predicted for Armageddon by the Book of Revelation. Apocalyptic killer cults and terrorist orga-nizations are not born, they evolve through stages. There were ample warnings about al-Qaeda's determined progress on the path to 9/11. In the heeding of warning signs lie the possible means for preventing what will otherwise be the certain destructiveness of the apocalyptic prophecy.

11

Serial Sexual Killers

Your Life
for Their Orgasm

While nothing is easier than to denounce the evildoer,
nothing is more difficult than to understand him.

—*Fyodor Mikhailovich Dostoyevsky*

Few passersby near the steps of the Rostov library noticed 44-year-old Andrei Romanovich Chikatilo, a bespectacled, respectably dressed Russian *apparatchik*. With briefcase in hand, he chatted good-naturedly with 17-year-old schoolgirl Larisa Tkachenko. While traveling on one of the many assignments that took him away from home each year, he enjoyed reading newspapers and literary journals at the local public libraries. Larisa, a pretty blonde waif from Moldavia, was on a school break, during which she had helped to bring in the crop at the Kirov state farm, not far from Rostov. She had lingered in Rostov for a few days to rest and was now waiting for the bus that would take her and all the other girls back to school. After some small talk, Chikatilo invited Larisa to take a walk to a relaxation station that contained restaurants, cafes, and recreational areas. It was understood between them that they would find refreshments and a private place to lie down together. Chikatilo appeared old and harmless to Larisa. She was unaware of the great strength in his shoulders that he hid beneath his respectable coat. She was not alarmed as he steered her into a hidden area at the center of the woods. She was not aware that the last day of

247

her life was winding toward an end. Nor was Chikatilo aware that it would be the first day of his later life, the product of a monstrous epiphany.

In the clearing, Chikatilo pounced on Larisa. He overpowered her easily, with his six-foot-tall, muscular body. He tore off her clothes and underwear. Larisa's futile struggle only sexually excited him more. To him, it was an aphrodisiac. Her terrified, anguished screams were like a siren's song to Chikatilo, transporting him into an erotic frenzy. This was nothing like the vapid, tiresome, unsatisfying sex that he had experienced with his wife in the privacy of their home. Larisa was prey to be eaten and consumed. She was, to him, no longer a human being with feelings and a life to live. Like a wild beast, he devoured his victim. She was his, totally. He could do anything he pleased with her.

Her last struggles were hopeless. Chikatilo muffled her screams by shoving dirt into her mouth. He punched her in the head, stunning her, and then, with all the animal power he possessed at that moment, began to strangle her. As Larisa Tkachenko twisted and thrashed, the power that Chikatilo exerted over her aroused him further. He experienced powerful sexual feelings, more arousal than he had ever achieved during ordinary sex. As her life ebbed, his sense of power and excitement heightened. In a moment of ecstatic release, Chikatilo ejaculated over Larisa as she lay dying under him. Then he tore at her dying body with his teeth and fingers. He ripped away flesh. From her dead body, he bit off one of her nipples.

With the mutilated body of Larisa Tkachenko crushed beneath him, Chikatilo launched into a primal celebration of acceptance. He picked up her rumpled clothes and ran around her body, whooping in ecstasy. He flung his arms wide and some of her blood-stained garments sailed high into the trees. He was intoxicated with emotion. This middle-aged, lifelong failure felt he had avenged and overpowered all the wrongs and humiliations that had been visited upon him by God, country, family, and the women who made him impotent. He was floating on air. For a moment, he sank to his knees before the defiled body. He felt tremendously empowered, as if he were one of his wartime heroes who had fought and killed the Nazis that had invaded the motherland. In that instant, he knew that Larisa had been sacrificed on the altar of his new identity. He had killed once before, but it had never been this satisfying. He had had fantasies, but had never completely realized them. Now he had found his true identity and his life's calling: forever after, he would become one of the most prolific and monstrous serial sexual killers of all time.

The lust murder of Larisa Tkachenko gave enormous impetus to Chikatilo in the acting out of his fantasies. For years, murderous, sadistic fantasies had grown in him, like a cancer in his mind, but he had not known precisely where they would lead. Now he did. When he had first killed little 9-year-old Yelena Zakatovna, he had been terribly shocked, vowing to never kill again. But this time, with Larisa, he felt almost nothing. Now he could kill other women without compunction.

From his earliest school days, Chikatilo had known he was different, an outcast who could not mix easily with the other children. In his first failed and mocked relationships with girls, he felt intense emotional pain. Later he married, but he was impotent and dissatisfied with married life. He felt a growing attraction to the children he taught as a schoolteacher. Meanwhile, in his other job as a faceless factory supply clerk, he experienced only continual abuse and humiliation.

Impotent with women, despised and shunned by everyone, he found his life was made tolerable only by his increasingly violent sexual fantasies. At first, in his acting out, he needed only to touch. Later he needed to have total power over the girls, to torture and to kill. He required that they suffer, and it was on this need that he became hooked, because his gratification came not from intercourse but from thrusting his knife into the bodies of his victims. He would masturbate over his victims, then frantically try to push his sperm into their bodies with his hands.

In his parodies of passion, Andrei Chikatilo managed to kill and mutilate at least 52 victims in 12 years before he was finally apprehended. Each lust murder was more grisly and sadistic than the previous one. His hunters later called him the Red Ripper because he slashed his victims' bodies and stabbed their eyes in a sort of mutilation that they came to know as his "signature" and distinctive trademark. As Chikatilo later told the world, "The purpose of life is to leave your mark on this earth."

Chikatilo lost an eleventh-hour appeal for clemency. He was taken from his prison cell and marched along a stone corridor to the execution room. Chikatilo was made to kneel as his sentence was read. The executioner drew a Makarov automatic and fired a single bullet into the back of the serial killer's head. Unlike his victims, Andrei Romanovich Chikatilo died quickly and mercifully.

In a terrible coda, Chikatilo became the model for Alexander Pichushkin, who, according to his confession, set out to murder 64 people—one for each square on a chessboard—to outdo Chikatilo. He was convicted of 48 murders and claimed a total of 61.

If Wishes Were Horses

When bad men do what good men dream, psychiatrists are called upon to explain why. Murder is the crime of crimes. Murder inspires the ultimate in feelings of repugnance, fear, and fascination about the violation of God's commandment, Thou shalt not kill. There are endless depictions of murder in songs, books, plays, movies, and video games. For many people, these representations of murder produce inexhaustible delights, thrills, and titillating horror.

Given the horrible circumstances of many murders, the neophyte forensic psychiatrist's first interview with a murderer is usually an astonishing experience. For the murderer is not a blood-dripping monster but is usually a quiet, reasonably cooperative, guy-next-door type of human being who is uncomfortably like any other person—including the psychiatrist. The comparison between the guy next door and the blood-dripping monster becomes even more unnerving when one realizes that even good men's consciences are regularly roiled by murderous fantasies and dreams. As Theodore Reik, a pioneering psychoanalyst once succinctly put it, "If wishes were horses, they would pull the hearses of our dearest friends and nearest relatives. All men are murderers at heart." In the O. J. Simpson murder trial, testimony was given by a longtime friend that Simpson had dreamed of killing his wife. The prosecution strategy was to expose Simpson's state of mind (i.e., that he was fatally obsessed with his wife, Nicole). The law, however, punishes criminal acts, not antisocial thoughts. If murderous thoughts and dreams were a capital crime, we all would be on death row.

The FBI defines murder as the *unlawful* taking of life for the purpose of achieving or expressing power, brutality, personal gain, and, occasionally, sexuality. In the criminal justice system, murder is considered to be a subset of homicide that also includes other forms of taking life such as an unpremeditated auto fatality (vehicular homicide), manslaughter, and criminal and noncriminal negligent homicide. In this book I use the terms *homicide* and *killing* interchangeably with murder.

In 1960, there were approximately 10,000 murders a year in the United States. From 1976 to 1992, according to the Uniform Crime Reports (UCR), the number of murders has fluctuated from a low of 16,605 in 1976 to a high of 24,703 in 1991 before dipping slightly in 1992. In 2006, the number of murders was 17,034. The murder rate had dropped significantly since the high of 1991, but increased by 1.8% for the second consecutive year in 2006. It is estimated that 50% of all violent crimes go unreported in the United States. These figures reflect the fact that murder is terribly common among us.

Despite a rising rate of random "stranger" murders—drive-by shootings and hate crimes—the UCR statistics show that two-thirds of homicide victims are family members, friends, or acquaintances of the murderer. In 2004, 3,233 victims were murdered by acquaintances, 1,694 by family members, and 1,046 by friends or neighbors. In 1993, for the first time, the FBI Uniform Crime Report revealed the chilling statistic that a stranger is just as likely to kill us as a family member or friend. The FBI reports that every American has a "realistic chance" of being murdered. In a survey of 25 countries, the homicide rate for infants was as high as or higher than the rate for adults. Most child murders are committed by women. Men who kill their children are usually found to be severely mentally retarded or to have an emotionally explosive disorder.

Overall, recent research has found an important but only modest correlation between violence and mental disorder. The National Institute of Mental Health Epidemiologic Catchment Area study estimated that 90% of persons with current mental illnesses are not violent within 1 year. If a person is not having a psychotic episode or if psychotic symptoms are not part of the psychiatric problems, then he or she is no more likely to be involved in violent behavior than the average person. In particular, though, mentally ill persons who become violent are more likely to kill family members or acquaintances than to kill strangers. Most murders of mothers are committed by schizophrenic sons who live with them alone. Of the people acquitted of murder by reason of insanity, a study shows a significant fraction had paranoid schizophrenia. These people are more likely to have killed a parent or a child than a spouse or a stranger.

In a study of adolescent killers, it was found that over two-thirds of the victims were family members or acquaintances. If the adolescents killed a family member, it was most likely to be the father, after pro-

longed conflict between father and son. The murder was most frequently committed with a gun. If the victim was an acquaintance, the
weapon more frequently used was a knife. The deed happened while
the murderer was in the throes of intense emotion or during the commission of another criminal act.

Homicide numbers make for difficult reading. Moreover, they lack
human detail. But also, homicide numbers are probably underreported. Every murder is unique, defying classification because of the
complexity of interwoven personal factors, motivations, and circumstances. Because the combined numbers of family and acquaintance
murders are so high, it is also clear that many murders occur within
the context of an existing relationship between perpetrator and victim.

The term *serial murderer* was coined by FBI Special Agent Robert K.
Ressler, an expert on serial killers, during the David Berkowitz "Son
of Sam" killings in New York in the 1970s. At that time, and for some
years before it, there were probably only a half-dozen such killers in
the United States. In recent years, estimates of them have run from 50
to 500. The FBI estimates that 500 serial killers are at large who kill
at least 3,500 people each year. Another, more conservative estimate
has the death toll from 200 serial killers at 2,000 people each year—
or approximately 10% of all murders. Gary Leon Ridgway, the Green
River Killer, likely the most prolific serial sexual killer in U.S. history,
admitted to strangling and sexually abusing the bodies of 48 young
women from 1982 to 1998. "I picked up prostitutes because I thought
I could kill as many of them as I wanted without getting caught," Ridgway told prosecutors.

Serial killers are rare—50 to 200 killers among the population is
not a large number of people. We do not need to run out and buy serial killer insurance. Still, their crimes frighten us because serial killers
murder more than their share of victims and because, for the most
part, they kill people who are total strangers. However, serial killers
differ from those who commit random or hate murders because serial
killers act out an intense fantasied relationship with their victims. In
fact, serial sexual murderers require their victims to be anonymous
props on whom they can inflict their lethal fantasies to achieve what
they desire: the exhilaration of orgasm.

Serial killers are classified by the FBI in a different group from
other mass murderers, who kill many people at one time. One of the
latter, Colin Ferguson, a 35-year-old Jamaican immigrant, walked

down the aisles of a Long Island Railroad train, firing into a car of 23 passengers, killing six and wounding many others before he ran out of ammunition. He was finally wrestled to the floor by several other passengers. Serial murders, by the FBI's classification and definition, are those that involve more than three victims and a cooling-off period between murders—something that indicates the premeditation of each one. A classic serial killer was Ted Bundy, who murdered more than 30 times over a period of 6 years and in at least five different states.

But premeditation is not the real difference between the mass murderer and the serial murderer. The common perception is that it is the ordinary guy who becomes the mass murderer, the guy who simply goes berserk one day and starts shooting. But contrary to popular perception, most mass murders are planned. Also, according to forensic psychiatrist Park Elliot Dietz, "It's never a normal person who snaps. It's always an abnormal person, often in a pressure situation. Generally, it's a sad toll of tragic proportions because the harm is so foreseeable." Mass murderers tend to suffer from a lethal combination of paranoia and depression. They feel despondent and hopeless while blaming others for their plight.

The mass murderer's fantasies tend to be common and unartful—revenge against his perceived persecutors—and his weapons tend to be military-style assault weapons that he uses at some distance from the victims. Serial killers have baroque fantasies, and they kill in an "up close and personal" way, by knifing or strangling their victims.

Serial Sexual Murderers: Lethal Recreational Predators

Serial sexual murderers, though not so named, first entered public consciousness in 1888, in London, when Jack the Ripper killed at least five prostitutes during a 10-week killing spree, slashing the victims' throats and slitting their bodies open. In the late 1920s, in Düsseldorf, Germany, Peter Kurten obtained his gratification by catching blood spurting from his victims' wounds into his mouth and swallowing it. The "Vampire of Düsseldorf" was convicted of nine murders and hanged in Cologne in 1931.

In the more modern era, there have been notable serial sexual murderers overseas—Dennis Nilsen killed 15 men who visited his London flat. Chikatilo killed at least 52 victims at various sites all over

Russia—but the United States produces more serial sexual murderers than any other country: an astounding 75% of them. It is likely that less sophisticated crime detection techniques in less industrialized countries contribute to the underreporting of serial sexual killers outside the United States. Nonetheless, the United States has the dubious distinction of leading the world in this category of serial murderers.

Serial sexual murderers are a distinct subcategory of serial killers. Not all serial murderers are serial sexual murderers. Some kill for reasons other than sex, such as money, jealousy, revenge, power, or dominance. For example, Aileen Carol Wuornos, a 34-year-old hitchhiking prostitute, became known as the "Damsel of Death" for robbing and murdering middle-aged men who stopped to give her a ride. Robbery was her chief motivation, though power and dominance may also have been factors. She pleaded guilty to seven murders and was sentenced to death. In October 2002 she was executed by lethal injection. Wuornos was not a female version of the Ted Bundy–type true predator serial sexual killer. She would likely be classified as a serial enterprise killer according to the FBI Crime Classification Manual. In other words, Wuornos killed for material gain, in this case money. In fact, most women do not appear to experience murderous, sexually sadistic fantasies. If they do experience them, they do not act them out in serial killings.

I do not know of any female serial sexual killer who operated alone. Women have collaborated with husbands in serial sexual killings. Fred and Rosemary West of Gloucestershire, England, tortured, raped, and murdered 12 young women including their 16-year-old daughter. In Canada, husband and wife Paul Bernardo and Karla Homolka teamed together to rape and kill 3 teenage girls; one was Karla's sister. Karla procured girls for Paul to rape, and videotaped the husband's rape of her sister. It seems that these women's selves were co-opted and fused with their husbands, who had these terrible sexual murder fantasies. The wish to psychologically fuse with others is a normal human tendency. Romantic love is a good example. But taken to an extreme, on one end of the scale it can result in participation in evil deeds, but on the other, it can lead to the ecstatic fusion with God experienced by saints.

No sexual fantasies were reported in the case of 64-year-old Sacramento landlady Dorothea Puenta, another criminal enterprise murderer, who was convicted of murdering three of her elderly tenants. Here the motive seems to have been greed. She was charged with nine killings in all, for poisoning her former tenants in order to get their government benefit checks. Seven bodies were unearthed from the yard of her Victorian boarding house. She received a life sentence.

Less than 5% of serial killers are women. When women commit multiple murders, they tend to do so in one episode. Sylvia Seegrist walked into a shopping mall near Philadelphia and opened fire with a rifle, killing three and injuring six others. Seegrist was found to be legally insane and was committed to a mental institution. Poisoning is a favored method of female killers. Usually, the degree of sadistic aggression is less in female murderers, perhaps due to acculturation of women against violence and the relative absence of the male hormone tied to aggression: testosterone. Women who do have murderous impulses more typically turn them on themselves and commit suicide. In every setting except where women are acutely psychotic, men have a higher incidence of violent behavior.

Serial sexual killers torture their victims for one reason only: to obtain a maximal orgasm that they are unable to achieve in any other way. That is to say, they capture, torture, and kill for recreational purposes. Killing is usually an integral part of the sexual turn-on. Sometimes, however, the killing is done to obtain a body for necrophilic purposes. At other times, the victim succumbs to the torture or the victim is killed to eliminate a witness.

It is difficult to understand serial killers because their acts seem to have nothing to do with the usual human motives that impel most ordinary crimes. They even have very little to do with the motives of most murders, which tend to be done out of passion, jealousy, and revenge, or to obtain money or power. This understanding of the killers' motivation is supported by the fact that the serial sexual killers' victims are usually unknown to them. The victims are or become mere objects or props on which the killers play out their lethal sexually sadistic and, frequently, necrophilic fantasies. Serial sexual killers do not want a partner; they crave a victim. The ultimate sexual gratification is the total domination and humiliation of helpless prey.

Serial sexual killers prey on the weak, the vulnerable, the confused, and the naïve. Their victims are people who happen to be in the wrong place at the wrong time. Often, there is very little resemblance among the victims of one serial sexual killer—although Ted Bundy did frequently choose young women who parted their long, dark hair down the middle of their heads.

Serial sexual killers are usually identified—when they are identified at all—because in the acting out of their fantasies, they leave their characteristic signatures on the bodies of their victims and on the other elements of the crime scene. It is these clues that have led the FBI's Behavioral Science Unit to success in deducing the general identity of serial sexual killers, as well as in arresting some killers.

Serial sexual killers have been studied psychologically. They usually hit their peak of killings in their late 20s, with a range in age from the early 20s to the mid-30s. Their fantasies, however, begin 10 or 15 years before the first killing, usually in their early to mid-adolescence. Serial sexual killers do not suddenly become psychotic and start killing. In fact, very few are out of touch with reality. As a group, they show certain striking characteristics. Serial sexual murderers become loners at an early age and show a marked preference for fantasy over reality. Their fantasies usually fuse violence and cruelty with sexuality. Many, though not all, were severely physically and sexually abused as children. A number of them, including Bundy and Berkowitz, were illegitimate or adopted; several were sons of prostitutes. Although they are deeply angry and full of malignant hatred, there is no evidence that a particular childhood trauma is being endlessly repeated in their crimes. Some serial sexual killers had intensely ambivalent, smothering relationships with their mothers that were fueled by both maternal abuse and sexual attraction to the mother.

The play of children who become serial sexual killers is joyless and shows repetitive and aggressively hostile patterns. They display a disregard for other children. They set fires, lie, steal, destroy property, and are cruel to animals as well as to other children. David Berkowitz set thousands of fires. They are rebellious and difficult to control. As adults, when they begin their criminal careers, they may start with assaultive behavior and escalate to burglary, arson, abduction, rape, and nonsexual murder. They finally reach the absolute depths with sadistic and necrophilic sexual murder. Some serial sexual killers like to impersonate police officers, are attracted to police work, and sometimes even insert themselves into the investigations of crimes they have committed. John Gacy, Edmund Kemper, Ted Bundy, Kenneth Bianchi, David Berkowitz, and Wayne B. Williams (who was convicted of murdering at least 28 known victims in Atlanta) were police buffs or impersonated police. Dennis Nilsen, who killed for company out of loneliness, actually served a year in the London police force.

Police work holds a certain fascination for many people, particularly because it exposes the titillating darker side of life. But serial sexual killers have their own unique set of motivations. Impersonating a police officer gains the serial sexual killers easy access to their victims by momentarily lowering the victims' guard. Police work lends itself to the killers' fantasies of power, domination, and submission. Some killers view their relationship with the police as a chess match, taking great pleasure at beating them at their own game. For others, the fear of being apprehended is an aphrodisiac, leading some serial killers to court police attention. Others still may want to have an inside track on the progress of police investigations into the murders. The line between police work and criminal behavior sometimes can be a very fine one.

Dennis L. Rader, the BTK murderer ("Bind them, Torture them, Kill them") started killing in 1974 and stopped in 1991. He killed at least 10 victims, men, women and children ranging in age from a woman in her 60s to a child of less than 10. Rader is the perfect example of a serial killer hiding in plain view. He was employed as a code enforcement officer, having a badge and carrying a gun, which gave him the power to control others. For 34 years Rader and his wife attended church. He became a member of his church's governing council, volunteered in his son's Boy Scout troop, and earned a college degree in criminal justice. When his wife told Rader she was afraid of the BTK killer, he told her to lock the doors and not to worry.

Dr. Jekyll and Mr. Hyde—Hiding in Plain View

As with Dr. Jekyll and Mr. Hyde, the famous fictional depiction of the two alternate sides of a single personality, most serial sexual killers can appear quite ordinary and indistinguishable from the rest of humanity. Parallel with their monstrous, murderous side, they also lead reasonably normal lives, at least in outward appearance. Serial sexual murderers share the same human condition with everyone else. They have to fill their cars with gas, pay their bills, make a living, and pay their taxes. So they take on the protective coloration of the guy next door—a coloration that makes it even more difficult to detect and apprehend them.

Like politics, most serial killers are local. A notable exception is Ted Bundy, who traveled through a number of states during his killing spree. Serial killers generally prowl within a specific area. Gary Ridgway, the Green River Killer, collected his prey from the red light districts of Seattle and Takoma and along Pacific Highway South.

It is much easier to live in a community and hide in plain view than to be a newcomer who attracts attention and thereby risks detection. Changing locations also requires adjustments to the killer's tried and true methods of stalking victims, thus increasing the likelihood of apprehension.

The most seemingly normal and prosperous of outward lives was that composed by John Wayne Gacy. As a serial sexual killer, he raped, sodomized, tortured, and strangled to death 33 young men. He did this while running a prosperous construction business, marrying twice, and becoming a public benefactor. The acute phase of his killings began about 7 months before his second marriage and continued through that marriage and afterwards. The gregarious Gacy buried most of his victims in the basement of the home where he lived with his wife and entertained their friends. These burials, with Gacy's use of the house as a cover for horrible activities, were a perfect metaphor of his dual life.

Gacy was active in community projects and belonged to several civic organizations. He was voted the local Jaycees' outstanding member for 1967. As a member of the Jolly Jokers Club, Gacy created the character of Pogo the Clown, and as Pogo he traveled to hospitals to bring cheer to sick children. As director of the Polish Constitution Day Parade in 1978, he was photographed with First Lady Rosalynn Carter. In referring to his antics as a clown—and perhaps to more of his other activities—he once said, "A clown can get away with murder."

When Gacy had victims alone in his home, he would ply them with alcohol and drugs and show them heterosexual and then homosexual porn films. He would immobilize them by tricking them into participating in handcuff and rope tricks. He would then strangle them to death, but slowly, tightening and loosening the ligatures many times in order to prolong the victim's agony and his own sexual pleasure.

In the movie about Gacy, *To Catch a Killer*, Gacy was played by actor Brian Dennehy. In a television interview about the role, Dennehy candidly admitted, "I learned about a part of myself."

Theodore Robert "Ted" Bundy, who killed 35 women, and possibly more, had an almost perfect cover. His mother considered him to be an ideal son. His political friends considered him to be on the fast track in the legal profession, heading toward being a future governor or senator. His girlfriends found him to be a woman's romantic dream come true, an attentive, tender lover who sent flowers and wrote love poems. He was engaged to marry at one point. At another time, he was dating one woman and killed 24 others, all of them strangers to him. His girlfriends did not satisfy his intense, predatory impulses. Most of them were unaware of those impulses, although at least one of them became aware of some of his desires for deviant sexual practices.

Bundy and Gacy used their covers to lure victims. Gacy attracted some young men with promises of jobs in his construction business, whereas Bundy lured women by smooth talking, and also by feigning an injury. With his arm in a cast, he would get them into his car, or to some isolated spot, and then bludgeon them with a short crowbar concealed in the removable arm cast. While the women were unconscious or semiconscious, he would then commit gross sexual acts, including anal assault. Bundy bit various body parts, sometimes biting off a victim's nipple or leaving bite marks on her buttocks. He killed the victims by strangulation. Bundy mutilated and decapitated their bodies and severed their hands with a hacksaw. He would leave the bodies in secluded spots and return to them after several days to commit necrophilic acts such as ejaculating into the mouth of a disembodied head.

More Bad Than Mad?

Serial sexual killers are sadistic sexual psychopaths. They are males, mostly white males, and of at least average intelligence. Some have demonstrated superior intelligence.

Sadistic. Sexual. Psychopaths. Each of these descriptive terms is important. Psychopaths have deviant personality and character flaws. They are detached from others. Their relationships with people have importance to themselves only insofar as these relationships provide them with pleasure; otherwise, they discard people like trash. Psychopaths' consciences are deformed or essentially absent—they are unwilling to restrain their antisocial aggressive and sexual impulses.

In serial sexual killers, the sexual and aggressive drives are fused together at an early age. Among sexual murderers, sadists are those who derive intense sexual pleasure from inflicting suffering upon a live victim. Some of these killers record the terrified screams of the tortured victims and play them back later for renewed pleasure. Kenneth

Bianchi and his cousin Angelo Buono, known together as the Hillside Strangler, would strangle women while having sex, bringing them back to life over and over again to heighten their own orgiastic ecstasy. Once the women had been strangled to death, they were no longer of interest to the cousins, who dumped them unceremoniously along hillsides in the Los Angeles area. Because both men also carried on plentiful sex lives during the period that they were committing their murders, it is clear that sex alone was not the motive for the murders. Sadism played a large part in it.

As with some other serial killers, Bianchi was fascinated by police work and wanted to join the Los Angeles police force. He even inserted himself into the Hillside Strangler investigation, asking the police to show him some of the sites where the women had been found. It is actions like these that permit us to understand that, unlike some psychotic killers, serial sexual murderers do know right from wrong. The perception that their sexually aggressive impulses are irresistible is an incomplete explanation of their behavior; instead, serial killers choose not to resist these impulses in their continuing quest for thrilling orgiastic pleasure. Even those serial sexual killers who claim to be compelled to kill by the sheer force of their deviant drives know what they are doing and that what they are doing is wrong. But they choose to do it anyway for the sexual gratification. Among human beings, knowing what is right does not necessarily lead to doing the right thing. It is necessary to *want* to do the right thing. Often we do not want something because it is good. It is good because we want it.

Serial sexual killers are always sadistic, sometimes necrophilic, often both. They all obtain sexual thrills from the hurt and terror they produce in their victims and from the total power they wield over their victims, alive or dead. In psychiatric terms, these killers are psychopaths who have a *paraphilia*. Paraphilias are characterized by acting out, or being distressed by, recurrent intense sexual urges and sexually arousing fantasies that involve either nonhuman objects or the suffering and humiliation of oneself or of children or other nonconsenting persons. A psychopath who does not also have a sadistic paraphilia might not kill; he or she could be satisfied with perpetrating various scams. And the sadist who is not a psychopath might confine his or her sexual desires to fantasy or to acting out the sadistic impulses with the aid of a consenting masochistic partner. So, too, the necrophile who is not a psychopath might be content to have sex with dead bodies that he digs out of a graveyard or with bodies that he works with in a mortuary. The disordered core of the serial sexual murderer requires that he have a lethal combination of psychopathy and sadism or necrophilia.

Edmund Emil Kemper III was a necrophilic killer. Such killers usually murder their victims quickly to obtain the object of their desire. The victim may be spared a slow, agonizing death. The necrophilic killer's sexual desires begin with the victim's death and are kindled by the dead body. Kemper wished to procure a dead body for his purposes, and later, after being imprisoned, he was quite clear about his intentions. "I'm sorry to sound so cold about this, but what I needed to have was a particular experience with a person, and to possess them in the way I had to, I had to evict them from their bodies." It was as though he was a landlord, getting rid of an unwanted tenant. Kemper also said,

> I have fantasies about mass murder—whole groups of select women I could get together in one place, get them dead, and then make mad, passionate love to their dead corpses. Taking life away from them, [from] a living human being, and then having possession of everything that used to be theirs—all that would be mine. Everything.

A small proportion of serial killers, though no less deadly, are driven to murder by psychosis (a break with reality), hallucinations (seeing or hearing things not there), and delusions (immutable false ideas). It is estimated that for every 10 sadistic sexual psychopathic killers, there is one psychotic serial killer. Richard Chase, "the Vampire of Sacramento," murdered six persons and drank their blood in order to replace his own, which he delusionally believed was turning to powder. David Berkowitz, the "Son of Sam" murderer in New York City, said he was tormented by howling voices and mad fantasies. Investigators were told that he had been commanded to kill by his demonic neighbor, 63-year-old Sam Carr, a semiretired owner of a local telephone answering service. Berkowitz may have raised this notion as a ruse during his trial and may not have been truly delusional during the murders, whereas Richard Chase was very deranged.

Generally, in psychotic serial killers, clear sexual motives and fantasies are absent or play only a minor role. These individuals are not serial sexual killers because sexual fantasies do not motivate them. That is evident from studies of the crime scenes that they leave behind. Whereas the crime scene of the serial sexual killer has been characterized as organized and ritualized, the crime scene left by a psychotic serial killer is recognizably disorganized and shows palpable evidence of his or her inability to think rationally.

It is possible for killers, driven by sadistic sexual fantasies, to kill without attempting penetration of their victims or without performing any overtly sexual acts with the victim. The *sexual* in the serial sexual killer refers to the presence of sexual fantasies that drive them to kill, not to sexual activity that may or may not occur before or after the victim's death. Most killers, however, demonstrate a pattern of escalation. In the beginning, just the death of the victim may be sufficient to gratify some key elements of the killer's sadistic sexual fantasies. Later on, in their series of killings, additional and more bizarre and baroque elements may enter into the murders.

After they are caught, most serial killers proclaim their innocence to the bitter end. John Wayne Gacy, for example, maintained his innocence despite overwhelming and irrefutable evidence that he had killed at least 33 men. Gacy was executed by lethal injection on May 10, 1994, after spending more than 14 years on death row. Some serial killers seek to exculpate themselves by pleading insanity. Insanity is a legal construct that does not correspond well to psychiatric definitions of mental disorder. There is often an imperfect fit between legal and psychiatric concepts and terminology. In the courts, a criminal defendant may be quite psychotic (that is, out of touch with reality) but still may not qualify for an insanity defense. Jeffrey Dahmer's counsel described his client as a "steam-rolling killing machine" that was out of control, a man on the track of madness. The prosecution, however, depicted Dahmer as a cold, calculating murderer who carefully planned his crimes and covered up their traces. Generally, in order to be relieved of criminal responsibility in the courts, the accused must suffer from a mental disease or defect that substantially interferes with the accused's ability to distinguish right from wrong or to conform his or her conduct to the requirements of the law. These requirements vary from jurisdiction to jurisdiction. In a few states, the insanity defense has been abolished altogether.

The law presumes that criminals choose to commit crimes rationally and of their own free will and therefore are deserving of punishment. Some offenders, however, are so mentally disturbed in their thinking and behavior that they are considered to be incapable of acting rationally. Under these circumstances, and with an eye toward fundamental principles of fairness and morality, civilized societies have deemed it unjust to punish a "crazy" person. Additionally, the punishment of a person who cannot rationally appreciate the consequences of his or her actions thwarts the two major aims of punishment: retribution and deterrence.

Neuroscience is confirming what psychiatrists have always known, that total free will is a fiction. Free will is a controversial notion, influenced by philosophical, political, cultural, religious, social, and psychological factors, as well as medical ones. For example, some bad choices are based on faulty brain circuitry and neuronal activity. These neural defects in turn may arise from childhood trauma, head injury, substance abuse, deprivation, genetic defects, or other causes. When psychiatrists examine the individual and the circumstances, they may discover that free will played a minor role or no role in the individual's choices and actions.

The Dahmer case displayed for a wide audience the mine field of legal sanity and insanity, and of making a forensic psychiatric diagnosis of the condition of such a murderer as Jeffrey Dahmer. Respected forensic psychiatrists testified for both sides. The prosecution experts found that Dahmer was not suffering from a mental illness that prevented him from distinguishing right from wrong, and that he could control his behavior. The defense experts disagreed, saying that in their opinion, Dahmer was indeed seriously mentally ill. His paraphilia, in their opinion, approached psychotic proportions. Furthermore, he could not control his murderous impulses even when he wanted to do so.

It was true that Dahmer had struggled hard against his aberrant sexual impulses in the 7 years that elapsed between his first and his second killing. Because Dahmer was able to plan his murders, and to systematically dispose of the bodies, the jury was convinced that he did have the ability to control his behavior. All the testimony bolstered the theory that, like most serial killers, Dahmer knew what he was doing and knew right from wrong. Finally, the jury did not accept the defense that Dahmer suffered from a mental illness to the degree that it had disabled his thinking or behavioral controls.

Most juries are outraged by the violent crimes of serial killers and seek to punish the killers severely, sometimes even when they are offered irrefutable evidence of severe mental illness present in the killer.

For example, in order to convict, juries may seize on the evidence that the murders were planned, even though the accused did not know that what he or she was doing was wrong because of a severe psychosis. The fact that murders may be planned in exquisite detail does not necessarily mean that the perpetrator appreciated the wrongfulness of his or her acts. In these cases, the juries invariably find the killers to be bad rather than mad, even though the commonsense view of the killers' outrageous behavior is that it is "crazy," that is to say, mentally deranged. Dahmer was sentenced to 15 consecutive life sentences, or about 950 years in jail without the possibility of parole. On November 28, 1994, Dahmer was beaten to death in a prison bathroom by another inmate.

In the case of Dahmer, experts agreed that one way or another, he should never be released from an institution—whether it was a jail or a confining psychiatric institution. This agreement reflects the common view, too, that such killers ought never to see freedom again. In fact, psychopathic sexual sadistic murderers are not treatable by any current psychological therapy or medicine. Proof of that comes from such cases as that of Edmund Kemper. As a huge 15-year-old, Kemper murdered his grandparents, was declared insane, and was committed for an indefinite period to the Atascadero State Hospital in California. Five years later, after his model behavior and psychological insights convinced the authorities that Kemper was ready to return to the outside world, he was released in the care of his mother. Three years after his release, he murdered eight more people, including his mother, before voluntarily surrendering. He has since told interviewers that he knows he must be kept incarcerated in one form or another because if he is not, he will kill again. Similarly, more than a year after Jeffrey Dahmer's trial and conviction, he admitted, "I still do have those old compulsions." Even 17 years after committing the Son of Sam murders, David Berkowitz still maintained to interviewers the belief, whether delusional or fabricated, that it was others in a satanic cult, and not he, who had killed on the streets of New York.

Some psychotic killers may experience a remission in their mental illness through medical treatment and thus escape the demons that pushed them to murder. Serial sexual killer psychopaths cannot escape their own murderous fantasies. While they are incarcerated, however, these psychopathic killers are affable, eager to please, helpful—and always manipulative.

Lost Childhoods and the Fantasy Inferno

The sad fact is that serial sexual murderers are created in their early childhoods, probably before the age of 5 or 6. Some experts say they are born killers; others assert that they develop into killers through their teens and young adulthood. In either case, a troubled environment only enhances inherited lethal tendencies. In an important FBI study that interviewed in depth 36 incarcerated serial killers, there were many findings that offer some insight into these killers' psychological development. Almost half of the biological fathers of these men left home before the boys were 12 years old. The absence of a solid male role model is a significant fact in their development as killers. But the presence of a father in the house is no guarantee of normality. For these boys, the presence in the house of a cruel, insensitive father may be worse for them than having an absent father. The fact remains that the vast majority of boys from troubled homes and backgrounds do not become serial killers. Moreover, in the midst of a caring, loving family, it is unlikely that a child will consistently prefer fantasy to real life.

But serial sexual killers do choose fantasies that are related in varying degrees to their uncaring, unloving families. Most serial killers experienced severe physical and sexual abuse as children. John Wayne Gacy was terrorized by a harsh, alcoholic, disciplinarian father. Gacy was sickly, overweight, unathletic, dreamy, and imaginative. As a young child, Gacy was sexually abused by a neighbor and by a family friend. His father whipped him with a belt kept expressly for that purpose and heaped on him a merciless barrage of emotional abuse. He never lost an opportunity to express disappointment in him, calling him "dumb" and "stupid." At around age 5, Gacy began to suffer from a form of psychomotor epilepsy (seizures with multiple sensory, muscular, and psychic components) for which he eventually was prescribed phenytoin and phenobarbital. As a preadolescent, Gacy became progressively more dependent on the mood-altering highs of his medication. His father expressed contempt for the son's illness, thought the boy was malingering, and accused his wife of pampering him. He warned his wife that John was "going to be a queer" and heaped scorn on his son by calling him a "he-she." Years afterwards, when he was killing his 33 victims, Gacy referred to them as "worthless little queers and punks."

Ted Bundy was an illegitimate child. His father's identity remained a mystery. The family situation was distinctly abnormal for that era, and his maternal grandparents created a cover story to hide Ted's illegitimacy. The grandmother suffered from recurrent depression that sometimes required electroshock treatment. Bundy's grandfather was an inflexible perfectionist given to easy verbal abuse and to the occasional physical abuse of cats, dogs, and his wife. Ted later denied that the grandfather or anyone else had physically or sexually abused him in his childhood.

Ted Bundy's own morbid tendencies were apparent from the time he was 3. When he was that age, and his Aunt Julia was 15, she later recalled, she woke up one morning to find little Ted lifting the blankets from her bed and quietly sliding in a butcher knife next to her. "He just stood there and grinned," she said of the incident. "I shooed him out of the room and took the implement back down to the kitchen, and told my mother about it. I remember thinking at the time that I was the only one who thought it [the incident] was strange. Nobody did anything."

In grade school, Bundy's innate intelligence was recognized, but the reports home about his good grades were invariably accompanied by notes from his teachers about the need for control of his ferocious temper. In junior high, still an excellent student, Ted was active in the Boy Scouts and continued to go to church regularly with his family. A female high school classmate remembered him as attractive, well dressed, and very well mannered. However, beneath such a facade of normalcy, Bundy was sneaking out of his home at night to peep on women as they undressed. It was part of his compulsive masturbating. Later on, during his high school years, Bundy shoplifted expensive clothes and ski equipment. He was picked up twice by the police on suspicion of burglary and auto theft, but nothing came of it. And so, beneath the all-American boy image, the psychopathic predator continued to develop, and so did his murderous fantasies.

As Bundy did, most serial sexual killers progress through an escalating series of antisocial acts before they begin killing. Such people do not simply wake up one morning to discover their monstrous identity. Considered odd since childhood, and habitually isolated socially, those who become future serial sexual killers turn inward and incubate sadistic sexual fantasies. The fantasy inferno raging within their minds throws off symptomatic sparks that assume the shape of compulsive masturbation, transvestism, voyeurism, exhibitionism, and other deviant acts.

During their childhoods, a number of serial killers also develop the triad of behaviors made up of bed-wetting, fire-setting, and cruelty to animals. Richard Chase displayed the full triad. David Berkowitz set, by his own admission in his journals, 1,411 fires. He also tortured and killed small animals. One early victim was his mother's parakeet, which he stealthily fed cleaning powder over a period of weeks until the bird dropped dead.

Jeffrey Dahmer was particularly remembered for his mutilation of dead animals. As a youngster, he would roam the woods adjacent to his home, collecting dead animals and often abusing their carcasses. He collected and placed into jars a large number of animals and animal parts. Once Dahmer came across a road-killed dog. He dismembered it, cut off the head, and impaled it on a stick. Andrei Chikatilo suffered from chronic bed-wetting. So did Kenneth Bianchi.

Edmund Kemper's cruelty to animals was enormous. He buried a kitten alive, dug it up, took it to his room, decapitated it, put the head on a spindle, and offered prayers to it. One of his favorite prayers—which he also offered in church—was that everyone in the world would die except himself. At around age 13, Kemper was killing neighborhood cats and other animals. When one cat seemed to prefer his sister to him, he sliced off the top of its head with a machete, exposing the brain. Then, as the cat went into convulsions, he stabbed it repeatedly until it died. Afterward, he burned the body, keeping some of its parts in his closet. He also cut off the hands and head of his sister's doll.

Kemper would repeat these actions as an adult in his murders. He decapitated one of his victims and kept her head in a box in a closet of his mother's apartment for a while before burying the head underneath a stepping stone near the back door, which faced his bedroom window. "I talked to it," he later told police; "I said affectionate things like you would say to a girlfriend or wife." One of his last victims was his mother. He cut off her head and right hand, and he cut out her larynx and put that in the garbage disposal. He put the head on his mantelpiece, so he could throw darts at it. In fantasy, as much as in other aspects of life, the child is father to the man.

As noted earlier, there are thousands upon thousands of children who have been bed-wetters and fire-setters and have been cruel to animals but who have not grown up to be serial sexual murderers. One expert observed that such children are statistically much more likely to become vice-presidents of corporations than to become serial killers. Nevertheless, this "terrible triad" of behaviors is usually a sure sign of a child who is in trouble. Psychologically caused bed-wetting usually implies emotional disturbance, together with poor impulse control. Torturing and killing animals demonstrates an ominous level of sadism and cruelty. Fire-setting by a child is usually a symptomatic expression of sexual and aggressive overstimulation. Fire often expresses the child's hyperactive excitement and deep-seated anger. The recognition and treatment of children who display these symptoms appears to be critical to the prevention of future violence of all kinds.

As for child abuse, which is also present in the backgrounds of most serial killers, its precise relationship to their killing remains a mystery. It may act as a trigger that later sets off murderous impulses in individuals predisposed toward violence. Very many thousands of children have been abused, and very few of them become serial killers. Nevertheless, the recognition and treatment of children who have been abused are also of potentially great importance to the prevention of future violence.

Deviant Fantasies, Lethal Orgasms

In the ideal, sexual love between two persons is the mutual, tender, intimate exploration of one another that ultimately becomes a joyful celebration of the couple's caring relationship. In real life, however, sexual relations may come to include elements of power, domination, deprecation, anger, and even cruelty. For some couples, these latter elements may add creativity and zest to their sexual experience. In all sexual relationships, both conscious and unconscious fantasies are played out. In other couples, however, these added elements serve to make their relationships unhappy.

Men who become serial sexual murderers are usually sexually dysfunctional. Most suffer from some form of impotence during "normal" sex. Whether they are heterosexual or homosexual, serial sexual murderers are unable to have and to maintain mature, consensual sexual experiences with other adults. Serial sexual killers can, however, achieve powerful orgasms if their extremely deviant sexual fantasies are fulfilled. Many of their sexual acts are regressive, sadistic parodies of sexual intercourse. Some, for example, insert objects into their victims and masturbate. Bundy raped one college girl vaginally and rectally with an aerosol can. The homosexual killers on record have shown a marked preference for sadomasochism, torture, and bondage.

The fantasies of serial sexual murderers link sexual and destructive acts. These powerful fantasies reflect themes of power, dominance, exploitation, and revenge. Most people have fantasies of sexual adventure. In serial killers, these are fused with ideas of degradation and humiliation of others. In most people's fantasies of sexual adventure, the partner experiences as much fun as the dreamer. Not so with sexual murderers: the more fun the serial sexual murderer is having during his fantasy, the more lethal danger the fantasy partner will experience. A common male fantasy is to have sex with a beautiful model or movie star. A common serial sexual murderer fantasy may begin with a beautiful model or movie star but goes on from there to fantasies of immobilizing and slashing her during sex. The more pain she suffers, the greater his enjoyment. The articulate and brutally perverted Ted Bundy described the moment of thrilling orgasm this way:

> You feel the last bit of breath leaving their body. You're looking into their eyes. A person in that situation is God! You then possess them and they shall be a part of you, and the grounds where you kill them or leave them become sacred to you, and you will always be drawn back to them.

As sexual killers go through puberty and adolescence, and experience sexual arousal, their deviant sexual fantasies deepen. The fantasies that they already have are supercharged by the upsurge in sex hormones and are further fed by the solitariness that they also cultivate. The lethal fantasies gain power and finally begin to drive not only the dreams of a potential murderer, but most of his waking thoughts, too. Ed Kemper remembered, "I knew long before I started killing that I was going to be killing, that it was going to end up like that. The fantasies were too strong. They were going on for too long and were too elaborate."

Once killers have had the fantasies spill out into reality, and have committed a murder based on them, they feel further empowered. The killing makes them feel invincible and, this too, feeds the fantasies. The elements of murder then become integrated into more and more elaborate, continually embellished and Byzantine sadistic sexual fantasies. Over time, the serial sexual murderers improve their homicidal techniques, learning from prior mistakes to become more efficient killing machines. Chikatilo, horrified by the murder of his first victim, vowed to himself it would never happen again. But when it happened for the second time, he accepted his murderous identity and rejoiced with a spontaneous celebratory dance. When Kemper cut off the head of one of his later victims, "There was almost a climax to it," he recalled. "It was kind of an exalted, triumphant-type thing, like taking the head of a deer or an elk or something would be, to a hunter."

Why would a person do such things as Kemper did—keep the heads and perform sexual acts with them, keep mementos of hair, skin, and personal belongings, keep Polaroid photos of the bodies and eat parts of his victims? "If I killed them," Kemper said of his victims, "they couldn't reject me as a man. It was more or less making a doll out of a human being, carrying out my fantasies with a doll, a living human doll." When he destroyed his victims, down to their individual parts, Kemper felt "a fantastic passion overwhelming me." Echoing Bundy, he said that he returned to one of his victims' burial site because "I visited there to be near her. I loved her and wanted her." The compulsion to come back to the murder site and relive those moments has been referred to by one expert as "rolling in it." During the time that the killings were taking place, Kemper was having a platonic relationship with a young woman to whom he eventually became engaged, and who later described him as a perfect gentleman. Today, in prison, Kemper feels he is not completely alone. At his trial, he chillingly explained, "I wanted the girls for myself, as possessions. They were going to be mine. They are mine."

Jeffrey Dahmer discussed his fantasies with several of the psychiatrists who examined him before his trial. He began compulsively masturbating two or three times a day at age 14, initially to a conventional though homosexual fantasy of having sex with a well-proportioned, muscular male. By his late teens, his fantasy had evolved into rendering his victims unconscious and exposing their viscera. His only delight and sense of feeling alive came from the all-consuming, relentless urge for sexual pleasure as his fantasy now defined it.

Dahmer desired a warm male body next to him that he could totally control and that would never leave him. He needed a compliant, nondemanding, unresisting, always available partner. And so, when a victim visited his apartment, Dahmer would furtively put him to sleep with a rum and coke drink spiked with a ground-up sleep medication. If the victim woke and tried to leave, Dahmer would strike and immobilize him. He would then come up close and listen to the victim's body sounds. What Dahmer really wanted sexually was hugging, genital fondling, mutual masturbation, lying together for long periods of time so he could listen to his partner's heartbeat and feel human warmth.

It is possible that Dahmer could have found consenting adults who would fulfill those parts of his fantasy having to do with being close and with bondage, but Dahmer had few social graces and even less confidence that he could meet someone who could gratify his sexual needs. So, to satisfy those needs, he immobilized and killed his victims. He performed primitive frontal lobotomies on two of them while they were still alive, boring holes into their heads with a small electric drill. He then used a turkey baster to inject weak muriatic acid into one victim, boiling water into the other, producing convulsions and, after a few hours, death in the latter victim. These failed experiments expressed his fantasy: that he would never be alone but would always possess compliant, zombie-like sex slaves upon whom he could perform his preferred sex acts.

Dahmer was not a true necrophile. He would rather have satisfied his sexual wishes with a live body, but he did not think anyone would cooperate with him, so he used dead bodies. That way, his victims did not awake to assault him or to escape and inform the police—or even to demand from Dahmer, in return for their sexual favors, sexual acts for themselves, particularly anal sex, which Dahmer detested. Although he committed monstrous acts on the bodies of his victims, Dahmer apparently was not a sadist. His goal was not to derive pleasure from torturing his victims but to create sex slaves through his demonic "zombie experiments." Dahmer defies definitive psychiatric diagnosis. This was quite apparent from the divergent diagnoses proffered by forensic psychiatric experts during his trial.

Once Dahmer had killed his victims, he felt it was a shame to waste their lives, so he kept various of their body parts, even though he disliked the act of cutting up the bodies. He decapitated 11 of the victims and kept some of the heads in a refrigerator, along with genitals and other parts that Dahmer used to enhance his masturbation. He also created a ghoulish temple of painted skulls and skeletons on a table flanked by incense urns and lit by blue globe lights.

If he ate his victims, Dahmer thought, they would provide him with strength and vitality, and they would live on through him. So he treated a victim's biceps and heart with meat tenderizer, fried them in cooking oil, and added steak sauce. Dahmer later said the biceps tasted like steak, but the heart was spongy and rather tasteless. While he dined, Dahmer watched a pornographic video and drank more and more alcohol. By consuming parts of his victims, Dahmer was living out primitive cannibalistic merger fantasies, perhaps an aberrational twist of the universal human wish to fuse with others.

Mind Murder and Sexual Murder

In the book *Sexual Homicide: Patterns and Motives*, Robert Ressler and colleagues note that "many [serial sexual killers] emphasize that they are doing exactly what everyone else thinks of doing." Well, not exactly. Most people do experience cruel, sadistic thoughts and feelings at some level and at some time, but it is highly unlikely that they grapple with the same intensity and elaboration of sadistic sexual fantasies as serial killers, much less put them into action. Lionel Dahmer, in speaking of his son's first victim, whom Jeffrey Dahmer had no memory of killing, chillingly revealed,

> He had awakened, as I had awakened at times in my youth, feeling a terrible certainty that I had committed murder. The only difference was that Jeff had actually done it, had actually done what I had only feared having done. I had awakened in a panic that consciousness had soon ended. Jeff had awakened into a nightmare that would never end.

For some, the fascination with the lurid crimes of serial sexual killers betrays a fear that within them the same violent demons lurk. Yet it is highly unlikely that "good" persons who harbor conscious, garden-variety sexually sadistic fantasies and impulses will ever slide down the slippery slope into serial killing. In my judgment, serial sexual killers are on the extreme end of our human dark side. They act out consciously the antisocial impulses that "normal" men and women keep locked way in the dark crevices of their mind. Yet bits and pieces of sadistic sexual fantasies may escape in the form of disguised dreams, symptoms, or quirky behaviors in almost everyone. Many years ago, Freud observed that the sexual life of so-called normal people often contained behaviors that were commonly found among what he called the sexual perversions. Freud said, "The conclusion now presents itself to us that there is indeed something innate lying behind the perversions but that it is something innate in *everyone*, though as a disposition it may vary in its intensity and may be increased by the influences of actual life." Given the complexity and vicissitudes of individual psychosexual development, Freud's observation that every man (and woman) is entitled to at least one perversion is certainly understandable.

Although many people imagine a piece of the serial killer's fantasies—such as the need to control or dominate another—their fantasies are not directed toward obtaining an orgasm at the cost of another person's life. Most people cannot derive intense sexual arousal by hurting another person. Nor are they psychopaths, totally devoid of conscience or empathy for others. The serial killer's sadistic sexual fantasies begin where most people's conscious fantasies end. The serial sexual killer's path is not a stroll through the garden of everyday cruel thoughts and feelings. Rather, the serial killer's fantasies relentlessly take him across a nightmarish mental landscape into the valley of death.

In their attempt to rationalize the murders they commit by stating that others have similar wishes but are afraid to act on them, serial killers do make an unintended point that tells us something about other people. There are many spouses and children in the world whose minds are raped and murdered sexually, and who in other ways are sadistically brutalized by their partners or parents. These cases never find their way to a court, to the authorities, or even into the headlines. Even when the outcome is not physical murder, all sorts of depredations and sadistic sexual acts are regularly perpetrated on unwilling but trapped victims. All over the world, every day, spouses and children are treated with utter contempt, used as objects solely for the pleasure of someone else, plundered, and thrown away. Although most victims do not die at the hands of their exploiters, they are mentally murdered, and often behind very respectable doors. The individuals who sadistically abuse and exploit—mind-rape—others are disturbingly ordinary, some are exemplary citizens, and they come from all walks of life. Some are our neighbors and, to varying degrees, some are ourselves.

Beyond Fantasy: Biology, Addiction, and Destiny

Beyond every deviant thought lies a deviant molecule, some say. But what causes the brain to act in a deviant manner? Do serial killers inherit their monstrous behaviors? Are their strong, aberrant sexual fantasies fueled by powerful, genetically determined aggressive and sexual drives? Are the genetic factors present at birth enough to condemn an individual to a life of lust and murder? Jeffrey Dahmer's father, Lionel Dahmer, writing in his book *A Father's Story*, fatalistically observes, "As a scientist, I further wonder if this potential for great evil also resides deep in the blood that some of us fathers and mothers may pass on to our children at birth." What about head injuries or the presence of covert or overt neurobiologic disorders—do these play a significant role in producing violence? For example, preliminary studies have found high levels of the elements cadmium and lead in the hair of some serial killers. Other research reveals significant differences in the brain chemistry of murderers compared with normal control subjects. How about mental injuries, for instance, those produced by parental deprivation of care, by physical or sexual abuse of a child? It is quite possible that bad experiences may cause bad brain chemistry. Jeffrey Dahmer's history revealed no physical or sexual abuse in his childhood. Could he have been a victim of aberrant genes?

As stated earlier, most serial sexual murderers were abused as children. Some forensic experts believe that being the victim of extreme child abuse ultimately causes the abused person to identify with his or her abuser. This accords with reports from sadistic sexual murderers that they became highly sexually excited by the fear they saw in their victims' faces. Some serial killers inflict terror, pain, and helplessness on their victims as a means of obtaining empowerment and mastery over their own terrifying child abuse experiences.

A most common attitude among serial killers is contempt for their victims. Bundy felt no compassion for his prey. In fact, he appeared genuinely surprised that such a fuss was being made over the murder of these "girls," or that their families would mourn their losses so deeply. "What's one less person on the face of the earth?" he shrugged, and derisively referred to his many victims as "cargo" and "damaged goods."

We know from other research that abused children tend to grow up with strong feelings of self-contempt. Treated with contempt in their childhoods, they frequently experience a depreciated view of themselves and others. Severely abused individuals often complain that they feel emotionally dead. Child abuse may lead the person to massive repression of all feelings as a means of continued survival.

This finding is pertinent to the ways in which serial murderers interact with their victims. Hating themselves, they view others with equivalent contempt. To the serial sexual murderer who uses his victim solely for the purposes of his own orgasm, the victim has no inherent value as a human being. Dennis Nilsen observed with inhuman detachment that the weight of a severed head when picked up by the hair was far heavier than one would imagine. The ever-present deprecation and humiliation of self that the perpetrators transfer to their victims may make it easier for serial sexual murderers to carry out their sadistic behaviors. In their actions of controlling, torturing, and killing a victim, murderers briefly relieve themselves of profound self-contempt. Moreover, it may be that only intensely sexually sadistic exploitation of their victims brings serial sexual killers out of an emotional deadness to life, temporarily allowing them to feel calm and relaxed. A number of serial sexual killers reported feeling "normal" for a period of time after committing a murder.

The fact that most serial killers escalate their level of killing over time has given rise to the suggestion that an addiction model may explain some things about their behavior. In Gacy, Kemper, Chikatilo, and Bundy, the killing pace not only quickened over time, but dramatically increased near the end as they spun out of control. "A compulsive obsession with doing what I was doing overpowered any feelings of revulsion," Dahmer told a psychiatrist. "I was dead set on going with this compulsion. It was the only thing that gave me satisfaction in life." Dennis Nilsen plaintively confessed, "I wished I could stop but I could not. I had no other thrill or happiness."

As in the story of Dr. Jekyll and Mr. Hyde, what happens to these murderers is that Mr. Hyde gradually takes over. It becomes harder and harder to bring back the kinder, gentler Dr. Jekyll. In many of these cases, the last, escalating phase was accompanied by drugs, alcohol abuse, depression, and utter depravity. As their devilishly deviant acts soared, the murderers experienced a concomitant, rapidly descending spiral in their personal lives and in their care of their own persons. The pattern overall followed that of a drug addict's descent into a living hell.

Serial sexual murderers also seem to follow that pattern in becoming addicted to the high they experience from the murders. They require ever more frequent "fixes"—that is, richer doses of sexually sadistic murder—to maintain that high. Dahmer agreed that the high was "almost addictive: it was almost a surge of energy I would feel." Kemper described it in a similar way: "The spilling of blood was not the point. What I wanted to see was the death, and I wanted to see the triumph, the exultation over the death. It was like eating, or a narcotic, something that drove me more and more and more." Gary Ridgway, the Green River Killer, described a similar experience, saying that killing prostitutes did for him "what drugs do to a junkie."

I believe that a biological theory of the behavior of serial killers is suggested by analogies from animal research into the phenomenon of *kindling*. Kindling is a word that is usually associated with the starting of fires, and a phenomenon analogous to fire starting is assumed to happen in the brains studied in this research. It was found that intermittent electrical stimulation of the brain has the effect of altering brain excitability to the point where repeated stimulation produces seizures. Over a period of time, the brain becomes more and more sensitive to this stimulation, until seizures are kindled spontaneously. In human beings, this model has been applied to explain the escalation of mood disorders over time, particularly manic-depressive disorder. What we think happens is that in vulnerable persons, repeated stressors may induce an initial, minor depression that soon remits. Subsequent life stressors produce progressively more severe cycles of depression. But later, life stressors produce a full-blown depression, and this takes longer to fade. Over time, manic-depressive symptoms appear more and more frequently. The mood-cycling progresses until the appearance of depression or manic phases seem to come about spontaneously, without obvious stressors being present. Each subsequent episode becomes more and more intractable to treatment.

Neurobiological disorders are amazingly common among criminal defendants. In one study, 15 death row inmates were chosen for examination. Evidence of neuropathology was not a criterion for selection. In each inmate, the researchers found evidence of severe head injury and neurological impairment. Other research, however, shows that there is no necessary connection between brain injury and violence, and no certain connection proven between other types of brain disorders and violence. Yet some of the serial sexual murderers have had such disorders and injuries. John Gacy had a form of psychomotor epilepsy as a child. Arthur Shawcross, another serial killer, had, in addition to his psychiatric disorder, psychomotor seizures related to temporal lobe damage.

My own speculation is that the kindling concept may have applicability to serial sexual murderers, although its ability to explain the mental life and behaviors of these murderers is unproven. Because of the escalating pattern of killings, the relief that some murderers feel after the killing, the quickening of the cycle, and the out-of-control feelings, the kindling model seems to fit. This is particularly true if the killings are understood as an aspect of recurrent depression or of manic-depressive disorder. It may be that some serial killers have an unrecognized, aberrant, or atypical form of mood disorder. One forensic psychiatric expert who examined Ted Bundy made the diagnosis of manic-depressive psychosis and attributed his murders to "uncontrollable manic rage."

Of course, that is only a theory, and no one really knows what complex of factors causes a person to become a serial sexual killer. There are tens of thousands, perhaps hundreds of thousands of children who are abused each year, but there are only 50 to 200 serial killers among us. We can classify serial killers into sadistic psychopaths or necrophiles. This may help us identify them and sometimes help us to catch them before they kill more people, but if truth be admitted, all explanations of the genesis of the serial killer are woefully inadequate. Psychiatrists and other mental health professionals must avoid becoming either "mindless" or "brainless" in their approach to understanding serial killers and the darker side of human behavior. The mindless mode dismisses psychological factors, whereas the brainless view rejects biological determinants of human behavior. Mind and body are inextricably one. In the meantime, we can perhaps better tolerate our state of ignorance concerning serial sexual killers by recalling the wisdom in Jeremiah 17:9: "The heart is deceitful above all things, and desperately wicked; who can know it?"

Jeffrey Dahmer demonstrated that the human mind is difficult to fathom, extremely plastic, and almost infinitely pliable. The capacity to fantasize is quintessentially a human experience. In fantasy, we can become anyone we choose, go anywhere, do anything. We can go forward or backward in time. We can love or hate anyone we want. Any imaginable (or unimaginable) wish can be indulged. And nobody need be the wiser. In considering Dahmer, we are reminded once again that the most important sex organ is the brain. Through fantasy, it can find almost anything sexually exciting—Dahmer was sexually aroused by the internal body sounds of his victims.

A few things can be said with certainty: serial sexual murderers have not been thoroughly studied genetically, medically, or psychologically. When the explanation for their actions is finally complete, it will turn out that their behavior can be traced to some combination of nature and nurture. Facilities and money do not exist for any project to study serial killers in a thorough way, so what we are left with is informed speculation based on the best data available. Dr. Park Elliot Dietz believes that serial killers are produced by the "right" genes in combination with the wrong parents. Asked to imagine what it would take to create another Bundy, Gacy, or Kemper, Dr. Dietz suggested:

> Start with an abusive, criminal father and a hysterical, alcoholic mother; torture the boy as erotically as possible; have the naked mother spank him and sleep with him until age 12; bind and whip him regularly; have the mother sexually arouse him and punish him for his erections; let the mother appear promiscuous while condemning prostitutes; leave detective magazines and bondage pornography around the house for him to find; and encourage him to watch R-rated slasher films and violence against glamorous women.

But for the genetic and parental luck of the draw, might you or I have become a serial killer? Yet as a practicing psychiatrist, I have been greatly impressed by patients who have been dealt a very difficult, if not impossible, hand by life. Nevertheless, these people have assumed full responsibility and have led productive and meaningful lives. A patient with a severe manic-depressive illness who was married and ran a successful business once told me, "Doc, it's not the cards you're dealt, it's how you play them." Becoming a serial killer, to some extent at least, is exercising a choice.

Ted Bundy, in his last days, made apocalyptic pronouncements against pornography, saying that it was responsible for his excesses. He opined that men progress from soft-core porn to hard-core, sadistic, bloody porn, to rape and serial murder. Dr. Dietz does not subscribe to this simplistic though popular "domino theory" of pornography addiction being the cause of serial murder. The cause lies far deeper, in the childhood that has been spent before the boy ever sees a pornographic magazine or video. Dr. Dietz observes:

> Paraphilia almost never originates after adolescence, and psychopathy never does. No sprinkling of images, however deviant, can render an

otherwise normal man either paraphilic or criminal. The leap from fantasy to action has much to do with character and the vicissitudes of life, and little or nothing to do with the objects of desire.

Perhaps Heraclitus had it right when he stated that character is destiny. The serial sexual killer's character is one so firmly formed that it fashions his destiny. We who live with a few of these killers in our midst can only hope that our destinies do not cross. But we cannot escape our human destiny. There is a bit of the sadist, the psychopath, the killer in all of us. The basic difference is that the character-driven destiny of bad men is to consciously do what good men are destined to unconsciously dream.

12

Character and Destiny

The Making of
Good Men and Women

A man's character is his fate.

—Heraclitus

Recently, one of my colleagues, an innovative thinker, posed to me the following question: Why do good men and women not act on their destructive dreams and fantasies? As is his habit, my colleague inverted the theme of my book and challenged me to examine the issue from a diametrically opposite position. The question is provocative, but I think it presumes too much—that we don't act at all on our darker impulses. Actually, good men and women manage to keep their dreams and their dark impulses under reasonable control, though not under perfect control. As I have said earlier in this book, there are no saints among us.

Based on my experience as a psychiatrist, I have found that in our lives we live out complex and powerful fantasies about ourselves and the world. Our choice of partners, the work we do, the friends we seek, the possessions we acquire, the way we dress, the cars we drive, all reflect both conscious and unconscious fantasies that we have about ourselves. One of my patients would destroy in a rage possessions of his that he felt were not perfect. He could not abide any aspersions being cast on the image of himself as perfect.

Why good men dream what bad men do is governed by environmental, biological, and genetic factors that carve our character early in life and drive our destiny. We are just beginning to appreciate the

281

importance of the genetic determinants of behavior. Lionel Dahmer's account of his own murderous dreams provides a chilling hunch that genetics played a significant part in his son Jeffrey's killings. Although we have learned a great deal, our understanding of human behavior is still limited. Much remains shrouded in mystery. A goal of this book is to stimulate a deeper interest in our good and bad behaviors.

As I have observed in earlier chapters, serial sexual killers are relentlessly and compulsively driven to kill by intense sadistic sexual fantasies. Their victims are only the means to a thrilling orgasm. In contrast, the mainstream fantasies of good women and men are life-affirming and generally enabling of others, no matter how dark the tributaries and side streams of their fantasies. Gary Ridgway, Jeffrey Dahmer, Ted Bundy, and other serial sexual killers took the lives of people for their own psychopathically selfish ends. Albert Schweitzer and Mother Teresa dedicated their lives to improve the lot of others—but even Mother Teresa, we now know from her diary and letters, was tormented by doubts and dark thoughts.

Most people who are considered "good" live their lives at various points along a broad spectrum between the extremes of good and bad. All of us, if we remained unsocialized, would act as bad men do—in antisocial ways. Feral children, those who have grown up in the wild, bereft of human warmth and care, behave more like animals than like human beings. That our nature is unregenerate is a tenet of many religions, reflected, for instance, in the concept of original sin. As Job sat on his dung heap, he observed, "Yet man is born unto trouble as the sparks fly upward."

As a psychiatrist who has sat and listened to patients for more than 45 years, I have been unable to answer the question, "What do people really want?" Beyond the easy generalizations—money, sex, power, and the need to love and be loved—I have discovered that people are immensely complex in ways that have been unforeseeable to me as well as to themselves. What do people really want? I have found in patients the most unimaginable desires, and patients have uncovered needs and conflicts they never imagined.

One could conclude from such discoveries that bad behavior is a fundamental part of our nature. But the ability to dream about bad actions and *not* to act on them is a mental capacity that can be highly developed, although it must be acquired. The achievements of civilization, hard won over the course of centuries, can be destroyed in a relative instant by a "bad" act, as the world saw with Hitler. Destruction may be truer to our basic nature than "good" acts—a state of affairs recognized by all developed societies, which always need to pass laws and maintain police forces to ensure order.

A benefit of bringing a psychological and medical perspective to the question of why bad men do what good men dream is that this perspective, though narrow in some ways, avoids the pitfall of construing men and women in terms of good and bad and instead refers to mental conditions as psychologically healthy or ill. But even after leaving the analysis of good and evil to philosophy and religion, the psychiatrist must still admit that the concept of mental health itself is elusive. Various professionals in the mental health field define that concept according to their training and theoretical bent. Nevertheless, there is substantial agreement among professionals as to the general aspects of what constitutes good mental health. From my perspective as a psychiatrist, why good men dream but do not translate their antisocial impulses into action, as bad men do, is, in large measure, a function of psychological health.

Sound mental health is inextricably bound to character. As I define *character,* it is a highly individual personality structure that expresses deeply held values and beliefs about oneself, others, and the world. It involves the typical enduring patterns of a person's functions. We know a person's character by his or her habitual ways of thinking, feeling, and speaking.

Serious character flaws invariably create psychological problems. Impaired mental health can adversely influence character development. Perfect character, like perfect mental health, is a fiction. "Good enough" character is a more realistic approximation. One's character is always on display, especially in the little things that we do, or do not do.

Mental Health—What Is It?

> Shallow men believe in luck.
> —*Ralph Waldo Emerson*

What constitutes the state of mental health of the hypothetically good man and woman? Over the years, psychiatry has deduced some answers to that question. To begin with, psychologically healthy persons like and accept themselves. They do not depend excessively on others for approval, nor are they severely wounded by others' criticism. Admiral James Stockdale, the highest-ranking military officer to be held captive during the Vietnam War, observed that many of the American prisoners who survived did not need or seek the approval of their captors. Moreover, a solid, integrated sense of self exists with relatively continuous, reasonably pleasant memories of the past. In psychologically healthy people, the "Who am I?" question arises only infrequently. Neither a grandiose nor a despised self is present. A healthy person does not have to diminish other people to maintain a positive self-view. This person acknowledges and accepts personal shortcomings, and seeks help from others when it is needed. The psychologically healthy person knows that one does not have to be perfect to find self-acceptance.

The healthy person has internalized loving, nurturing parental figures that provide sustenance during times of crisis and inner support at times of failure. This person intrinsically rejects suicide as a solution to life's vicissitudes. In the examples cited in this book, many physically and sexually abused children internalize hostile, sadistic parents and repeat the cycle of abuse with their own children. In both the adults and the children who suffer abuse, memories of the past are painful and often discontinuous.

Another measure of psychological health is the presence of values and standards that throughout life provide the mentally healthy person with a moral rudder. The conscience of the healthy person is firm but fair and adaptive, not harsh and punitive. Absent is any cruel, unbending righteousness; present is a clear but reasonably flexible sense of right and wrong. In the face of human suffering, the healthy person does not insist on compliance with trivial formalities. He or she accepts guilt when it is appropriate without experiencing panic or immobilizing depression. The healthy person's conscience works in harmony with other aspects of the personality. It is not a conscience full of holes that permits the acting out of destructive behaviors that are inconsistent with the person's consciously held value system.

The reader can assess the true nature of his or her own conscience by answering the following question: If you had at your command a genie who could grant you any wish without personal consequences, what would you request? Would your wishes benefit or harm others? Would antisocial wishes emerge? The point of the question is to help discover to what extent are we guided by inner principles of right and wrong that function relatively independently of external constraints, or to what extent do we need a policeman at our elbow? The true measure of a person's integrity is tested by what he or she would do or not do if there were no possibility of getting caught or punished. At the extremes, we come full circle when we realize that both truly good men and truly bad men are indifferent to external constraints.

The healthy individual's value system emphasizes becoming proficient at one's work while aiming at realistic goals. The healthy person is willing to work hard to achieve success, to learn from failure, and to forge ahead. Debilitating perfectionist standards that guarantee failure are absent. The perfect is the enemy of the good. I have worked with patients who have felt psychologically deprived and hungry because they have pursued pie-in-the-sky goals, unaware of the sumptuous meal present before them. Many of the disturbed individuals described in this book had a deviant, utopian vision, one that required the relentless pursuit of money, possessions, power, sex, and love.

The healthy person values cooperation and collaboration with others, enjoying competition, though not at the expense of humiliating one's competitors or deriving satisfaction if bad things happen to them. As Schopenhauer pointed out, "the worst trait in human nature is *Schadenfreude* [taking pleasure in another's misfortune], for it is closely related to cruelty." Although almost all of us have glimmers of such feelings now and then, for mentally healthy people they usually pass quickly. A mentally healthy person views life not as a dog-eat-dog struggle but as a positive challenge. By contrast, the psychopath has no moral core and acts at all times in accordance with maximizing his or her pleasure. To the psychopath, the damaging of others is of no consequence.

Healthy and nonhealthy people can be determined by their relationships. Psychologically healthy people enjoy their relationships with others. They place appropriate trust in others as well as themselves acting in a trustworthy manner. They are empathetic toward others, accepting those who manifest conflicts and problems similar to their own. Support and empowerment of friends and acquaintances is their hallmark. They curb feelings of envy and jealousy in deference to the importance of maintaining relationships. They do not desire domination of others. By contrast, most rapists and all serial killers are power-mad in the extreme. They use people as objects for their selfish purposes; the serial sexual killer, for instance, kills for the sole purpose of having a thrilling orgasm. The healthy person esteems other individuals in their own right and appreciates that we all must bear the vicissitudes of the human condition. He or she seeks no personal advantage. Indeed, while healthy people pursue their own self-interests, they do so with empathetic regard to the consequences that these actions might have on others.

The psychologically healthy person maintains good personal boundaries, knowing where he or she stops and another individual begins. The erotomanic stalker has lost personal boundaries, fusing with the object of his or her erotic delusion. A total self-absorption and disregard for others is the sign of the psychopath, and, in my opinion, the origin of what much of the world calls evil. Pathological self-centeredness is roughly equivalent to Christianity's pride, one of humankind's chief sins and greatest evils. In the chapter on sexual misconduct of professionals, persons in positions of power and trust can abuse their standing to exploit others for their own gratification. The healthy person does not do this. He or she feels regret or guilt if others are unnecessarily harmed by his or her own actions, and if they are, the healthy person makes efforts at reparation. The ability to feel remorse, sadness, regret, and guilt in appropriate measure is based on toleration and acknowledgment of our own failings. The healthy person does not shift blame to others, as we find with some of the workplace killers. The person with good character makes liberal use of two phrases in nurturing her or his relationships: "I am sorry" and "Thank you." It is amazing how difficult it is for some people to apologize and to express appreciation.

Psychologically healthy persons are able to accept the darker side of their humanness—their conflicts, their unbridled desires, and even their antisocial impulses—without undue emotional distress. An essential quality of being human is the ability to fantasize. Animals do not have this capacity. Good men and women are able to contain antisocial impulses within fantasy, exercising the option to act or to continue dreaming. Bad men and women, like young children, live in the present and act for the moment. The mature person can enjoy childish pleasures, but at the appropriate time and within measure.

A strong indicator of emotional health is the ability to withstand anxiety that arises from internal or external conflict without falling apart or launching into drastic action. During a crisis, our internalized loving family relationships sustain us. Those persons who have experienced hate and rejection from their caretakers find that in a crisis, these abusive relationships emerge to once again tear at their hearts and minds. They feel abandoned in the present as they were in the past. Some of the mass murderers described in the chapter on workplace violence were unable to contain and control their feelings of anger and vengeance without descending into a lethal paranoid depression. The ability to delay gratification and to tolerate frustration, when appropriate, is a critical developmental step that is accomplished by the psychologically healthy person. Primitive, unsocialized personalities cannot perform this fundamental psychological delaying action. A sure sign of psychological dysfunction is the inability to defer gratification without becoming angry, anxious, or depressed. When frustrations arise, the less than healthy person uses others as "whipping boys." Critical to health is the ability to think before acting and to modulate impulses in the way that one adjusts the volume control on a television set.

The capacity to sublimate—that is, to transform and redirect basic impulses deriving from sexuality and aggression toward higher goals—speaks of mental health. The abilities to compete, to succeed against odds, and to be a winner all borrow energy from redirected aggression. Rechanneled sexual energy may find expression in music, art, and literary creativity.

The psychologically healthy person is able to love—that is, to value and care for another person beyond oneself. Love nurtures the independence and growth of others. The ability to love another person has nothing to do with Hollywood's version of love. The lovers whose moonlight gazes sparkle on the silver screen mirror only the illusion of each other's perfection. We are all imperfect. To love someone requires that we first accept ourselves, despite our weaknesses and foibles. To truly commit to another person, we must first authentically value ourselves. Perfectionists cannot do that and often end up hating themselves. When we acknowledge our dark side, we take our first transcendent steps toward discovering the miracle of love.

In the chapter on stalking, I described individuals who terrorized former partners out of feelings of rage, vengeance, and the inability to emotionally let go of the former partner. In the healthy person, feelings of jealousy, anger, hate, and rejection are tempered by an overriding concern for the person who is loved. The most difficult relationships are with the people whom we love, not those we un-equivocally hate. We may hate a Hitler or a Ted Bundy, but it is not the same as simultaneously hating someone we love. Except when hate feelings are overwhelming, love usually softens the conflict to a tolerable level. The ability to preserve our relationships amidst such contrary feelings is a hallmark of psychological health.

Sex for the healthy person is not merely a spasm of physiological release or just another form of masturbation. If sexuality enters the healthy person's relationship, it does so in an empowering way, through a mutually loving, physical, and mental exploration of one another. In searching for a mate, the emphasis is less on finding the right person than on being the right person.

Healthy people have many satisfying facets to their lives. They work to make a living, but work is not the only source of satisfaction for them. Work is a source of creative emotional growth and mental refreshment rather than a primary way of obtaining or maintaining self-esteem. I have treated patients undergoing serious personal cri-ses whose positive work experience helped sustain them through a very difficult time. Professional goals are folded into a broader fabric of life that is rich in sustaining relationships, recreation, hobbies, and spiritual quests. The healthy person is capable of experiencing awe, joy, and wonder about the world, finding a sense of fulfillment in a life not beset by regret or bitterness.

A firm commitment to relationships and to work or professional goals enriches the mentally healthy person. Money, though impor-tant, pales in comparison to these commitments. Money is a means to an end but not an end in itself. Money has extrinsic value; that is, what it can buy. Problems arise when money is sought for its intrin-sic value, for example, as an important source of self-esteem. Joy is felt with the "small" things in life: a sunset, the smell of a spring, a sense of awe about the world, a moment with a friend, morning's first light. The ability to laugh and cry, to have one's feelings avail-able, is a distinct sign of mental health. One of my depressed patients put it well when she anguished, "I would just like to *be*!" Emily Dick-inson wrote, "To live is so startling it leaves time for little else."

It's the Little Things...

> The man who has not conscience in small things
> will be a scoundrel in big things.
> —*Arthur Schopenhauer*

People often throw away their hard-won careers, their families, and their lives over some small thing, a trivial matter. Persons in positions of great trust and power betray the most sacred trust placed in them, often for a peccadillo, or 30 pieces of silver—and in full knowledge that if they are caught, dishonor and disgrace will follow. This is an affliction of all humankind, not just of prominent persons.

Why do we cross the line? The better question is, why doesn't it happen to all of us much more than it does? For most people, gross antisocial behaviors are inhibited by the policeman at the elbow. But although they believe that major breaches will be discovered, they also feel that minor transgressions will go unnoticed. The psychiatrist knows that character can be best discerned in such "little things," which reflect serious character flaws just as major transgressions do. Character is what we display when we think no one is watching.

Yet no one can escape the consequences of character. Emerson stated that "All infractions of love and equity in our social relations are speedily punished." As a psychiatrist, I hold that the "punishment" is instantaneous, even though the person may be unaware of it, because at the moment of the infraction, destructive character traits are reinforced that further ensnare one in a troubled destiny. Thus, some of us, when reacting to the slings and arrows of everyday life, find that exacting revenge on an individual for hurts we have suffered is superfluous, because punishment of the offender is instantaneous, an inevitable consequence of his or her character and destiny. In other instances, we may need to call the police, file a lawsuit, or go to war. The progression is summed up in an anonymously written verse:

> Sow a thought, and you reap an act;
> Sow an act, and you reap a habit;
> Sow a habit, and you reap character;
> Sow a character, and you reap a destiny.

Character, Perceiving Reality, and Accepting Limitations

Reality is perceived reasonably clearly by the psychologically healthy person. Personal needs and conflicts do not usually interfere with a reasonably accurate perception of the world. The reality principle is harmoniously melded with the pleasure principle. For the most part, the healthy person confronts the threat of internal and external dangers and only denies them when it becomes necessary for survival, say, in an acute crisis or emergency. Anger has a realistic place in the person's palette of feelings and is expressed in an appropriate, adaptive manner. But no person totally leaves behind his or her childish feelings of complete self-absorption, of the rageful intolerance to frustration, of the insistent need for the immediate gratification of all wishes. Some of life's comedy and much of its tragedy arises when infantile strivings clash with reality.

From my perspective as a psychiatrist, I know that individuals who can accept that they have emotional problems that go beyond their ability to cope, and who seek professional help for them, can achieve a significant measure of maturity and mental health. The Dahmers, Bundys, and Kempers never think of obtaining help. Their deviant acts and fantasies provide them with too much pleasure. Both Dahmer and Kemper received court-ordered treatment for earlier offenses but obviously did not obtain any benefit, since they went on to commit many murders based on their horrific fantasies.

One of the measures of a parent's success at the child-rearing task is that his or her children recognize their limitations and know that it is reasonable to ask for help from others when necessary. The ability to depend on others should not be confused with a pathological state of dependency. On the other hand, rigid independence is as emotionally limiting as an intractable dependence on others.

Psychological treatments aimed at developing insight into our darker side are not meant for everyone. Analyzing our actions before rushing to critically judge ourselves is a responsible course—but difficult for many people. For example, I have treated patients whose harsh self-criticism, though very painful, was easier for them to bear than facing their dreaded inner demons. Often with such patients, the therapy was unsuccessful. A prickly conscience provided excellent cover against self-discovery.

Insight psychotherapy is just one of many therapies available. Currently, there are over 450 different psychotherapies that individuals can choose from. Psychotherapies have been scientifically proven to be effective.

The purpose of insight psychotherapy is to identify conflicts and develop new ways of coping and resolving problems. When successful, it frees the individual from being stuck with automatic, reflexive reactions to life's stresses. A fundamental tenet of insight therapy holds that, in general, the more realistic a person's perception of oneself and the world, the more harmonious that person's adaptation to life. When a person has experienced an important insight, she or he is never the same. However, much depends on how the person uses the insight, if it is used at all. One patient analogized the psychotherapeutic process to a worm that enters a cocoon, and, in time, emerges as a beautiful butterfly that flies away free. Another patient, an intractable curmudgeon, used the same metaphor to insist that his transformation process in therapy was from a worm to an ugly moth with a flame fixation. Individuals who respond favorably to insight therapy are able to replace reflexive responses by choices. Also, positive changes in character structure generally improve prospects for a more inner-driven destiny.

The list of attributes of the hypothetical healthy person could go on and on, but ultimately any such list must end with the succinct summation about mental health once made by William Sloane Coffin, former Chaplain of Yale University, who said, "I'm not okay, you're not okay, and that's okay." Perfect mental health is a fiction. It is also undesirable and downright inhuman. Mental health and illness exist on a continuum, and in delicate, dynamic balance—and perfection is entirely off the scale. Much depends on the context. A noise that barely catches our attention in the morning after a good night's sleep can, later that evening, when we are tired, frighten us terribly.

Born Unto Trouble

As can be readily appreciated, much hard work, sustained effort, and loving care go into raising good women and men. Socialization and character appear to develop best within an intact family providing *good enough* care, preferably with both parents present. In many instances, good parenting can overcome or inhibit inherited antisocial tendencies. In others, the best parenting and family situation available may not be sufficient to control innate destructive behaviors, particularly if alcohol and drug abuse are involved. So even under optimal circumstances, parenthood is an impossible task. There are neither perfect parents nor perfect children.

Many of the mentally healthy attributes previously described play a role in the fashioning of sound character. No one can go beyond his or her character. In many ways, our character foretells our future. In this sense, character is destiny—who we marry, if we marry, our relationships, what sort of work we do, how we live, who we are, whether we are good or bad. Obviously, many things happen in life over which we have no control. But how we respond, whether adaptively or dysfunctionally, is directly related to our character. The murderers, rapists, and psychopaths in this book represent the end stage of character development gone awry. The answer to prevention of antisocial behavior does not reside in adding more police and building more jails. These solutions can only address the end-stage problem, which, of course, is still important. But effective prevention will occur only when society undertakes to provide and protect those elements that foster the development and continuity of stable, caring families.

It is also quite clear that the bad men and women depicted in this book failed miserably in the areas of character, conscience, impulse control, reality testing, and interpersonal relationships. Compared with people with the hypothetically "normal" character profile, these bad men and women are riddled with debilitating emotional and mental deficiencies. When a psychiatrist has the opportunity to examine these persons, their severe psychological conflicts and developmental problems are displayed in excruciating detail. They hardly are the stuff for even the lowest grade of Hollywood movie.

Why bad men do what good men dream is explained to a certain degree when one has the opportunity to psychiatrically examine antisocial persons. But the answer to the good men–bad men conundrum must go beyond psychiatric examination. Even when the psychiatrist has been able to spot glaring psychological conflicts and deficiencies that led to a destructive act, the origins of these dysfunctions often remain obscure. The need for certainty where none is possible unrealistically places unfounded reliance on psychological theories. We are all born with a darker side. Good men—for reasons only some of which are known—are able to contain that dark side. Bad men live it.

Empathy

> Taught by time, my heart has learned to glow
> for other's good, and melt at other's woe.
> —*Homer*

One difference between bad and good people may have to do with empathy. This is a core character trait that enables us to understand our fellow human beings and to feel compassion. It has something to do with an anatomical structure that has been found in monkey brains and human brains, called mirror neurons. The cells are located in the brain's motor cortex, where muscle movement and control are initiated. The mirror neuron circuitry allows us to step into the shoes of others, to feel their pain. The more empathetic the person, the stronger is their mirror neuron response. Although science has discovered this neuronal basis for empathy, it can only be a foundation upon which personal experiences of love and caring build. Adverse life experiences can interfere with or disable the functioning of mirror neurons. Psychopaths, for instance, do not feel empathy. Presumably their mirror response is very weak or nonexistent.

The lack of empathy may be an important reason why psychopaths are untreatable. In previous chapters that have analyzed all sorts of "bad men," from serial killers to heads of state, we have seen how spectacular failures in empathy drive the engines of evil.

For psychotherapists and other providers of health services to be effective, they must be empathetic. But excessive empathy may cause these providers to live too much in another's shoes, and thus share the patient's destiny. To be truly effective, the healthcare provider must also be able to step *out* of those shoes.

Empathy allows us to feel the pain of others, but also to experience their joy. As such, empathy can combat envy, a pernicious character flaw that can destroy relationships and make life miserable for everyone.

Are We Hard-Wired for Trouble?

What causes our destructive behaviors? Is it genetics, one's family of origin, terrible experiences, bad brain chemistry, or all of these? Have our brains been hard-wired through the evolutionary process for inevitable trouble? Is dysfunctional behavior attributable to factors that are beyond our control? And how much of good mental health is the blind luck of the draw? For example, what does the future hold for children who are born addicted to cocaine and whose mothers are teenaged and unwed? What opportunities will these children have to learn how to channel or control their antisocial impulses?

What we do know is that the brain of every individual—his or her "computer hardware"—is genetically distinct from all others. The human genome (an organism's complete set of DNA) contains 3.1 billion DNA pairs. The opportunities for genetic aberrations are great. J.D. Watson, the codiscoverer of the double helix structure of DNA, observed, "We used to think our fate was in our stars. Now we know, in large measure, our fate is in our genes." Adding yet another level of complexity, environmental and other factors may also influence the gene expression. As in a computer, the brain's capacity to process information correctly and to adequately perform various complex psychological tasks depends on the circuitry. It is estimated that the human brain contains approximately 30 billion neurons that have 100 trillion interconnections. Into this "hardware" goes important "software"—for instance, the individual's personal experiences with caregivers and with the world in general. The possible combinations of a person's unique hardware with the permutations of this software are infinite. We know this because even identical twins with identical brain hardware and the same parents have different software experiences. These twins appear identical on the surface, but their characters are not identical. Suffice it to say that malfunctions in either or both modalities, hardware and software, are what lead to psychological limitations and to trouble. With all this genetic and neuronal complexity, it is incredible that most of us come out reasonably whole.

Good computer hardware combined with good software allows good men to dream. But again there are no perfect computers, and there is no perfect software. In fact, even apart from our inherent limitations as human beings, there are too many places for things to go wrong, to even contemplate the possibility of a hypothetically "normal" person who has all of the attributes described in this chapter. Our dark side is a fundamental part of our personality—of our brain-computer hardware. In so many instances, it is the software of our personal experiences with our parents, family, and the world that fashions our character and our destiny. Many of the persons depicted in this book were destined for trouble by aberrations in both their brain-computer hardware and their software experiences. Many of us may escape a similar harsh fate because we have either good enough hardware or good enough software, but not necessarily both. For the troubled, modern psychiatry has developed a wide variety of beneficial treatments for mental disorders, which can help substantially in controlling destructive, antisocial ideas and impulses.

Fortunately, the majority of humankind does tolerably well in rising above the inherent limitations that we have as human beings. I find it truly remarkable that we have so many good people in this world, even if they are all limited in their goodness. Although, as Job says, we are all born unto trouble, we are not condemned to miserable lives. Good people are able to dream and to contain the impulses that bad people act out. Taming our demons and acknowledging our humanity with its attendant dark side can be empowering. Those who become psychologically resourceful may be able to put the demons to useful work, in the same way as humankind has learned how to tame and use fire, though the sparks inevitably fly upward. It is the essence of the human condition that we struggle against our dark demons, that our spirit strives to harness these demons in the pursuit and the fulfillment of our human destiny.

Bibliography

Chapter 1: Illuminating the Darker Side

Brute force can never subdue the basic human desire for freedom. The Washington Post, October 21, 2007, B1

Dreifus C: The Dalai Lama. The New York Times Magazine, November 28, 1993, pp 52–55

Drukteinis AM: Serial murder: the heart of darkness. Psychiatric Annals 22:532–538, 1992

Freud S: Civilization and Its Discontents. New York, WW Norton, 1962

Golding W: Lord of the Flies. New York, Perigee, 1954

Herman JL: Trauma and Recovery. New York, Basic Books, 1992

Lorenz K: On Aggression. New York, Harcourt, Brace & World, 1967

Pope KS, Keith-Spiegel P, Tabachnick BG: Sexual attraction to clients. Am Psychol 41:147–158, 1986

Staub E: The Roots of Evil: The Origins of Genocide and Other Group Violence. New York, Cambridge University Press, 1989

True Crime: Compulsion to Kill. Alexandria, VA, Time-Life Books, 1993

U.S. Department of Justice: U.S. Annual Crime Statistics, 2005. http://www.ojp.usdoj.gov/bjs. Accessed January 31, 2008

Chapter 2: Human Killing Machines and Us

Dahmer L: A Father's Story. New York, William Morrow, 1994

Goldberg C: The Evil We Do. Amherst, NY, Prometheus, 2000

Koehn D: The Nature of Evil. New York, Palgrave Macmillan, 2005

Ressler RK, Shachtman T: Whoever Fights Monsters, New York, St. Martin's, 1992

Simon RI: Should forensic psychiatrists testify about evil? J Am Acad Psychiatry Law 31:413–416, 2003

Singular S: Unholy Messenger. The Life and Crimes of the BTK Serial Killer. New York, Scribner, 2006

Wenzl R, Potter T, Hurst L, et al: Bind, Torture, Kill: The Inside Story of the Serial Killer Next Door. New York, HarperCollins, 2007

A writer's lust for life—and death. The Washington Post, November 13, 2007, G1

Chapter 3: Psychopaths

American Psychiatric Association: Diagnostic and Statistical Manual: Mental Disorders. Washington, DC, American Psychiatric Association, 1952

American Psychiatric Association: Diagnostic and Statistical Manual of Mental Disorders, 2nd Edition. Washington, DC, American Psychiatric Association, 1968

American Psychiatric Association: Diagnostic and Statistical Manual of Mental Disorders, 4th Edition. Washington, DC, American Psychiatric Association, 1994

American Psychiatric Association: Diagnostic and Statistical Manual of Mental Disorders, 4th Edition, Text Revision. Washington, DC, American Psychiatric Association, 2000

Andrew C, Gordievsky O: KGB: The Inside Story of Its Foreign Operations From Lenin to Gorbachev. New York, HarperCollins, 1990

Black DW, Baumgard CH, Bell SE: The long-term outcome of antisocial personality disorder compared with depression, schizophrenia, and surgical conditions. Bull Am Acad Psychiatry Law 23:43–52, 1995

Cleckley H: The Mask of Sanity, 5th Edition. Augusta, GA, Emily S. Cleckley, 1988

Dinitz S: The Antisocial Personality in Forensic Psychiatry and Psychology. Edited by Curran WJ, McGarry AL, Shah SA. Philadelphia, PA, FA Davis, 1986, pp 391–408

Earley P: Family of Spies: Inside the John Walker Spy Ring. New York, Bantam, 1988

Freud S: Some character-types met within psycho-analytic work (1916), in The Standard Edition of the Complete Psychological Works of Sigmund Freud, Vol 14. Translated and edited by Strachey J. London, Hogarth Press, 1968, pp 311–333; see pp 332–333

Hare RE: Without Conscience: The Disturbing World of the Psychopaths Among Us. New York, Pocket Books, 1993

Heilbroner D: Death Benefit: A Lawyer Uncovers a Twenty-Year Pattern of Seduction, Arson, and Murder. New York, Crown, 1993

Kernberg OF: Aggression in Personality Disorders and Perversions. New Haven, CT, Yale University Press, 1992, pp 67–84

Lewis DO: Adult antisocial behavior and criminality, in Comprehensive Textbook of Psychiatry, 5th Edition. Edited by Kaplan HI, Sadock BJ. Baltimore, MD, Williams & Wilkins, 1989, pp 1400–1405

McGrath P, Horrock NM, Shannon E, et al: A family of spies. Newsweek, June 10, 1985, pp 32–33

Milgram S: Behavioral study of obedience. J Abnorm Soc Psychol 67:371–378, 1963

Olsen J: The Misbegotten Son: A Serial Killer and His Victims: The True Story of Arthur J. Shawcross. New York, Delacorte, 1993

Perry JC, Vaillant GE: Personality disorders, in Comprehensive Textbook of Psychiatry, 5th Edition. Edited by Kaplan HI, Sadock BJ. Baltimore, MD, Williams & Wilkins, 1989, pp 1373–1377

Person ES: Manipulativeness in entrepreneurs and psychopaths, in Unmasking the Psychopath: Antisocial Personality and Related Syndromes. Edited by Reid WH, Dorr D, Walker JI, et al. New York, WW Norton, 1986, pp 256–273

Reid WH: Antisocial personality in forensic psychiatry, in Principles and Practice of Forensic Psychiatry. Edited by Rosner R. New York, Chapman & Hall, 1994, pp 427–431

Reid WH, Dorr D, Walker J, et al (eds): Unmasking the Psychopath: Antisocial Personality and Related Syndromes. New York, WW Norton, 1986

Sanchez J: Social crises and psychopathy: toward a sociology of the psychopath, in Unmasking the Psychopath: Antisocial Personality and Related Syndromes. Edited by Reid WH, Dorr D, Walker J, et al. New York, WW Norton, 1986, pp 78–97

Shannon E, Blackman A: The Spy Next Door: The Extraordinary Secret Life of Robert Philip Hanssen, the Most Damaging FBI Agent in U.S. History. New York, Little, Brown, 2002

Skodol AE, Gunderson JG: Personality disorders, in American Psychiatric Publishing Textbook of Psychiatry, 5th Edition. Edited by Hales RE, Yudofsky SC, Gabbard GO. Washington, DC, American Psychiatric Publishing, 2008, pp 821–860

Wise D: Nightmover: How Aldrich Ames Sold the CIA to the KGB for $4.6 Million. New York, HarperCollins, 1995

Chapter 4: Why Do They Rape?

American Psychiatric Association: Diagnostic and Statistical Manual of Mental Disorders, 4th Edition, Text Revision. Washington, DC, American Psychiatric Association, 2000, pp 573–574

Dietz PE: Social factors in rapist behavior, in Clinical Aspects of the Rapist. Edited by Rada RT. New York, Grune & Stratton, 1977, pp 59–115

Dietz PE, Hazelwood RR, Warren J: The sexually sadistic criminal and his offenses. Bull Am Acad Psychiatry Law 18:163–178, 1990

Douglas JE, Burgess AW, Burgess AG, et al: Crime Classification Manual: A Standard System for Investigating and Classifying Violent Crimes. New York, Macmillan, 1992

Graverholz E, Koralewski MA: Sexual Coercion: A Sourcebook on Its Nature, Causes and Prevention. Lexington, MA, DC Heath, 1991

Hazelwood RR: Practical Aspects of Rape. Boca Raton, FL, CRC Press, 1993

Hazelwood RR, Warren J: The serial rapist: his characteristics and victims. FBI Law Enforcement Bulletin, January–February 1989, pp 3–16

Klama J: Aggression: The Myth of the Beast Within. New York, Wiley, 1988

Koss MP, Harvey MR: The Rape Victim: Clinical and Community Interventions, 2nd Edition. Newbury Park, CA, Sage, 1991

Nadelson CC, Notman MT, Hilberman E: The rape experience, in Modern Legal Medicine, Psychiatry and Forensic Science. Edited by Curran WJ, McGarry AL, Petty CS. Philadelphia, PA, FA Davis, 1980, pp 509–531

New York City Alliance Against Sexual Assault. http://www.nyc-againstrape.org. Accessed August 28, 2007

Prentky R, Cohen M, Seghorn T: Development of a rational taxonomy for the classification of rapists: the Massachusetts Treatment Center System. Bull Am Acad Psychiatry Law 13:39–70, 1985

Pressley SA: Rapist asked to use condom gets 40 years. The Washington Post, May 15, 1993, A3

Rape, Abuse and Incest National Network. http://www.rainn.org. Accessed August 28, 2007

Rose DS: Worse than death: psychodynamics of rape victims and the need for psychotherapy. Am J Psychiatry 143:817–824, 1986

Rosenberg R, Knight RA, Prentky RA, et al: Validating components of a taxonomic system for rapists: a path analytic approach. Bull Am Acad Psychiatry Law 16:169–185, 1988

Seghorn TK, Cohen ML: The psychology of the rape assailant, in Modern Legal Medicine, Psychiatry and Forensic Science. Edited by Curran WJ, McGarry AL, Petty CS. Philadelphia, PA, FA Davis, 1980, pp 533–551

Shields WM, Shields LM: Forcible rape: an evolutionary perspective. Ethology and Sociobiology 4:115–136, 1983

Simon RI: Posttraumatic Stress Disorder in Litigation: Guidelines for Forensic Assessment, 2nd Edition. Washington DC, American Psychiatric Publishing, 2003

Sullivan K, Sevilla G: Serial rapists: varied profiles, similar patterns. The Washington Post, August 22, 1993, A1, A20

Sullivan T: Unequal Verdicts: The Park Jogger Trials. New York, Simon & Schuster, 1992

Thornhill R, Palmer CT: Why men rape. The Sciences, January/February 2000, pp 30–36

Van der Kolk BA: Physical and sexual abuse of adults, in Comprehensive Textbook of Psychiatry, 8th Edition. Edited by Sadock BJ, Sadock VA. Baltimore, MD, Williams & Wilkins, 2005, pp 2393–2398

Chapter 5: Stalkers

American Psychiatric Association: Diagnostic and Statistical Manual of Mental Disorders, 4th Edition, Text Revision. Washington, DC, American Psychiatric Publishing, 2000

Centers for Disease Control and Prevention: Injury Center. http://www.cdc.gov/injury. Accessed February 2, 2008

Chance S: If not our business, then whose? Psychiatric Times, December 1993, p 41

Dietz PE: Defenses against dangerous people when arrest and commitment fail, in American Psychiatric Press Review of Clinical Psychiatry and the Law, Vol 1. Edited by Simon RI. Washington, DC, American Psychiatric Press, 1990, pp 205–219

Dietz PE, Matthews DB, Van Duyne C, et al: Threatening and otherwise inappropriate letters to Hollywood celebrities. J Forensic Sci 36:185–209, 1991

Douglas JE, Burgess AW, Burgess AG, et al: Crime Classification Manual. New York, Lexington Books, 1992

Ellis D, Blackman J, Sellinger M, et al: Nowhere to hide. People, May 17, 1993, pp 63–66, 68, 71–72

Jones J: Let Me Take You Down: Inside the Mind of Mark David Chapman, The Man Who Shot John Lennon. New York, Villard, 1992

Lardner G: Federal task force suggests states make stalking a felony offense. The Washington Post, September 12, 1993, A19

Lesson F: Inside the mind of a star stalker. Crimebeat, April 1992, pp 20–25, 57

Lystad M: Violence in the Home. New York, Brunner/Mazel, 1986

Meloy JR: Violent Attachments. Northvale, NJ, Jason Aronson, 1992

Meloy JR: Demographic and clinical comparison of obsessional followers and offenders with mental disorders. Am J Psychiatry 152:258–263, 1995

Revelations on John Lennon's assassination. Larry King Live, transcript #721, December 17, 1992

Segal J: Erotomania revisited: from Kraepelin to DSM-III-R. Am J Psychiatry 146:1261–1266, 1989

Stalking Resource Center: Stalking fact sheet. http://www.ncvc.org/src. Accessed February 2, 2008

Wolfe L: Double Life: The Shattering Affair Between Chief Judge Sol Wachtler and Socialite Joy Silverman. New York, Pocket Books, 1994

Chapter 6: Workplace Violence

American Psychiatric Association Task Force Report on Clinician Safety. Washington, DC, American Psychiatric Association, 1992

Baron SA: Violence in the Workplace. Ventura, CA, Pathfinder, 1993

Bureau of Labor Statistics, U.S. Department of Labor: Survey of Workplace Violence Prevention 2005. October 27, 2006. http://www.bls.gov/iif/osh_wpvs.htm. Accessed February 4, 2008

Centers for Disease Control and Prevention: National Institute for Occupational Safety and Health Topics: Occupational violence. http://www.cdc.gov/niosh/topics/violence. Accessed February 4, 2008

Douglas JE, Burgess AW, Burgess AG, et al: Crime Classification Manual. New York, Lexington Books, 1992, pp 111–115

Ex-doctor charged with hospital murders. July 18, 2000. http://archives.cnn.com/2000/LAW/07/18/doctor.killings. Accessed February 12, 2008

Fox JA, Levin J: Overkill: Mass Murder and Serial Killing Exposed. New York, Plenum, 1994

Gold LH: Sexual Harassment: Psychiatric Assessment in Employment Litigation. Washington, DC, American Psychiatric Publishing, 2004

Malmquist CP: School violence, in Textbook of Violence Assessment and Management. Edited by Simon RI, Tardiff K. Washington, DC, American Psychiatric Publishing, 2008, pp 537–554

Samenow E: Inside the Criminal Mind. Crown, 2004

Schouten R: Workplace violence and the clinician, in Textbook of Violence Assessment and Management. Edited by Simon RI, Tardiff K. Washington, DC, American Psychiatric Publishing, 2008, pp 501–520

Simon RI: The myth of "imminent" violence in psychiatry and the law. University of Cincinnati Law Review 79:631–644, 2006

Simon RI, Tardiff K (eds): Textbook of Violence Assessment and Management. Washington, DC, American Psychiatric Publishing, 2008

Sperry L: Psychiatric Consultation in the Workplace. Washington, DC, American Psychiatric Press, 1993

Spotswood S: Prominent NIMH psychiatrist slain. http://www.usmedicine.com. Accessed September 19, 2007

Tardiff K: Clinical risk assessment of violence, in Textbook of Violence Assessment and Management. Edited by Simon RI, Tardiff K. Washington, DC, American Psychiatric Publishing, 2008, pp 3–18

True Crime: Mass Murderers. Alexandria, VA, Time-Life Books, 1992

Worker Health Chartbook 2004. http://www.cdc.gov/niosh/docs/chartbook. Accessed September 19, 2007

Chapter 7: Multiple Personality and Crime

American Psychiatric Association: Diagnostic and Statistical Manual of Mental Disorders, 3rd Edition, Revised. Washington, DC, American Psychiatric Association, 1987

American Psychiatric Association: Diagnostic and Statistical Manual of Mental Disorders, 4th Edition, Text Revision. Washington, DC, American Psychiatric Association, 2000

Brown SJ: Unusual rape case draws attention to culpability in multiple personality disorder. Clinical Psychiatry News, January 1995, pp 4, 13

Coons PM: Iatrogenesis and malingering of multiple personality disorder in the forensic evaluation of homicide defendants. Psychiatr Clin North Am 14:757–768, 1991

Daro D, McCurdy K: Current Trends in Child Abuse Reporting and Fatalities: The Results of the 1991 Annual Fifty State Survey. Chicago IL, National Committee for Prevention of Child Abuse, 1992

Dinwiddie SH, North CS, Yutzy SH: Multiple personality disorder: scientific and medicolegal issues. Bull Am Acad Psychiatry Law 21:69–79, 1993

Fox JA, Levin J: Overkill: Mass Murder and Serial Killing Exposed. New York, Plenum, 1994

Halleck SL: Dissociative phenomena and the question of responsibility. Int J Clin Exp Hypn 38:298–314, 1990

Herman JL: Trauma and Recovery. New York, Basic Books, 1992

Hypnotic misrecall. Sci Am 252:73, June 1985

Kluft RP: The simulation and dissimulation of Multiple Personality Disorder. Am J Clin Hypn 30:104–118, 1987

Kluft RP (ed): Incest-Related Syndromes of Adult Psychopathology. Washington, DC, American Psychiatric Press, 1990

Levitt S, Sider D, Wescot G: Portrait of a killer: even after confessing to the shocking drowning of her two small sons, Susan Smith remains an enigma. People, November 21, 1994, pp 54–59

Lewis DO, Bard JS: Multiple personality and forensic issues in multiple personality disorder. Psychiatr Clin North Am 14:741–756, 1991

Maldonado JR, Spiegel D: Dissociative disorders, in The American Psychiatric Publishing Textbook of Clinical Psychiatry, 4th Edition. Edited by Hales RE, Yudofsky SC. Washington DC, American Psychiatric Publishing, 2003, pp 721–729

McHugh PR: Psychiatric misadventures. American Scholar 61:497–510, 1992

Orne MT, Dinges DF, Orne EC: On the differential diagnosis of multiple personality in the forensic context. Int J Clin Exp Hypn 32:118–169, 1984

Perr IN: Crime and multiple personality disorder: a case history and discussion. Bull Am Acad Psychiatry Law 19:203–214, 1991

Putnam FW: Diagnosis and Treatment of Multiple Personality Disorder. New York, Guilford, 1989

Shechmeister BR, French AP: The multiple personality syndrome and criminal defense. Bull Am Acad Psychiatry Law 11:17–25, 1983

Shengold L: Soul Murder: The Effects of Childhood Abuse and Deprivation. New York, Fawcett Columbine, 1991

Spiegel D (ed): Dissociation: Culture, Mind, and Body. Washington, DC, American Psychiatric Press, 1994

Steinberg M, Bancroft J, Buchanan J: Multiple personality disorder in criminal law. Bull Am Acad Psychiatry Law 21:345–356, 1993

True Crime: Compulsion to Kill. Alexandria, VA, Time-Life Books, 1993

U.S. Department of Health and Human Services, Children's Bureau: Child Maltreatment 2005. http://www.childwelfare.gov/systemwide/statistics/can.cfm. Accessed September 16, 2007

Watkins JG: The Bianchi (L.A. Hillside Strangler) case: sociopath or multiple personality? Int J Clin Exp Hypn 32:67–101, 1984

Weissberg M: The First Sin of Ross Michael Carlson. New York, Delacorte, 1992

Widom CS: The Cycle of Violence. Washington, DC, National Institute of Justice, Research in Brief, October 1992

Chapter 8: The Ultimate Betrayal

American Psychiatric Association: The Principles of Medical Ethics With Annotations Especially Applicable to Psychiatry. Washington, DC, American Psychiatric Association, 1993

Bates CM, Brodsky AM: Sex in the Therapy Hour. New York, Guilford, 1989

Brabant E, Falzeder E, Giampieri-Deutsch P (eds): The Correspondence of Sigmund Freud and Sandor Ferenczi. Boston, MA, The Belknap Press/Harvard University Press, 2001

Chafetz GS, Chafetz ME: Obsession: The Bizarre Relationship Between a Prominent Harvard Psychiatrist and Her Suicidal Patient. New York, Crown, 1994

College of Physicians and Surgeons of Ontario: The Final Report of the Task Force on Sexual Abuse of Patients: An Independent Task

Force Commissioned by the College of Physicians and Surgeons of Ontario. Toronto, ON, Canada, November 25, 1991

Epstein RS: Keeping Boundaries: Maintaining Safety and Integrity in the Psychotherapeutic Process. Washington, DC, American Psychiatric Press, 1994

Epstein RS, Simon RI: The Exploitation Index: an early warning indicator of boundary violations in psychotherapy. Bull Menninger Clin 54:450–465, 1990

Epstein RS, Simon RI, Kay GG: Assessing boundary violations in psychotherapy: survey results with the Exploitation Index. Bull Menninger Clin 56:1–17, 1992

Firestone MJ, Simon RI: Intimacy vs. advocacy: attorney-client sex. Tort and Insurance Law Journal 27:679–692, 1992

Freud S: Observations on transference-love (1915), in the Standard Edition of the Complete Psychological Works of Sigmund Freud, Vol 12. Translated and edited by Strachey J. London, Hogarth Press, 1958, pp 159–171; see pp 160–161, 166

Gabbard GO: Sexual Exploitation in Professional Relationships. Washington, DC, American Psychiatric Press, 1989

Gartrell N, Herman J, Olarte S, et al: Psychiatrist-patient sexual contact—results of a national survey, I: prevalence. Am J Psychiatry 143:1126–1131, 1986

Graverholz E, Koralewski MA: Sexual Coercion: A Sourcebook on Its Nature, Causes and Prevention. Lexington, MA, DC Heath, 1991

Gutheil TG: Borderline personality disorders, boundary violations, and patient-therapist sex: medicolegal pitfalls. Am J Psychiatry 146:597–602, 1989

Gutheil TG: Patients involved in sexual misconduct with therapists: is a victim profile possible? Psychiatric Annals 21:661–667, 1991

Gutheil TG: Between the chair and the door: boundary issues in the therapeutic "transition zone." Harv Rev Psychiatry 2:269–277, 1994

Gutheil TG, Gabbard GO: Obstacles to the dynamic understanding of therapist-patient sexual relations. Am J Psychother 256:515–525, 1992

Gutheil TG, Gabbard GO: The concept of boundaries in clinical practice: theoretical and risk management dimensions. Am J Psychiatry 150:188–196, 1993

Gutheil TG, Simon RI: Non-sexual boundary crossings and boundary violations, the ethical dimension. Psychiatr Clin North Am 25:585-592, 2002

Maltsberger JT: A career plundered. Suicide Life Threat Behav 23:285–291, 1993

McNamara E: Breakdown: Sex, Suicide and the Harvard Psychiatrist. New York, Pocket Books, 1994

Noël B: You Must Be Dreaming. New York, Poseidon Press, 1992

Peterson MR: At Personal Risk: Boundary Violations in Professional-Client Relationships. New York, WW Norton, 1992

Pope KS: Sexual Involvement With Therapists: Patient Assessment, Subsequent Therapy, Forensics. Washington, DC, American Psychological Association, 1994

Pope KS, Keith-Spiegel P, Tabachnick BG: Sexual attraction to clients. Am Psychol 41:147–158, 1986

Schoener GR, Milgrom JH, Gonsiork JC, et al: Psychotherapists' Sexual Involvement With Clients: Intervention and Prevention. Minneapolis, MN, Walk-In Counseling Center, 1989

Shengold L: Soul Murder: The Effects of Childhood Abuse and Deprivation. New York, Fawcett Columbine, 1991

Simon RI: The psychiatrist as a fiduciary: avoiding the double agent role. Psychiatric Annals 17:622–626, 1987

Simon RI: Sexual exploitation of patients: how it begins before it happens. Psychiatric Annals 19:104–112, 1989

Simon RI: Psychological injury caused by boundary violation precursors to therapist-patient sex. Psychiatric Annals 21:614–619, 1991

Simon RI: Transference in therapist-patient sex: the illusion of patient improvement and consent: I. Psychiatric Annals 24:509–515, 1994

Simon RI: Transference in therapist-patient sex: the illusion of patient improvement and consent: II. Psychiatric Annals 24:561–565, 1994

Simon RI: Treatment boundaries in psychiatric practice, in Principles and Practice of Forensic Psychiatry, 2nd Edition. Edited by Rosner R. London, Arnold, 2003, pp 156–164

Simon RI, Sadoff RL: Psychiatric Malpractice: Cases and Comments for Clinicians. Washington, DC, American Psychiatric Press, 1992

Simon, RI, Williams I: Maintaining treatment boundaries in small communities and rural areas. Psychiatr Serv 50:1440–1446, 1999

Stone AA: Law, Psychiatry, and Morality: Essays and Analysis. Washington, DC, American Psychiatric Press, 1985

Vinson JS: Use of complaint procedures in cases of therapist-patient sexual contact. Professional Psychology: Research and Practice 18:159–164, 1987

Walker E, Young PD: A Killing Cure. New York, Henry Holt, 1986

Wisconsin Task Force on Sexual Misconduct: Making Therapy Work for You. Madison, WI, Wisconsin Task Force on Sexual Misconduct, 1986

Chapter 9: You Only Die Once— But Did You Intend It?

Botello TE, Weinberger LE, Gross BH: Psychological autopsy, in Principles and Practice of Forensic Psychiatry, 2nd Edition. Edited by Rosner R. London, Arnold, 2003, pp 89–94

Litman R: Psychological autopsies, mental illness and intention in suicide, in The Suicide Case: Investigation and Trial of Insurance Claims. Edited by Nolan J. Chicago, IL, Tort and Insurance Practice Section, American Bar Association, 1988, pp 69–82

Maris RW, Berman AL, Maltsberger JT, et al: Assessment and Prediction of Suicide. New York, Guilford, 1992

Mooar B: Tests contradict U.S. story of man's suicide. The Washington Post, July 12, 1994, B1, B8

Simon RI: Silent suicide in the elderly. Bull Am Acad Psychiatry Law 17:83–95, 1989

Simon RI: You only die once—but did you intend it? Psychiatric assessment of suicide intent in insurance litigation. Tort and Insurance Law Journal 25:650–662, 1990

Simon RI: Clinical risk management of suicidal patients: assessing the unpredictable, in American Psychiatric Press Review of Clinical Psychiatry and the Law, Vol 3. Edited by Simon RI. Washington, DC, American Psychiatric Press, 1992, pp 3–66

Simon RI: Murder Masquerading as Suicide: Postmortem assessment of suicide risk factors at the time of death. Journal of Forensic Sciences 43:1119–1123, 1998

Simon RI: Murder, suicide, accident, or natural death, in Retrospective Assessment of Mental States in Litigation. Edited by Simon RI, Shuman DW. Washington DC, American Psychiatric Publishing, 2002

Simon RI: American Psychiatric Association practice guideline for the assessment and treatment of patients with suicidal behaviors. Am J Psychiatry 160 (11, suppl), 2003

Simon RI: Assessing and Managing Suicide Risk. Washington, DC, American Psychiatric Publishing, 2004

Simon RI: Naked suicide. J Am Acad Psychiatry Law (in press)

Simon RI, Hales RE (eds): American Psychiatric Publishing Textbook of Suicide Assessment and Management. Washington, DC, American Psychiatric Publishing, 2006

Spoto D: Marilyn Monroe: The Biography. New York, Harper Collins, 1993

Thornhill R, Palmer CT: Why men rape. The Sciences, January/February 2000, pp 30-36

Chapter 10: Messianic Madness

American Psychiatric Association: Diagnostic and Statistical Manual of Mental Disorders, 4th Edition. Washington, DC, American Psychiatric Association, 1994

Bugliosi V, Gentry C: Helter Skelter. New York, Bantam, 1978

Cult Hotline and Clinic. http://www.cultclinic.org. Accessed September 13, 2007

Duffy JF: Stone criticizes FBI in cult assault report. Psychiatric Times, February 1994, pp 1, 41

Galanter M: Cults: Faith, Healing and Coercion. New York, Oxford University Press, 1989

Galanter M (ed): Cults and New Religious Movements: A Report of the American Psychiatric Association from the Committee on Psychiatry and Religion. Washington, DC, American Psychiatric Press, 1989

Goldstein WN: Clarification of projective identification. Am J Psychiatry 148:153–161, 1991

Goodstein L: "Free will" was the price of belonging to cult. Washington Post, March. 30, 1997, A1, A15

Hoffman B: The logic of suicide terrorism. http://www.theatlantic.com/doc/200306/hoffman. Accessed September 13, 2007

James W: The Varieties of Religious Experience. New York, Modern Library, 1929

Kahaner L: Cults That Kill. New York, Warner, 1988

Kernberg OF: Aggression in Personality Disorders and Perversions. New Haven, CT, Yale University Press, 1992, pp 159–174

Kildoff M, Javers R: The Suicide Cult. New York, Bantam, 1978

Lanning KV: Satanic, Occult, Ritualistic Crime: A Law Enforcement Perspective. Quantico, VA, National Center for the Analysis of Violent Crime, 1989

Marvasti JA: Physicians as killers? http://www.clinical_psychiatrynews .com. Accessed September 13, 2007

Mass suicides in recent years. http://www.cnn.com. Accessed September 9, 2007

Melton JG: Encyclopedic Handbook of Cults in America, Revised and Updated Edition. New York, Garland, 1992

Messianic madness of nuclear Osama. http://www.wnd.com. Accessed September 13, 2007

Timmerman KR: Iran's nuclear zealot. http://www.kentimmerman.com. Accessed February 12, 2008

Volkan VD: Suicide bombers. http://www.healthsystem.virginia.edu. Accessed September 13, 2007

Wright L: The Looming Tower. New York, Vantage, 2006

Chapter 11: Serial Sexual Killers

Apsche JA: Probing the Mind of a Serial Killer. Morrisville, PA, International Information Associates, 1993

Cheney M: The Coed Killer. New York, Walker, 1976

Conradi P: The Red Ripper. New York, Dell, 1992

Dahmer L: A Father's Story. New York, William Morrow, 1994

Darrach B, Norris J: An American tragedy. Life, August 1984, p 58

Dietz PE: Mass, serial and sensational homicides. Bull N Y Acad Med 62:477–490, 1986

Douglas JE, Burgess AW, Burgess AG, et al: Crime Classification Manual. New York, Lexington Books, 1992

Drukteinis AM: Serial murder: the heart of darkness. Psychiatric Annals 22:532–537, 1992

Elliott F: Violence: a product of biosocial interactions. Bull Am Acad Psychiatry Law 16:131–143, 1988

Felthous AR, Kellert SR: Violence against animals and people: is aggression against living creatures generalized? Bull Am Acad Psychiatry Law 14:55–69, 1986

Fox JA, Levin J: Overkill: Mass Murder and Serial Killing Exposed. New York, Plenum, 1994

Freud S: Three essays on the theory of sexuality (1905), in The Standard Edition of the Complete Psychological Works of Sigmund Freud, Vol 7. Translated and edited by Strachey J. London, Hogarth Press, 1968, pp 135–243; see p 171

Gilmore M: Shot in the Heart. New York, Doubleday, 1994

Jones V, Collier P: True Crime: Serial Killers and Mass Murderers. Forestville, CA, Eclipse, 1993

Kennedy D: On a Killing Day: The Bizarre Story of Convicted Murderer Aileen "Lee" Wuornos. Chicago, IL, Bonus, 1992

Kernberg OF: Aggression in Personality Disorders and Perversions. New Haven, CT, Yale University, 1992

Levin J, Fox JA: Mass Murder: America's Growing Menace. New York, Plenum, 1985

Lewis DO, Pincus JH, Feldman M, et al: Psychiatric, neurological, and psychoeducational characteristics of 15 death row inmates in the United States. Am J Psychiatry 143:838–845, 1986

Markman R, Boslo D: Alone with the Devil: Famous Cases of a Courtroom Psychiatrist. New York, Bantam, 1989

Masters B: Killing for Company: The Story of a Man Addicted to Murder. New York, Random House, 1993

Mednick SA: Congenital determinants of violence. Bull Am Acad Psychiatry Law 16:101–109, 1988

Meloy JR: Violent Attachments. New York, Jason Aronson, 1992

Michaud SG, Aynesworth H: The Only Living Witness. New York, Signet, 1989

Murder—Crime in the United States 2004. U.S. Department of Justice, Federal Bureau of Investigation. http://www.fbi.gov. Accessed September 21, 2007

Murder—Crime in the United States 2006. U.S. Department of Justice, Federal Bureau of Investigation. http://www.fbi.gov. Accessed September 21, 2007

Nelson P: Defending the Devil: My Story as Ted Bundy's Last Lawyer. New York, Morrow, 1994

Newton M: Hunting Humans: The Encyclopedia of Serial Killers, Vol 1. New York, Avon, 1992

Newton M: Hunting Humans: The Encyclopedia of Serial Killers, Vol 2. New York, Avon, 1993

Norris J: Serial Killers. New York, Anchor, 1989

Olsen J: The Misbegotten Son: A Serial Killer and His Victims—The True Story of Arthur J. Shawcross. New York, Delacorte, 1993

Post RM, Weiss SRB, Rubinow DR: Recurrent affective disorders: lessons from limbic kindling. Current Topics in Neuroendocrinology 8:91–115, 1988

Prentky RA, Burgess AW, Rokous F, et al: The presumptive role of fantasy in serial sexual homicide. Am J Psychiatry 146:887–891, 1989

Ressler RK, Shachtman T: Whoever Fights Monsters. New York, St. Martin's Press, 1992

Ressler RK, Burgess AW, Douglas JE: Sexual Homicide: Patterns and Motives. Lexington, MA, DC Heath, 1988

Rule A: The Stranger Beside Me: Ted Bundy. New York, Signet, 1989

Schreiber RF: The Shoemaker: The Anatomy of a Psychotic. New York, Signet, 1989

Schwartz AE: The Man Who Could Not Kill Enough: The Secret Murders of Milwaukee's Jeffrey Dahmer. Secaucus, NJ, Carol Publishing Group, 1992

Simon RI: Type A, AB, B murderers: their relationship to the victims and to the criminal justice system. Bull Am Acad Psychiatry Law 5:344–362, 1977

Sullivan T: Killer Clown: The John Wayne Gacy Murders. New York, Pinnacle, 1983

Swanson JW, Holzer CE, Ganju UK, et al: Violence and psychiatric disorder in the community: evidence from the Epidemiologic Catchment Area surveys. Hosp Community Psychiatry 41:761–770, 1990

True Crime: Compulsion to Kill. Alexandria, VA, Time-Life Books, 1993

True Crime: Mass Murderers. Alexandria, VA, Time-Life Books, 1993

Uniform Crime Reports, 1976–89: Crime in the United Sates. Washington, DC, U.S. Government Printing Office, 1989

Yarvis RM: Homicide: Causative Factors and Roots. Lexington, MA, DC Heath, 1991

Chapter 12: Character and Destiny

Brown D: How science is rewriting the book on genes. The Washington Post, November 12, 2007, A8

The mind's mirror. Monitor on Psychology 36:48, 2005. http://www.apa.org. Accessed September 24, 2007

Index

*Page numbers printed in **boldface** type refer to tables or figures.*